Introduction to
Healthcare
Informatics

Editors
Susan H. Fenton, PhD, RHIA, FAHIMA and
Sue Biedermann, MSHP, RHIA, FAHIMA

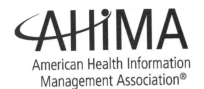

American Health Information
Management Association®

ISBN: 978-1-58426-281-7
AHIMA Product No.: AB120011

AHIMA Staff:
Jessica Block, MA, Assistant Editor
Jason O. Malley, Director, Creative Content Development
Ashley Sullivan, Production Development Editor
Diana M. Warner, MS, RHIA, CHPS, FAHIMA, Reviewer
Lydia M. Washington, RHIA, MS, CPHIMS, Reviewer

For more information, including updates, about AHIMA Press publications, visit http://www.ahima.org/publications/updates.aspx.

American Health Information Management Association
233 North Michigan Avenue, 21st Floor
Chicago, Illinois 60601-5809
ahima.org

Table of Contents

Detailed Contents

Chapter 3

Chapter 4

Chapter 5

Chapter 6

Chapter 10

Chapter 11

Chapter 12

Chapter 13

Consumer Health Informatics   321

Chapter 14

About the Editors and Authors

Dr. Susan H. Fenton, PhD, RHIA, FAHIMA, is an assistant professor at The University of Texas Health Science Center School of Biomedical Informatics in Houston, Texas. Prior to this position, she was an assistant professor in the HIM department at Texas State University. Dr. Fenton has worked in the health information management field for more than 20 years, including as a researcher and practice leader at AHIMA. Dr. Fenton received the 2012 AHIMA Foundation Triumph Award for Research, as well as the Texas State College of Health Professions 2011 Award for Research. Dr. Fenton is the Principal Investigator for the $5.4 million Professional University Resources and Education for Health Information Technology grant, as well as a Texas HIT Workforce Development Wagner-Peyser grant. Dr. Fenton is a member of the Perspectives in Health Information Management review panel, a CAHIIM accreditation reviewer, and a reviewer of SBIT/STTR grants for the National Institutes of Health. She was the Director of Health Information Management for six years in the Veterans Health Administration Headquarters, responsible for national patient record policy. Dr. Fenton has authored or coauthored multiple refereed publications and book chapters. She presents frequently at state and national meetings on various HIM-related topics. Dr. Fenton's research interests are health information workforce development, clinical classifications, and data quality.

Sue Biedermann, MSHP, RHIA, FAHIMA, is the chair of the HIM department at Texas State University. She has served the Texas Health Information Management Association in various appointed and elected positions including President. At the national level, she has been an accreditation site visitor for more than 15 years with additional past service including the Professional Conduct Committee, Nominating Committee, AOE Strategy Task Force, and Project Manager for the Professional Resource Task Force. Ms. Biedermann completed the AHIMA Research Institute and was most recently funded by the Texas Higher Education Coordinating Board for a project preparing for HIT students to advance to baccalaureate level education. She has been author or coauthor on a number of publications and reports and presents frequently at state and national meetings. During her tenure as a faculty member, she has received the College of Health Professions Faculty Excellence Award and was selected as an Alpha Chi Favorite Professor.

Contributors

Dr. Juliana Brixey, MSN, PhD, is an assistant professor at the University of Texas Health Science Center School of Biomedical Informatics. Previously, she served as the Manager of Outreach and Education Gulf Coast Regional Extension Center, was an adjunct assistant professor at the University of Texas Health Science Center at Houston, and was an assistant professor at the University of Kansas School of Nursing. For 10 years, she was in the Nursing Informatics Working

Group at AMIA. Dr. Brixey earned her PhD in health information sciences from The University of Texas Health Science Center at Houston and BSN and MSN degrees in nursing from The University of Texas Medical Branch at Galveston.

Dr. Christopher G. Chute, MD, is the chair of the ICD Revision Steering Group at the World Health Organization. Dr. Chute received his undergraduate and medical training at Brown University, internal medicine residency at Dartmouth, and doctoral training in Epidemiology at Harvard. He is board certified in internal medicine, and a Fellow of the American College of Physicians, the American College of Epidemiology, and the American College of Medical Informatics. He was the founding Chair of Biomedical Informatics at Mayo in 1988, a position he held for 20 years. He is now Professor of Medical Informatics, and is PI on a large portfolio of research including the Office of the National Coordinator (ONC) SHARP (Strategic Health IT Advanced Research Projects) on Secondary EHR Data Use, the ONC Beacon Community (Co-PI), the LexGrid projects, Mayo's CTSA Informatics, Mayo's Cancer Center Informatics including caBIG, and several NIH grants including one of the eMERGE centers from NGHRI, which focus upon genome-wide association studies against shared phenotypes derived from electronic medical records. Dr. Chute serves as Vice Chair of the Mayo Clinic Data Governance for HIT Standards and on Mayo's enterprise IT Oversight Committee. He is presently Chair, ISO Health Informatics Technical Committee (ISO TC215) and chairs the World Health Organization (WHO) ICD-11 Revision. He also serves on strategic advisory panels to NCRR and NHGRI within NIH, and the HIT Standards Committee for the ONC. Recently held positions include Chair of the Biomedical Computing and Health Informatics study section at NIH, Chair of the Board of the HL7/FDA/NCI/CDISC BRIDG project, on the Board of the Clinical Data Interchange Standards Consortium (CDISC), ANSI Health Information Standards Technology Panel (HITSP) Board member, Chair of the US delegation to ISO TC215 for Health Informatics, Convener of Healthcare Concept Representation WG3 within the (TC215), Co-chair of the HL7 Vocabulary Committee, Chair of the International Medical Informatics Association (IMIA) WG6 on Medical Concept Representation, and American Medical Informatics Association (AMIA) Board member.

Diane Dolezel, MSCS, RHIA, is a senior lecturer at Texas State University. She has many years of experience in the information technology field as a senior developer, technical lead, and consultant.

Desla Mancilla, DHA, RHIA, is the Senior Director of Academic Affairs in the AHIMA Foundation. In her HIM career prior to joining the AHIMA Foundation, she held a variety of academic- and practice-based positions including HIM Program Director, Assistant Professor, Regional Director of Information Protection Services, and EHR Project Manager. Dr. Mancilla's doctoral dissertation was on patient acceptance of biometrics methods for identity verification. She has also published several articles and presentations on medical identity theft. Dr. Mancilla has served as a principal investigator and secondary investigator on grants funded by The

Office of Minority Health, the AHIMA Foundation, and Texas State University. Dr. Mancilla is a frequent speaker at the local, regional, and national conferences on topics related to medical identity theft, electronic health records, privacy and security, and AHIMA's Reality 2016 initiative. As a Past-President of the Indiana Health Information Management Association and through various other state and national HIM leadership positions, Dr. Mancilla has demonstrated her knowledge of and commitment to the HIM profession. Prior to working at the AHIMA Foundation, Dr. Mancilla was appointed to and served on the privacy workgroup for the Chicago Health Information Exchange through the Metropolitan Chicago Healthcare Council.

William Kelly McLendon, RHIA, is the president and founder of Health Information Xperts, a consulting firm for electronic health records, electronic document management, and health information automation; and president and founder of Information Evolution Management, which provides EHR consulting and educational services to healthcare entities and vendors. At Eclipsys Corporation, McLendon served as VP, Clinical HIM Strategies; Director, Record Manager Domain; and Sales Executive. Prior positions include VP, Health Information Management; and Program Manager, Data Management Division, at MedPlus. McLendon is the author of the AHIMA publication *The Legal Health Record*, 2nd ed. His involvement with AHIMA spans 30 years, during which he has authored many articles, presented at national conventions, and served on several committees and task forces. He received the AHIMA Visionary Award in 2003.

Jackie Moczygemba, MBA, RHIA, CCS, FAHIMA, is an associate professor at Texas State University. She was recently appointed to the AHIMA exam construction committee for the Certified Coding Analyst (CCA) credential. Moczygemba is currently a secondary investigator in an exploratory foundational study to examine current practices used by acute healthcare facilities in response to medical identity theft. In addition, Moczygemba served on the board of the Texas Health Information Management Association as the Public Relations Director from 2002 to 2004. She also served as secretary for the Alamo Area Health Information Management Association from 2001 to 2002. Jackie's past awards include Faculty of the Year Award in the College of Health Professions from 2000 to 2001, Favorite Professor Award from the Alpha Chi National Honor Scholarship Society in 1997, and Guest Coach for the Texas State University Department of Athletics Guest Coaches Program in 1997. She has authored and coauthored several refereed publications and has given scholarly presentations at national and state conferences.

Kim Murphy-Abdouch, MPH, RHIA, FACHE, is a clinical assistant professor at Texas State University. Murphy-Abdouch has a broad base of healthcare leadership, hospital operations, health information management, and finance experience and has held a variety of healthcare operational positions from Director of Health Information Management to Hospital Chief Executive Officer. She is board certified in healthcare management as a Fellow in the American College of Healthcare Executives.

Joanne D. Valerius, MPH, RHIA is the Director, Health Information Management Graduate Programs at the Oregon Health and Science University in Portland, Oregon. Her current qualitative research for her doctoral dissertation focuses on the experience of health information managers who have worked with paper-based and electronic-based health records spanning more than 20 years in the field. Ms. Valerius' interest centers on human resource development in healthcare settings and the impact of the electronic health record. Her focus is on the holistic approach to the workplace and how diversity impacts the workplace. Ms. Valerius is a published writer, as well as a national and international speaker. She has 36 years of experience in HIM field.

Susan White, PhD, CHDA, is an Associate Professor of Clinical Health and Rehabilitation Sciences in the Health Information Management and Systems (HIMS) Division at The Ohio State University. Dr. White teaches classes in statistics, data analytics, healthcare finance, and computer applications. She has written numerous articles presented to national audiences regarding the benchmarking of healthcare facilities and appropriate use of claims data. Dr. White has also published articles covering outcomes assessment and risk adjustment using healthcare financial and clinical data analysis, hospital benchmarking, and claims data mining. She is the author of AHIMA's Healthcare Financial Management for Health Information and Informatics text. Dr. White received her PhD in Statistics from The Ohio State University. She is a member of AHIMA, the American Statistical Association, and the Healthcare Financial Management Association. Prior to joining OSU, Dr. White was a Vice President for Research and Development for both Cleverley and Associates and CHIPS/Ingenix. She has 15 years of experience in the practice of healthcare financial and revenue cycle consulting in addition to her academic experience.

The American Health Information Management Association (AHIMA) has an envisioned future: *Drive the Power of Knowledge—Health Information Where and When It's Needed*. In order to realize this dream, today's health information management professional must move from simply collecting and managing data to translating data into information and then into knowledge. If you want to be part of this exciting vision and assist in leading the country to a new future, then this book is for you.

For many years, healthcare providers have relied on paper-based records to tell the patient's story. With the rapid implementation of electronic health records, the process of organizing, storing, integrating, and retrieving medical and patient information has become antiquated and inefficient. Today we must rely on numerous computer systems to manage enormous amounts of patient information. Susan Fenton and Sue Biedermann tell us that the study of informatics is for professionals who are interested in learning how to work with all aspects of health data and information through the application of computers and computer technologies. By providing health intelligence through informatics, you will be able to make a significant difference to your organization.

From providers to associations supporting quality of care, information management and informatics has never been more important. Knowledge management is emerging as an important aspect of achieving excellent organizational performance as outlined in an article analyzing applications of healthcare organizations that received the Malcolm Baldrige National Quality Award from 2002 to 2008. "Knowledge management in these organizations is a deliberate effort to keep all relevant knowledge at the fingertips of every worker, characterized by frequent communication, careful maintenance of content accuracy, and redundant distribution" (*Journal of Healthcare Management* 2013, 58(3)). Simply stated, healthcare organizations will depend on informatics to drive administrative and clinical decision making in day-to-day activities to achieve continuous quality improvement.

Richard Umbdenstock, the President and Chief Executive Officer (CEO) of the American Hospital Association, spoke to the AHIMA Board of Directors and shared that CEOs are focused on performance and are concerned about quality and safety at a reduced cost. He went on to say that to *get to the table* with decision makers, health information managers must *go to the table* with results. You will become indispensable by providing information to decision makers that can be used to lower costs, increase revenue, improve safety and quality, focus on service, and improve population health (AHIMA Board minutes, May 2013). As stated in the AHIMA strategic plan, "Health information management professionals will need to be competent in creating clinical analytics and business intelligence processes that grant stakeholders better value through improved longitudinal coordination and quality of care" (AHIMA strategic plan 2014–2017).

According to the Agency for Healthcare Research and Quality (AHRQ), whose goal is to improve the quality, safety, efficiency and effectiveness of healthcare for all Americans, "meeting these expectations has often been difficult because systems to organize, store, and retrieve medical and patient information had not been developed. But today, computer systems exist that can help clinicians meet each of these challenges" (AHRQ 2013). AHRQ has stated that they support medical informatics to meet their goals.

Introduction to Healthcare Informatics is a compendium of information that will help to introduce the reader to an emerging and changing field. The editors and authors have provided information about computer science, technology, the provision of care, education, and research aspects of medicine. These knowledge clusters provide a background for jobs in transition and new emerging roles that do not yet exist.

Editors Susan H. Fenton, PhD, RHIA, FAHIMA, and Sue Biedermann, MSHP, RHIA, FAHIMA, wrote and compiled this text to develop the next wave of leaders in this exciting new field. Experts in their own right, they sought others throughout the country to represent the informatics field with outstanding credentials, training, education, experience, and professional knowledge.

Whether you are a college student, a young careerist, or a seasoned professional, informatics is a way to make a difference in the healthcare field through knowledge management. Health intelligence is the new asset for providers and will not only improve care now and in the future but health intelligence will become a competitive edge and driving force. Susan Fenton and Sue Biedermann tell us that this is a field of science concerned with the management of all aspects of health data and information through the application of computers and computer technologies. When successful, AHIMA and the health information management profession will have assisted in creating a framework in which huge amounts of healthcare data can be appropriately aggregated, analyzed, and leveraged using real-time algorithms and functions to provide a true asset to decision makers in the healthcare arena. This will make a difference to all patients and improve the care they receive.

Lynne Thomas Gordon, MBA, RHIA, CAE, FACHE, FAHIMA
Chief Executive Officer
American Health Information Management Association

Acknowledgments

I want to acknowledge my coeditor, Sue Biedermann, as well as all of our chapter authors and coauthors. This could not have been done without your dedication. I also want to thank my son, AJ, for his support.

Susan H. Fenton

I would like to thank Susan Fenton for including me as coeditor in this project and appreciate the commendable work done by all of the chapter authors and coauthors. Our students and graduates continue to be an inspiration and this book was written to support their educational needs. I am thankful for the continued support from my husband, Jim, and daughter, Amy.

Sue Biedermann

Both editors wish to thank the AHIMA Press staff and practice staff who supported us during the process of writing this book. We hope our fellow faculty and students find this book to be of benefit.

AHIMA Press would like to thank Donald W. Kellogg, RHIA, FAHIMA, PH.D, CPEHR for his review and feedback on this book.

Online Resources

For Instructors

AHIMA provides supplementary materials for educators who use this book in their classes. Materials include PowerPoint notes for lectures, case studies, and discussion questions, as well as syllabi for bachelor and master's level classes. Visit http://www.ahimapress.org/Fenton2817 and click the link to access the materials. These materials are *only* available for approved instructors. For more information on how to become an approved instructor, see http://ahima.org/publications/educators.aspx. If you have any questions regarding the instructor materials, contact AHIMA Customer Relations at (800) 335-5535 or submit a customer support request at https://secure.ahima.org/contact/contact.aspx.

Chapter

1

Foundations of Health Informatics

By Sue Biedermann

Learning Objectives

- To understand the evolution of the field of health informatics
- To consider the health informatics core competencies
- To recognize the terms related to health informatics
- To compare the methods associated with health informatics
- To appreciate the need for current policies to support electronic health records and use of the data
- To identify ethical issues associated with health informatics
- To understand the major roles associated with the field of health informatics

KEY TERMS

Biomedical informatics
Chief information officer (CIO)
Chief knowledge officer (CKO)
Chief medical informatics officer (CMIO)
Chief nursing informatics officer (CNIO)
Clinical decision support
Clinical informatics
Computer-aided diagnosis (CAD)
Computerized provider order entry (CPOE)
Consolidated Health Informatics (CHI)
Consumer informatics
Data mining

Decision analysis
Digital Imaging Communication in Medicine (DICOM)
e-Health
Genetic Information Nondiscrimination Act of 2008 (GINA)
Genomics
Health informatics
Health information technology (HIT)
Health Insurance Portability and Accountability Act (HIPAA)
Health Level 7 (HL7)
Human Gene Nomenclature (HUGN)

Informatics
Imaging informatics
International Classification of
    Functioning and Disability (ICF)
Interoperability
Logical Observation Identifiers Names
    and Codes (LOINC)
Meaningful use of information
Medical informatics
Medical scribe
National Drug File–Reference
    Terminology (NDF–RT)

Nursing informatics
Personal health record (PHR)
Protected health information (PHI)
Probability
Public health informatics
RxNORM
Systematized Nomenclature
    of Medicine–Clinical Terms
    (SNOMED CT)
Telehealth
Telemedicine
Translational medicine

⊙ Introduction

With the rapid advancement of the use of computers and technology in maintaining and utilizing patient information, the health informatics field is in a significant state of transition. New professional roles are emerging as a result of the increased focus on patient information as well. As a means of introduction, it can be said that **informatics** is using technology to acquire, manage, maintain, and use information as a basis for the plethora of decisions that must be made in a cost-effective manner. **Health informatics** is the field of information science concerned with the management of all aspects of health data and information through the application of computers and computer technologies (AHIMA 2012, 189). **Health information technology (HIT)** includes the technical aspects of processing health data and records including classification and coding, abstracting, registry development, and storage. The health informatics domain includes computer science, technology, and the provision of care, education, and research aspects of medicine. While these are the basic components that comprise health informatics, there is no one consistently accepted definition of it. Differences exist due to the frame of reference under which health informatics is being considered. Even the frame of reference continues to change as new health informatics applications continue to emerge across the healthcare disciplines. This first chapter of this book provides an introduction to health informatics by reviewing briefly its history, some of the relevant definitions, and associated methods and roles.

⊙ Definitions, Policies, Methods, and Ethics

New terms often emerge and the uses of these terms evolve as new technologies and fields are developed. It is important to understand the terminology that defines a concept or activity to truly be able to comprehend it. Many new health informatics terms are explored in this section, which covers the history of health informatics, core competencies, specific health informatics applications, methods for creating systems, and ethics.

History of Health Informatics

Health informatics is often referred to as a new discipline due to increased attention in recent years. The emphasis on the HIT movement is primarily due to federal legislation enacted to promote the use of technology in healthcare and the **meaningful use of information**. Meaningful use of information is using systems with certified software to enhance the use of data contained in and obtained from health records. The goals for the use of this data are to improve quality, safety, and efficiency; reduce health disparities; improve the engagement of patients and families; improve care coordination; and support population and public health while maintaining privacy and security. The significant increase in awareness of the field of health informatics has led to the belief that it is a new field, but the term health informatics was coined a number of years ago. References can be found in the literature in the early 1950s for topics such as the use of computers in the provision of healthcare, information processing, and data management in medicine, as well as the use of the terms "computer technology" together with "medicine" and "healthcare." As the capabilities of computer technology continued to evolve with more applications and opportunities for utilization to support the provision of healthcare, the need for a recognizable name for the new domain was desired but very difficult due to the diversity of science, technology, engineering, and healthcare that were the key components of the domain. There were early references to the term **medical informatics** documented in the early 1970s "to cover both the information and data parts as well as the controlling and automatic nature of data processing itself" (Anderson 1987). In the ensuing years as additional working definitions were considered, the terms that were consistently a part of the definition included computer science, information science, engineering, technology with relation to the fields of health and medicine to include practice, education, and research. The US government was instrumental in supporting and developing the medical informatics movement through the initial funding for academic medical centers in medical informatics in the 1960s. **Computer-aided diagnosis (CAD)** was a result of initial work to use computers and information science in the provision of care with the goal to improve the outcomes of the practice of medicine. CAD is the incorporation of computer images with aspects of artificial intelligence to detect and identify potential disease factors. Disease information such as symptoms, duration, medical history, and diagnostic information from numerous cases is stored in CAD systems. When similar information is entered on a patient it is compared to that which is in the system using computer algorithms. Following this processing, a list of probable diagnoses is generated for the physician to consider.

As health informatics continued to develop, the need for standards became apparent. Definitions of standards that would be appropriate for the discussion of the health informatics movement include such phrases as "A scientifically based statement of expected behavior against which structures, processes, and outcomes can be measured" or "A model or example established by authority, custom, or general consent or a rule established by an authority as a measure of quantity, weight, extent, value, or quality" (AHIMA 2012, 390). The need for models or examples and for the measurement of quality are vital for valid outcomes when health informatics is incorporated in the delivery of healthcare.

In recent history, the US government has sponsored or approved standards programs such as

- **Health Level 7 (HL7)**, an international organization of healthcare professionals dedicated to creating standards for the exchange, management, and integration of electronic information. It sets acceptable vocabulary standards for clinical documentation

- **Systematized Nomenclature of Medicine–Clinical Terms (SNOMED CT)**, by the College of American Pathologists, a processable collection of medical terminology covering most areas of clinical information such as lab results, nonlab interventions and procedures, anatomy, diagnosis and problems, and nursing

- **Logical Observation Identifiers Names and Codes (LOINC)**, a standardization of electronic exchange of laboratory test orders and drug label section headers

- The **Health Insurance Portability and Accountability Act (HIPAA)**, which addresses standards for transactions and code sets for electronic exchange of health-related information to perform billing or administrative functions; and standards for terminologies related to medications including the Food and Drug Administration's names and codes for ingredients, manufactured dosage forms, drug products, and medication packages

- **RxNORM**, (normalized names for clinical drugs), by the National Library of Medicine, for describing clinical drugs

- **National Drug File–Reference Terminology (NDF-RT)**, by the Veterans Administration, for specific drug classifications

- The **Human Gene Nomenclature (HUGN)** for exchanging information regarding the role of genes in biomedical research in the federal health sector

- The Environmental Protection Agency's Substance Registry Services for nonmedical chemicals of importance to healthcare

Additional standards were adopted to allow for the electronic exchange of clinical information across the federal government. Designed to build on the previous standards, these will be used to support the implementation of new information technology systems.

The new standards to support the electronic exchange of data include

- **Digital Imaging Communication in Medicine (DICOM)**, which enables the exchange of multimedia information

- RxNORM for the exchange of medication allergy information

⊙ HL7, **International Classification of Functioning and Disability (ICF)**, and related **Consolidated Health Informatics (CHI)** endorsed vocabularies for the exchange of Clinical Assessments and Disability and Functional Status. The ICF includes a list of body functions and structure, and a list of domains of activity and participation. The CHI initiative is a collaborative effort of the federal government to adopt standards.

While computers can easily be utilized in many industries to compile, manage, and utilize large quantities of information, applications related to the provision of healthcare provide unique challenges in the use of technology. Much of healthcare is subjective and hard to define with terms such as pain, feelings, and perceptions used to describe the condition of the patient. This is coupled with the sheer amount of information generated for the individual and in the aggregate for groups of patients which also presents challenges to the system and those who work with it. Being proficient in computer science and information systems is not adequate to design systems that will enhance the delivery of healthcare, contribute to quality of care, and facilitate cost-effective means of delivery. One must also be familiar with how the delivery of healthcare is carried out. When considering the information generated in the provision of care, the who, what, where, when, why, and how must be taken into consideration. Then, just as important but even more challenging to understand, is where the information is needed and used, how it is transmitted, and the form and format required for the transmissions while continuing to protect the confidentiality of the patient's information throughout the process. Technology professionals are knowledgeable in computer science and computer information systems. Healthcare providers are knowledgeable in the aspect of care that they provide and are familiar with the health information that they use and generate. The various other providers and other staff members who use health information are familiar with the aspects of care they provide and the associated information, and the use of technology in carrying out these functions. Health information management (HIM) professionals are experts in understanding the regulations for patient records, recognizing who is responsible for documenting in the record, and knowing the majority of the uses of the patient information since access is controlled and facilitated through the HIM Department. Healthcare informatics brings together all of these aspects to enhance patient care through the use of technology. The following statement summarizes all that health informatics encompasses:

> The apparent information overload and imperfection of medical decision making motivate the use of information systems for medical decision support. Health informatics provides tools to control processes in healthcare, acquire medical knowledge and communicate information between all people and organizations involved with healthcare . . . development of systems often lags behind possibilities (Imhoff 2001, 179–186).

Health informatics will provide the tools to enable the production of the right information to the right people in the right format at the right time. The evolving science of health informatics will provide for the continued development of the supporting, necessary systems.

Check Your Understanding 1.1

Instructions: Answer the following questions on a separate piece of paper.

1. What are the unique challenges associated with the use of computers related to health information?

2. Why is standardization important in the documentation of clinical data?

Match the following terms with the appropriate phrase.
   a. Health Level 7
   b. SNOMED CT
   c. LOINC

3. _____ Processable collection of medical terminology covering most areas of clinical information such as lab results, nonlab interventions and procedures, anatomy, diagnoses, problems, and nursing

4. _____ Vocabulary standards for clinical documentation

5. _____ A standardization of electronic exchange of laboratory test orders and drug label section headers

Core Competencies

Within the last 15 years, the movement to utilize information systems in healthcare has experienced varying degrees of success for a variety of reasons. The lack of a trained workforce throughout all levels in an organization from the highest levels in administration and technological positions to those less skilled data entry and scanning employees has been an issue. Other industries have recognized that education and training to support the deployment and utilization of systems are vital for success. There has been very little development of educational and training programs specific to preparing users for healthcare applications. Health services throughout the world have been relatively uninterested in, and in some cases reluctant about, or even resistant to the development of education and training programs to accompany the considerable investment in IT in healthcare (Brittain and Norris 2008, 117–128). Training has usually been developed by individual healthcare entities to meet their immediate needs as they arise or the training has been vendor specific to support the acquisition of their specific product. The increased reliance on computer technology and the increasingly more sophisticated software and systems requires the continued development of training methods.

The reasons for the reluctance and lack of workforce development to support health informatics are complex and include many contributing factors. With the rapid evolution of information systems and advancement within systems and procedures already developed for use in other industries it would seem that deployment in the healthcare environment would be occurring at a more rapid pace. The diversity and magnitude of the healthcare workforce is huge. Nearly all healthcare workers will be required to interact with the computerized information systems in some manner. In addition to learning new technical skills, the workforce must also become familiar with a new lexicon of terms and acronyms that have emerged as systems have emerged. The terminology in question is related to HIM, medical or clinical informatics, and health informatics. This is compounded by the plethora of applications utilized within one system within a facility. Another contributing factor is the varying degrees of implementation of information systems across the full spectrum of healthcare facilities. For all of these reasons, attention must be given to technical training programs and formal educational programs from the associate degree to the doctoral levels. The need for a skilled workforce at all levels was addressed by the federal government with the funding made available through the American Recovery and Reinvestment Act of 2009 (ARRA) for the creation of many programs. These programs included certificate programs at the associate, baccalaureate, and master's degree levels and as continuing education course offerings. These funds were limited and for a defined period of time. These programs were also envisioned before training needs were clearly understood, so many areas were not addressed. A number of the programs were focused primarily on assessing user needs, making a purchase decision, and implementing the systems. Data analytics is now a key function in the health informatics field whereby data is turned into useful information. Skills needed to support these positions include an understanding of issues and challenges related to data collection, assessing the data for correctness and reliability, using statistical software to abstract information from the data, and presenting the information in the most effective format, especially for decision making.

In 2008, the Joint Work Force Task Force of the American Medical Informatics Association (AMIA) and the American Health Information Management Association (AHIMA) published the report *Health Information Management and Informatics Core Competencies for Individuals Working with Electronic Health Records*. The Electronic Health Record Core Competency domains identified by this task force are

I. Information literacy and skills

II. Health informatics skill using the EHR

III. Privacy and confidentiality of health information

IV. Health information/data technical security

V. Basic computer literacy skills (AHIMA and AMIA Joint Work Task Force 2008, 8)

Core competencies for each of the domains were identified and a matrix tool was developed to provide guidance for the competencies needed by a variety of disciplines. For example, all healthcare workers need an awareness of privacy and security regulations for keeping patient information confidential. However, the privacy officer, often an HIM professional, will require an in-depth understanding of the HIPAA Privacy Rule.

Domain II specifically addresses the health informatics skill set, but many competencies from the other domains are applicable to informatics-related roles directly or indirectly depending on the role. The model presented by this group was intended to be used to encourage the development of models of health information and informatics education and training programs and to serve as a resource for policy makers when considering funding for such programs. For health informatics skills using the electronic health record (EHR) and personal health record (PHR), needed skill sets and knowledge are the following:

1. Create and update documents within the EHR and the PHR
2. Locate and retrieve information in the EHR for various purposes
3. Perform data entry of narrative information
4. Locate and retrieve information from a variety of electronic sources.
5. Differentiate between primary and secondary health data sources and databases
6. Know the architecture and data standards of health information systems
7. Identify classification and systematic health-related terminologies for coding and information retrieval
8. Know the policies and procedures related to populating and using the health-care content within primary and secondary health data sources and databases
9. Apply appropriate documentation management principles to ensure data quality and integrity
10. Use software applications to generate reports
11. Know and apply appropriate methods to ensure the authenticity of health data entries in electronic information systems
12. Use electronic tools and applications for scheduling patients (AHIMA and AMIA Joint Work Task Force 2008, 9)

Definitions and Terms

Over the years, HIT-related definitions and terms have continued to emerge because of the increased interest of healthcare and governmental leaders, policy makers, and healthcare providers. The terms "health information technology" and "health informatics" are still not clearly defined or understood. The acronym HIT is also used to refer to health information technician programs, the associate-level HIM educational programs, which causes additional confusion when using HIT. Federal legislation brought the term "health information technology" (health IT or HIT) to the forefront, as legislators and other policy makers used the term to describe the application of computers and technology in a healthcare setting (Hersh 2009). Informatics has been defined as the discipline focused on the acquisition, storage, and use of information in a specific setting or domain with others continuing to provide similar but varying definitions (Hersh 2009). While consensus can generally be achieved on the definition of informatics, more specificity can be implied with the use of descriptive terms attached to the term "informatics." These include biomedical informatics, health or medical informatics, nursing informatics, and clinical informatics, all of which further define or indicate subcategories of the field of health informatics.

Biomedical informatics has multiple definitions and can be considered from several perspectives. Publications from the Stanford School of Medicine allude to the fact that modern science has given us tools for scientific research but produces a preponderance of data that is impossible to analyze with traditional methods. However, the biological data are key to learning the causes of disease and developing new treatment modalities. A clear definition or statement of the meaning of biomedical informatics is important to provide a perspective from which to consider the topic. One example of such a definition is presented here.

> Biomedical informatics, by definition, incorporates a core set of methodologies that are applicable for managing data, information, and knowledge across the translational medicine continuum, from bench biology to clinical care and research to public health (Sarkar 2010, 22).

Translational medicine can be thought of as taking the scientific knowledge gained from basic advances in research to the bedside by developing new procedures and modes of treatment to improve healthcare. Biomedical informatics is a broad category of informatics and within its continuum includes areas from **imaging informatics** to **clinical informatics**. Imaging informatics, synonymous with radiology informatics or medical imaging informatics, utilizes the radiology information gathered from individual patients to enhance patient care by finding ways to efficiently and reliably use the collected data.

Clinical informatics is part of the biomedical continuum, as outlined above. It is focused on information systems to ensure they support patient care that is safe, efficient, effective, timely, patient-centered, and equitable (Detmer, 2009, 167–168). A more specific definition for clinical informatics would infer that it is the scientific study of patient care, clinical research, and medical education and the effective use of information to support these activities, establish standards, and set policy. The goal of clinical informatics is to provide healthcare practitioners with timely, accurate data to support the delivery of care efficiently to improve quality of care in a cost-effective manner. The users of clinical information systems include all providers of care and may include consumers as well.

In **nursing informatics**, the practice of nursing intersects with computers and information science. The concept of nursing informatics has been in existence in some capacity for about three decades. At the basic level it is using technology to improve patient care. The more advanced level is with the nurse scholar conducting research to validate practice and identify means of improving nursing practice to achieve enhanced outcomes and greater patient satisfaction. In 2011, a nursing informatics workforce survey was conducted that supports the evolution of the role and contributions of the nurse informaticist. In this study, the top two job responsibilities reported were systems implementation and systems development with involvement in quality initiatives reported as the next most common job responsibility (Murphy 2011). Related to nursing informatics, the **chief nursing informatics officer (CNIO)** is a position that seems to be emerging in larger healthcare facilities and organizations. The typical responsibilities in this position are related to the implementation and utilization of HIT systems for clinical care.

Consumer informatics is consistent with other kinds of healthcare informatics in that it is the intersection of health, computers, and information management. In this case, the focus is on the interest of the consumer. A goal of consumer informatics is to support and inform consumers to facilitate the management and participation in their own care. Activities within this subset of health informatics may include evaluating the information needs of the consumers, and developing means of providing accessible and meaningful information to the patient or family consumer of the healthcare. Another important aspect of consumer informatics is utilization of consumer input and preferences in the development of information systems to maximize their perspective and promote usability. The gamut of information to be made available to the consumer includes that for prevention, wellness, and treatment options. Consumer informatics should be distinguished from patient education information, which is more commonly considered to be the instructions provided by a healthcare provider to instruct and communicate specific information for a specific treatment option. Examples of patient education include the instructions provided by the healthcare provider for activity restrictions, special diets to be followed, signs and symptoms to monitor, wound care, and the drug information that is provided to the patient with new prescriptions. Consumer informatics could include things such as interactive health communication. An example of this is where a consumer can access a website to seek information on a specific symptom or condition and possibly even be able to submit questions to be answered. Physicians who provide a portal on their website where their patients can develop and maintain a **personal health record (PHR)** is another example of consumer informatics. A PHR is an electronic or paper health record maintained and updated by an individual for himself or herself, a tool that individuals can use to collect, track, and share past and current information about their health or the health of someone in their care (AHIMA 2012). E-mail exchanges between a provider of care and a patient or a patient portal for the EHR would also fall in the category of consumer informatics.

Public health is "a state of complete physical, mental, and social well-being and not merely the absence of disease of infirmity" (WHO 2013). Discussions of public health commonly include topics such as disease prevention, health promotion, increasing life expectancy, and threats or health perils, along with terms such as population analysis, biostatistics, and monitoring of diseases, all of which require large amounts of information. **Public health informatics** is then the systematic application of this information and utilization of computer technology to support public health initiatives as related to research, education, and delivery of public health services. The focus of public health is not on the individual patient but rather large groups of individuals and communities. A large amount of deidentified aggregate data is collected and analyzed. The data are on all members of the population under study to include the healthy as well as those suffering from illness and other health conditions. With the increased use of technological advances to aggregate and analyze public health data, it is predicted that public health data will be a key component with health exchange initiatives. This information can also play a greater role in the treatment of conditions such as cancer with the potential for IT-supported surveillance and care.

Genomics is a biological science in which the structure and function along with the evolution and mapping of genomes is the focus. Genomic mapping, or the creation of a genetic map, is where the DNA fragments are assigned to chromosomes. Studies of genomic maps can identify major risk factors for certain illnesses at the individual level, and can also assess a person's risk of inherited diseases. In 1990, the US Human Genome Project was started in the United States. The project, coordinated by the US Department of Energy and the National Institutes of Health, was originally planned to take 15 years. The project was completed after only 13 years due to the acceleration of the project because of technological advances moving forward at an unexpected rate. While the focus of the project was to identify an estimated 20,000 to 25,000 genes and the sequences of three billion pairs that comprise human DNA, the storing of the associated information in databases and designing improved data analysis tools were also established goals of the project. The final goals of the project were to make the use of the technology available in the private sector and to address the ethical, legal, and social issues that were anticipated to arise from the project. The Human Genome Project provided a significant impact on the kinds and amount of health information maintained and was part of the motivation for the emergence of health informatics as a separate discipline rather than a part of medical or clinical informatics, which tend to be more oriented towards the actual management of disease. Health informatics includes all of the information starting with the genomic and clinical data of an individual patient, to the study of complex diseases, to the many types of comparative studies which can be done with the enhanced data analysis applications. The consequences of the advances in genomics are the ability to study the precursers, markers, and presentations of disease over time. The issue that discrimination might occur due to knowledge of genetic information does present an ethical challenge, which led to the **Genetic Information Nondiscrimination Act of 2008 (GINA)**. This law provides the legal standard to be followed for the collection, use, and disclosure of genetic information. In general, Title I of GINA prohibits health plans from discriminating against covered individuals based on genetic information (National Human Genome Resarch Institute 2013). The law further clarifies that genetics is health information. As health information it is then considered **protected health information (PHI)**, which according to the HIPAA Privacy Rule is that which could be used to identify the patient and therefore must be protected.

Telemedicine is the remote delivery of healthcare services over the telecommunications network. Although used interchangeably, use of the term **telehealth** tends to include both medical and nonclinical elements of care to include education, monitoring, and administration to facilitate the prevention or treatment of medical conditions. In either case, it is the use of technology that allows the service to be provided when the patient and the healthcare provider are remote from each other, which has caused a paradigm shift in the provision of healthcare. The technology for telehealth and telemedicine range from e-mail and videoconferencing, to the use of imaging and monitoring devices with results recorded and transmitted to the provider, to the transmission of health information for the use of diagnosis and treatment.

E-health is an emerging field at the intersection of medical informatics, public health, and business, referring to health services and information delivered or enhanced through the Internet and related technologies.

> In a broader sense, the term characterizes not only a technical development, but also a state-of-mind, a way of thinking, an attitude, and a commitment for networked, global thinking, to improve health care locally, regionally, and worldwide by using information and communication technology (Eysenback 2001).

Simply stated, e-health is the use of the Internet and other electronic media to provide access to health-related information including that for specific medical conditions and services as well as for information related to lifestyle information and services. E-health is not telemedicine where there is a healthcare provider of some sort at one or both sides of the electronic communication. The increased utilization of e-health services is the result of a number of factors that have made it possible and it has become a popular option for certain services with a growing number of individuals. Consumerism and patient expectations are a key factor in the increased use of e-health resources with the desire to have immediate and more information and to become more engaged in their care and self-management of medical conditions. E-health sites are becoming more sophisticated, linking much information together in one place on an easily navigable site. Some healthcare providers are encouraging the use of e-health via their own sites where patients are directed to a number of services including disease and treatment information, links to sites such as governmental sites that allow access to needed forms and information, scheduling, and payment options, and for some a portal to a PHR. These kinds of sites not only support the needs of the patient but also aid in staffing issues for the provider.

Check Your Understanding 1.2

Instructions: Answer the following questions on a separate piece of paper.

1. What is the difference between biomedical informatics, clinical informatics, and nursing informatics?
2. What is the relationship between biomedical informatics and translational medicine?
3. What is the specific focus of public health informatics?
4. What specific ethical issue arises out of the advancement of genomics?
5. What are key factors to the importance of e-health for the future of healthcare?

Policies

With the implementation of the EHR and subsequent use of the information, a facility must ensure that effective policies are in place to address the new way of maintaining patient information and the expanded use of the data available in an electronic system. All policies related to the health record must be reviewed to determine whether changes need to be made once the record is electronic rather than in the paper format. Hybrid record systems must be reviewed to determine the needed policy changes for this interim step to a fully functioning EHR. Key policies relating to privacy and security, compliance with HIPAA, and the assurance that the needed information is available to support the federal meaningful use requirements are of prime importance. An example of a new policy that might need to be developed relates to systems that utilize alerts such as **computerized provider order entry (CPOE)**. CPOE systems are applications that allow providers to write orders for medications or other treatments and transmit them electronically. A policy would need to address the requirements for alert monitoring to guide the provider in the appropriate way to respond to alerts. Policies that might need to be changed are those that relate to privacy and security and HIPAA compliance. A facility should already have policies in place to address these, but a review will need to be done to see how these functions have changed in the electronic environment. Examples of this would include how access to the system is granted to employees and what specific information can be accessed by each employee. Another related policy would be one which outlines sanctions for employees inappropriately accessing information relating to patients not under their care.

Methods

Technical aspects of creating systems include programming HIT systems to recognize the language of healthcare. One key application requiring this ability is **clinical decision support**, which uses codified information from a patient record and aids in diagnosis and treatment. The multiple ways that medical information can be stated presents significant challenges in creating these systems. The work of informaticists is to define the way information is represented in HIT systems. This can be done by interpreting the data, codifying it, and identifying relationships between the data. An example of the outcome of the work of a health informaticist is a system for CPOE. These systems usually contain error prevention software that provides the user with prompts to warn against the possibility of drug interaction, allergy, or overdose and other relevant information to assure that the order is correct before it is processed and administered to the patient (AHIMA 2012, 95). Incorporated into such a system would be the relevant drug information including the different names the drug could be identified by, the typical dosage protocol, contraindications for taking the drug, symptoms of untoward events such as allergies, and interactions with other drugs. This drug data would be codified, which reduces words to codes of numbers and letters. Once the codes are assigned, the relationships are identified. There are a multitude of relationships that would need to be identified to reflect the potential interactions that could occur between the data elements. For example, for one drug, alternate names of the drug, the standard dosage, common side effects, and the names of other drugs that are contraindicated need to be identified, to name a few. An example of how this CPOE system could then contribute to improved patient care is a scenario where the standard dosage is keyed in incorrectly, such as 25 milligrams versus 75 milligrams. In this instance in most CPOE systems, the physician would receive an immediate prompt questioning this order as entered. Available for the physician to review would be manufacturer information that indicates the normal drug dosage with a request for the physician to confirm the correct dosage to be prescribed. A defined vocabulary to identify clinical conditions is imperative in creating the system. The difficulty in healthcare is exacerbated by multiple terms meaning the same thing; that is, lacerations and cut, compounded by all the words that can then be used to further describe such a term. Coding systems which use specific clinical terminologies provide a means for providing specific definitions with more standardized terms. The transition to ICD-10-CM/PCS provides an expanded lexicon for enhanced standard terminology. There is a lack of specificity of what the code number represents with many of the ICD-9 codes. For example, an ICD-9 code for a laceration on the leg would not distinguish whether it was on the right or the left leg, where on the leg, or if the laceration is being treated for the first time or as a follow-up. The issue of first or subsequent visits could raise issues by third-party payers in processing the claims. This situation could also provide confusion with compiling data from this patient's record with not all encounters considered. The ICD-10 diagnostic codes would distinguish between the first encounter or return visits, whether on the right or the left leg, and other clinical information to identify initial treatment or follow-up treatment of the wound.

Health informatics also must consider the development of standards for software to be used in the EHR and the exchange of data. Compatibility and **interoperability**, allowing different health information systems to work together within and across organizational boundaries in order to advance the effective delivery of healthcare for individuals and communities, are a key focus in health informatics. Vendors have a vested interest in the establishment of standards to assure their products are compatible and competitive with the multiple applications required to build an EHR system.

Using the information to make decisions relies on the technology, the defined vocabulary, and the standards, as mentioned previously. These are tools to achieve the ultimate goal of having useable, meaningful information to facilitate the decision-making process. Informatics processes utilized to support this include **probability** and making predictions. Probability in this instance would be to use patient-related data to determine the likelihood of various occurrences in the disease process and modes of treatment. Informaticists must apply probability modes numerous times when developing systems to assist with making treatement decisions, often while utilizing incomplete, minimal, or even conflicting information. The various methods of decision analysis may be incorporated to identify the course to be taken in treatment or in making administrative decisions and setting policies. **Decision analysis** is a systematic approach to decision making under conditions of imperfect knowledge; it is a practical application of probability theory that is used to calculate the optimal strategy from among a series of alternative strategies. The results of this process are often expressed graphically in the form of a decision tree. With the wealth of data that can be transformed into information, opportunities exist to create new knowledge through numerous statistical applications and activities such as **data mining**, which involves searching, analyzing, and summarizing large data sets from different perspectives to identify trends and other useful information.

Check Your Understanding 1.3

Instructions: Answer the following question on a separate piece of paper.

1. Why is it difficult to create a vocabulary to identify clinical conditions?

Instructions: Choose the best answer.

2. Using patient-related data to determine the likelihood or various occurrences in the disease process and modes of treatment is an example of
   a. Reliability
   b. Probability
   c. Standardization
   d. Decision analysis

3. Intraoperability can best be described as
   a. A certified system
   b. Where multiple users can be accessing and using a system at the same time
   c. When there is complete standardization of data that can be accessed in a system
   d. Where there is the ability to exchange and use data between components of a system

4. Data mining is
   a. Searching, analyzing, and summarizing large data sets from different perspectives to identify trends and other useful information
   b. A statistical analysis software program
   c. Abstracting and categorizing large amounts of information
   d. Building flags into systems to automatically identify certain data elements

5. Under conditions of imperfect knowledge, a practical application of probability theory that is used to calculate the optimal strategy from among a series of alternative strategies is
   a. Strategizing
   b. Alternative analysis
   c. Decision analysis
   d. Data mining

Ethics

Ethics involves the standards of moral practice, values, and a code of conduct. Ethical issues with EHRs and health informatics are inherent due to the nature of the information involved, the confidential patient information. The goal of health informatics is to convert the patient-related data into information that can be used to make treatment decisions and to compile information that can be used to enhance the care of large populations of patients. This information is valuable for administration and policy making. To support this activity the information must be compiled, shared, transmitted, and reviewed by a variety of entities. As more patient data is generated and used across the spectrum of healthcare, the potential for ethical challenges arise. Probability and predictability of the incidence of a medical condition and/or potential survival with a meaningful life could influence who receives healthcare and to what extent the services are provided. The hybrid state of the majority of health information systems can lead to the potential for medical care errors due to system issues with incomplete, incorrect, or unavailable information when part of the record is in an electronic system and part is in paper form. The difficulty in keeping the patient information secure and confidential is a continuing problem whether the records are electronic, paper, or hybrid. Quality issues exist as well with occurrences such as poor quality of images transmitted via an electronic system, medical errors when protocols are inadequate to support quality care, and lack of staff or inability to use the system appropriately. Ethical issues could potentially arise from the empowerment of the patient consumer with online resources and the consequences of making an incorrect self-diagnosis. With regard to telemedicine, there is also the reliance on the technology and the inherent problems of availability and quality of the information and the electronic transmission and storage of information. For aggregate data reported on large groups of patients, the selective use and distribution of the analysis of the information, privacy concerns, and unscrupulous use of data for commercial gain are all of concern from an ethical standpoint.

Ethical issues are not new in the provision of healthcare. It must be recognized that for all of the positive outcomes that technological advances can bring, such as the amount of and enhancement of patient data with the ability to transmit and share it, the potential for ethical issues still exists and such issues are arguably more complex than with the paper record.

⊙ Roles

As alluded to previously, there are a number of different individuals who play a key role with health informatics from HIM professionals, to physicians and other providers of healthcare, to information technology specialists, to those in administrative positions in the facility such as the **chief information officer (CIO)** and the **chief medical information officer (CMIO)**. The CIO is a senior manager responsible for the overall management of information resources in an organization (AHIMA 2012, 73). The CMIO is an emerging position, typically a physician with medical informatics training, that provides physician leadership and direction in the deployment of clinical applications in healthcare organizations (AHIMA 2012, 73).

Additionally, health information managers are filling the role of **chief knowledge officer (CKO)**, the person who oversees the entire knowledge acquisition, storage, and dissemination process and identifies subject matter experts to help capture and organize the organization's knowledge assets (AHIMA 2012, 73). Each role contributes to the success of the health informatics initiatives with their specific area of expertise but the diversity of the roles illustrates the breadth of knowledge and skills necessary to meet the goals and realize the potential of informatics in the healthcare environment. An introduction to several of the primary roles and how professionals in a variety of existing roles will play an important part in the informatics movement utilizing their knowledge and skills from their perspective is shown below. These existing roles will inherently continue to evolve in relation to the influence of health informatics and as advances continue to be made.

Health Information Professional

The foundation of the HIM profession has always been to ensure the integrity of patient information through its life cycle while maintaining confidentiality. As the regulations, laws, technology, and payment methods have evolved over the years, the HIM professional domain of knowledge and skills has evolved. But the advances and utilization of technology within the past few years have resulted in a fundamental change in the functions and resulting roles of all levels of HIM professionals. These will continue to evolve with the continued deployment of computer systems throughout the healthcare enterprise, which results in the creation of much more data than in the past with new means of evaluating and using the resulting data. The selection, acquisition, and implementation of systems requires the ongoing input of HIM professionals for this endeavor to be successful. HIM roles that have supported this process include those related to project management, work redesign, and privacy concerns. HIM professionals transitioning in these roles will require the acquisition of IT knowledge and leadership capabilities. Numerous other new roles continue to emerge to include those related to data analysis, research activities, information exchange, consumer health informatics related primarily to the PHR, and the previously mentioned CKO, to name a few.

Physician

The role the physician plays in the adoption and utilization of the EHR is vital and therefore key to generating the information utilized in any informatics-related activity. An understanding of how technology can benefit their patients and the appropriate level of use is the key to success. E-prescribing was one of the initial applications that many physicians experienced. One of the programs of the American Recovery and Reinvestment Action (ARRA) of 2009 was to promote the adoption and use of EHRs. In this law the Health Information Technology for Economic and Clinical Health (HITECH) Act refers to the HIT components of the stimulus package that was a part of the ARRA bill. "One of HITECH's most important features is its clarity of purpose. Congress apparently sees HIT—computers, software, Internet connection, telemedicine—not as an end in itself but as a means of improving the quality of health care, the health of populations, and the efficiency of healthcare systems" (Blumenthal 2009, 1477–1479).

Information Technology Specialists

The role of information technology specialist cannot be well defined based on job title or role alone. This generalist title can be interpreted or designed to meet the specific needs of a facility or defined based on a specific perspective or frame of reference. Within the scope of this job title or domain would be the knowledge and ability to use computers for the collection, maintenance, and use of patient health information. Aspects of using hardware and software would be key as would the ability to utilize the data that could be obtained from the systems that maintain patient care data, along with the skills to then use that data to enhance the quality and efficiency of healthcare. Using a job description posted on the National Institutes of Health (NIH) as a guide, figure 1.1 illustrates a job description indicative of the current role of the information technology specialist.

CIO, CMIO, and The C-level Positions

The chief administrative positions related to health informatics may vary from facility to facility and may not even be present in some facilities as a named position. In this instance the related responsibilities are shared by many throughout the

Figure 1.1   Sample job description for health information technology specialist

Job Title	Health Information Technology Specialist
Job Description	Health Information Technology (HIT) Specialists are experts in the development, implementation, management, and support of systems and networks. HIT specialists plan and carry out complex assignments and develop new methods and approaches in a wide variety of IT specialties.
Job Specialties	Bioinformatics Systems analysis Customer support Information security Applications software Data management Internet applications Network services Operating systems Systems administration
Job Requirements	Knowledge of IT principles, concepts and methods Systems testing and evaluation principles, methods, and tools IT security principles and methods COTS (Commercial Off-the-Shelf) products (nondevelopmental items such as computer software and hardware systems) Internet technologies Emerging technologies

Source: NIH 2012.

organization, mostly to carry out the tasks within their domain and area of expertise. Over the past few years the scope of information technology within a facility has increased significantly and permeates every aspect of the delivery of healthcare. The statement below indicates the prevalence of health informatics tasks throughout healthcare organizations.

> Whether it involves sending laboratory test results and appointment reminders to patients on their smart phones, giving nurses earlier warnings that a patient's vital signs are trending in a dangerous direction, or developing the paradigm-changing clinical and financial systems needed to put an accountable care organization into place, health information technology's (HIT) presence is pervasive. And it has become integral to virtually every process and operation within the healthcare field, from clinical decision making to materials management (Birk 2007).

While job descriptions for CIOs would vary significantly for those holding this position from one facility to another, the required knowledge and skills for the position would probably include technical skills, but just as important would be the need for strategic planning and thinking, leadership, and the ability to predict and prepare for the future.

The CMIO provides that vital link between the medical aspect of care and the information technology or systems departments within the healthcare facility. The individual who holds this title may either be a physician who has a particular interest or knowledge of the use of technology or an individual with a technology background specifically in health informatics, utilizing information in medical treatment and research. Common requirements for a CMIO position would include the ability to integrate systems to support the delivery of healthcare, the ability to evaluate and analyze the outcomes of using technology on patient care, and the more administrative-related tasks of planning, setting standards, project management, and being an advocate of the use of technology with the members of the medical staff.

The CKO is someone who has a broader view of the effective use of the information in ways that contribute to the knowledge of workers and the organization. An effective CKO can help utilize improved technology and expanded data assets to efficienctly convert data into knowledge and strategically meet an organization's needs in regards to cost reductions, clinical outcomes, pay-for-performance, competitive advantage, and best practices (Cassidy 2011).

Scribes

The term scribe alludes to one who authors or writes. A **medical scribe**, many times a medical student, nurse practitioner, or physician's assistant, assists the physician with the required documentation in the patient's medical record. The benefits to direct patient care are two-fold with improved productivity of the physician in terms of time and ability to focus more directly on the patient and the ability of the scribe to support the treatment by providing the physician with needed information. This could include updates on diagnostic information and other information from the patient's record to enhance the encounter with the patient by providing timely and comprehensive information. With the increased use of the EHR, scribes are instrumental in incorporating the documentation into the EHR system thus again freeing up the physician's time and ensuring that required fields and other documentation requirements are met. A more comprehensive record will enhance the aggregate use of data in research and meaningful use activities and in making administrative decisions. The Centers for Medicare and Medicaid Services (CMS) regulations allow for the use of scribes, with the stipulation that the physician is clearly the one providing the service, with the scribe serving to record the spoken words of the practitioner. Notation must be made attesting to the involvement of the scribe with the practitioner authenticating the information with signature upon completion of the report. Improved patient care may be one of the benefits when scribes are utilized. Other benefits documented in various studies include the increased productivity of physicians in seeing a greater number of patients, increased physician morale with the significant burden for documentation lifted, improved compliance with core measures, and enhanced reimbursement with improved capture of the data elements to support the billing function. Limitations in the use of scribes include the acceptance of providers to utilize them appropriately and the cost to the organization.

Check Your Understanding 1.4

Instructions: Choose the best answer.

1. The benefits of using scribes include
   a. Relieving the physician from the responsibility for completing documentation in the record
   b. Providing medical students the opportunity to learn to document
   c. Providing entries that are legible and easier to read
   d. Freeing up physician time and providing comprehensive documentation

2. The primary role of the CMIO is to
   a. Be a physician
   b. Provide a vital link between the medical aspect of care and the information/systems departments
   c. Ensure that all necessary perspectives are represented when health information technology is implemented
   d. Design the EHR system

3. With the advances in genomic information, the probability and predictability of medical conditions can be determined in many instances. What potential ethical issues arise out of this?
   a. It could influence who receives healthcare.
   b. It can lead to medical errors due to incomplete information.
   c. It would require documentation for such a patient to be filed separate from the rest of the record.
   d. Whether or not to tell the patient about the information.

4. The person charged with the primary functions of strategic planning, leadership, and ability to predict future technology needs would be the
   a. Facility administrator
   b. CIO
   c. CMIO
   d. Informatacist

Instructions: Answer the following question on a separate piece of paper.

5. What are common skills and knowledge that would be needed across the various roles of those involved with health informatics?

⊙ Summary

This chapter introduces the topic of health informatics and its evolution to illustrate the current state of the field and provide background and perspective for the remainder of the chapters in this text. Presented as a means of introduction were the basic competencies needed to support the field and the current major roles, along with the associated terms and other key concepts of healthcare informatics to illustrate the complexity of the informatics work throughout an organization. It is apparent that the most prevalent challenges in health informatics are related to the complexity of healthcare, the establishment of associated policies, the issues with potential new ethical dilemmas promulgated by informatics-facilitated data, acceptance by the various stakeholders, and the acquisition and appropriate use of the technology. This evolution and the challenges will continue and a knowledgeable, well-trained work force is vital. It is well accepted that despite the challenges and concerns, embracing health informatics will result in increased quality of care in a cost-effective manner due to having needed information in a timely manner. This information can serve as the basis for making decisions in all aspects of care and supports the analysis and research associated with the effective and efficient provision of healthcare.

REFERENCES

AHIMA. 2012. *Pocket Glossary for Health Information Management and Technology*, 3rd ed. Chicago: AHIMA Press.

AHIMA and AMIA. 2008. Joint Work Force Task Force, Health Information Management and Informatics Core Competencies for Individuals Working with Electronic Health Records.

Anderson, J. and S. Jay, eds. 1987. *Use and Impact of Computers in Clinical Medicine, Invited Volume in the Computers and Medicine Series*. New York: Springer-Verlag Publishing.

Blumenthal, D. 2009. Perspective: Stimulating the adoption of health information technology. *New England Journal Of Medicine*. 360:1477–1479.

Brittain, J. and A. Norris. 2008. Delivery of health informatics education and training. *Health Libraries Review* 17(3):117–128.

Birk, S. 2011. The evolving CIO: From IT manager to key healthcare delivery strategist. *Healthcare Executive* May/June, 20–27.

Cassidy, B.S. 2011. Teaching the future: An educational response to the AHIMA core model. *Journal of AHIMA* 82(1):34–38.

Eysenback, G. 2001. What is e-health? *Journal of Med Internet Research.* 3(2):e20. Published online June 18, 2001. doi: 10.2196/jmir.3.2.e20.

Hersh, W. 2009. A stimulus to define informatics and health information technology. *BMC Medical Informatics and Decision Making* 9(24). doi:10.1186/1472-6947-9-24.

Imhoff, M., A. Webb, and A. Goldschmidt. 2001. Health informatics. *Intensive Care Medicine* 27:179–186

Joint Work Force Task Force. 2008. *Health Information Management and Informatics Core Competencies for Individuals Working With Electronic Health Records.* AHIMA and AMIA.

Murphy, J. 2011. The nursing informatics workforce: Who are they and what do they do? *Nursing Economics* 3(29).

National Human Genome Research Institute. 2013. http://www.genome.gov.

National Institutes of Health. 2012. NIH: Jobs@NIH-Job Descriptions-Information Technology Specialist.

Sarkar, I. 2010. Biomedical informatics and translational medicine. *Journal of Translational Medicine* 8(22).

World Health Organization. 2013. www.who.int/en/.

RESOURCES

Arya, R., D. Salovich, P. Ohman-Stricklan, and M. Merlin. 2010. Impact of scribes on performance indicators in the emergency department. *Academy of Emergency Medicine* 17(5):490–494.

Betts, H. and G. Wright. 2009. Observations on Sustainable and Ubiquitous Healthcare Informatics from Florence Nightingale. *Connecting Health and Humans.* Edited by K. Saranto et al. Amsterdam: IOS Press.

Brandt, M. 2000. Health informatics standards: A user's guide. *Journal of AHIMA* 71(4):39–43.

Campbell, R. 2005. Getting to the good information: PHRs and consumer health informatics. *Journal of AHIMA* 76(10):46–49.

Carter-Templeton, H. R. Patterson, and C. Russell. 2009. An Analysis of Published Nursing Informatics Competencies. *Connecting Health and Humans.* Edited by K. Saranto et al. Amsterdam: IOS Press.

Cassidy, B. 2011. Stepping into New e-HIM roles: The e-HIM transition changes HIM roles and responsibilities. *Journal of AHIMA* 83(9):10.

Cesnik, B. and M. Kidd. 2010. History of health informatics: A global perspective. *Studies in Health Technology Information* 151:3–8.

Collen, M. 1986. Origins of medical informatics. *Medical Informatics* (Special Issue). 145:778–785.

Detmer, D.E., J.R. Lumpkin, and J.J. Williamson. 2009. Defining the medical subspecialty of clinical informatics. *Journal of the American Medical Informatics Association* 16(1):167–168.

Dolan, M, J. Wolter, C. Nielsen, and J. Burrington-Brown. 2009. Consumer health informatics: Is there a role for HIM professionals? *Perspectives in Health Information Management.*

Embi, P. S. Kaufman, and R. Payne. 2009. Biomedical informatics and outcomes research: Enabling knowledge-driven healthcare. NIH Public Access. December 8; 120(23):2393. doi:10.1161/CIRCULATION AHA. 108.795526.

Expanded scribe role boosts staff morale and templates help organize care. *ED Management.* July 2009; 21(7):75–77.

Eysenbach, G. 2000. Consumer health informatics. *British Medical Journal.* 320(7251):1713–1716.

Forgey, D. and J. Vickrey. 2005. Informatics: How an emerging field of study benefits HIM. *Journal of AHIMA* 76(6):46–49.

Fox, L. 2004. Health Record Paradigm Shift: Consumer Health Informatics. *IFHRO Congress & AHIMA Convention Proceedings.* October.

Georgiou, A. 2002. Data, information and knowledge: The health informatics model and its role in evidence-based medicine. *Journal of Evaluation in Clinical Practice* 8(2):127–130.

Houston, T., B. Chang, S. Brown, and R. Kukafka. 2001. Consumer Health Informatics: A Consensus Description and Commentary from the American Medical Informatics Association Members. AMIA, Inc.

Hovenga, E. 2010. National Standards in Health Informatics. *Health Informatics.* E. J. S. Hovenga et al. (Eds.). Amsterdam: IOS Press, Ch. 11.

Jesse, W. 2011. Healthcare IT is more than EHRs. *MGMA* Connexion, 5–6.

Kampov-Polevoi, J. and B. Hemminger. 2011. A curricula-based comparison of biomedical and health informatics programs in the USA. *Journal of American Medical Informatics Association* 18:195–202.

LaTour, K., S. Eichenwald-Maki, and P. Oachs. 2013 *Health Information Management: Concepts, Principles, and Practices.* Chicago:AHIMA.

Layman, E. 2009. Research and policy model for health informatics and information management. *Perspectives in Health Information Management* 6.

Macpherson, B. 2010. The role of a health information manager in creating data fit for purpose. *Health Information Management Journal* 39(3). 58–59.

Martin-Sanchez, F., V. Maojo, and G. Lopez-Campos. 2002. Integrating genomics into health information systems. *Methods in Informatics Medicine* 41:25–30.

McKinney, M. 2010. Most wired CMIOs steadily on the rise. *Hospital and Health Networks* 84(3):41–42.

Murphy, G. and M. Brandt. 2001. Health informatics standards and information transfer: Exploring the HIM role (AHIMA Practice Brief). *Journal of AHIMA* 72(1):68A–D.

Norris, A. 2002. Current trends and challenges in health informatics. *Health Informatics Journal* 8:205.

Russo, M. 1998. Consumer health informatics: The medical librarian's role. *Journal of AHIMA* 69(8): 38–40.

Scribes. 2009. ER please docs, save $600,000. *ED Management* 21(10):117–118.

Sethi, P. and K. Theodos. 2009. Translational bioinformatics and healthcare informatics: Computational and ethical challenges. *Perspectives in Health Information Management* 6, Fall.

Smith, S., L. Drake, J. Harris, K. Watson, and P. Pohlner. 2011. Clinical informatics: A workforce priority for 21st century healthcare. *Australian Health Review* 35:130–135.

Tegen, A. and J. O'Connell. 2012. Rounding with scribes: Employing scribes in a pediatric inpatient setting. *Journal of AHIMA* 83(1):34–38.

US Department of Energy Genome Programs. Human Genome Project Information. http://genomics.energy.gov.

Yasnoff, W., P. O'Carroll, D. Koo, R. Linkins, and E. Kilbourne. 2000. Public health informatics: Improving and transforming public health in the information age. *Journal of Public Health Management Practice* 6(6):67–75.

Zeng, X., R. Reynolds, and M. Sharp. 2009. Redefining the roles of health information management professionals in health information technology. *Perspectives in Health Information Management* 6, Summer.

Zhang, Y., X. Yang, X. Han, and R. Xia. 2010. The Research of Data Management Technology in Telemedicine Diagnosis System Based on Multimedia. *2010 International Conference on Computer Application and System Modeling (ICCASM 2010).*

The Electronic Health Record

By Kim Murphy-Abdouch and Sue Biedermann

Learning Objectives

- Review the evolution in the development of the electronic health record
- Articulate the issues surrounding the deployment and implementation of the electronic health record
- Compare the differences in electronic health record systems
- Describe HITECH funding
- Compare the advantages and disadvantages of the electronic health record
- Consider the current status and documented outcomes of EHR utilization

KEY TERMS

American Recovery and Reinvestment Act (ARRA)
Continuity of care document (CCD)
Clinical decision support system (CDSS)
Clinical data repository (CDR)
Clinical decision making
Clinical documentation
Clinical information systems (CIS)
Computer-based patient record (CPR)
Computerized provider order entry (CPOE)
Electronic health record (EHR)

Electronic medication administration record (EMAR)
Electronic medical record (EMR)
Episode of care
E-prescribing
Evidenced-based medicine
Health information exchange (HIE)
Health information system (HIS)
Health information technology (HIT)
Healthcare Information and Management Systems Society (HIMSS)

Health Information Technology for Economic and Clinical Health (HITECH) Act	Meaningful use
Institute of Medicine (IOM)	Office of the National Coordinator for Health Information Technology (ONC)
Integration	Practice management system (PMS)
Interface	Picture archiving and communication system (PACS)
Interoperability	
Laboratory information system (LIS)	Regional Extension Center (REC)

⊙ Introduction

The evolution of the field of informatics cannot be fully understood or appreciated without consideration of the introduction and advancement of information systems in healthcare and the continued emphasis on the implementation of the **electronic medical record (EMR)** and **electronic health record (EHR)** along with the subsequent analysis and use of the health information. The EMR is an electronic record of health-related information on an individual that can be created, gathered, managed, and consulted by authorized clinicians and staff within a single healthcare organization. The EHR is an electronic record of health-related information that conforms to nationally recognized **interoperability** standards and can be created, managed, and consulted by authorized clinicians and staff across more than one organization (Latour et al. 2013, 912). Interoperability standards allow different health information systems to work together within and across organizational boundaries in order to advance the effective delivery of healthcare for individuals and communities (HIMSS 2005).

Paper medical records and EMRs contain basically the same patient information, including the notes of the physicians, nurses, therapists, and all healthcare professionals who provided direct care to the patient. Also recorded in the patient records, whether paper or electronic, are consent for treatment and other consent forms; lab, imaging, and other diagnostic reports; reports of procedures; and medication records, all of which provide complete documentation of the medical care provided to a patient. Paper records provide a record of the **episode of care**, which is the specific instance of a condition or illness with a defined time frame with the beginning and ending times of care identified. An episode of care can apply to ambulatory encounters at a physician's office, outpatient clinic, ambulatory surgery center, or standalone laboratory and imaging facilities. An episode of care can also be an inpatient stay where the patient is admitted to a hospital or other healthcare facility for comprehensive care with multiple services provided within one setting. The limitation of the record in paper form is that the documentation is of just that episode of care, a well-defined, time-limited encounter. A paper record is initiated with the patient arriving at a physician's office or being admitted to a hospital and ends when the patient leaves the physician's office or is discharged from the hospital. Access to the information in paper form is limited to its location or by being copied and distributed to others via delivery, fax, or mail.

Compare the paper medical record environment to that of the electronic health record. Initially the patient information for the EHR is collected for an individual episode of care. However, once the information is maintained electronically all episodes of care can be accessed at one time and in different formats than the original record. With the EHR, the individual data elements in the record become searchable across visits. For example, a patient's medication history for a period of time rather than a single episode of care could be accessed without reviewing each individual record of care to compile the information. Other benefits of the EHR are the ability of multiple authorized individuals to access it at the same time as opposed to a paper record, which can only be accessed by one person at a time. EHRs also provide alerts and reminders about preventative services and provide information to support diagnostic and therapeutic decision making. To better understand the EHR systems of today, it is important to review the history of the evolution of the use of technology for maintenance of patient health information.

⊙ History

EHRs have evolved over time, beginning in the 1960s. Early applications were software based with several large healthcare systems developing applications for specific uses within their facilities. These early adopters included Latter Day Saints Hospital, and Harvard and Duke Medical Schools. Utilization of early applications also included collecting information for decision support. The development of software applications evolved with the development and the adoption of **health information systems (HIS)**. A health information system can be defined as a "set of components and procedures organized with the objective of generating information which improve health care management decisions at all levels of the health system" (Lippeveld et al. 2000, ch. 11).

With the anticipated potential of electronic systems for maintaining and utilizing patient information, there were multiple driving forces supporting the continued development and implementation of such systems. Physicians supported the movement due to concern for care of their patients as medical care increased in complexity and there was a growing need for critical patient information to be available in a timely manner. Healthcare administration supported HIS implementation with early systems developed to support billing and financial services. The transactional nature of the hospital's billing and financial services allowed the development of systems similar to those used in banking systems and by other early adopters of information technology (IT) to support business processes. Moving beyond software applications, the early applications of IT in the 1960s relied on mainframe computers, which were very large and expensive.

The availability of smaller computers in the 1970s enabled the development of early **clinical information systems (CIS)** to support individual clinical departments such as pharmacy, radiology, and laboratory. These clinical information systems were designed to facilitate the management of the activities of the clinical departments and to provide electronic charge capture and results reporting (McCullough 2007). Each department's CIS functioned as a stand-alone system within the department but could also be connected with other systems using an interface. **Interfaces** are hardware or software that enable disparate CIS and HIS software systems to communicate with each other. For example, interfaces eliminated the need to enter patient demographic information multiple times into separate laboratory, radiology, or pharmacy systems, and also enabled users to have a single sign-on to access information from any of the stand-alone clinical information systems. The single sign-on to access patient demographic and clinical information facilitated access to data, but interfaces could be expensive and time-consuming to develop. A significant milestone in the development of these early systems in the 1970s was the implementation of a **computerized provider (physician) order entry (CPOE)** system. The CPOE system allowed providers the ability to directly enter medication, other orders, and medical instructions electronically. The utilization of CPOE systems reduces medical errors that may result from handwritten orders. CPOE applications coupled with decision support applications became an important tool to reduce medical errors, improve healthcare quality, and provide efficient care.

One of the first comprehensive electronic medical record (EMR) systems was developed in the 1970s by the Regenstrief Institute in Indianapolis, Indiana. Samuel Regenstrief was an industrial production expert who founded the Regenstrief Institute in 1968 because he thought healthcare was inefficient and could benefit from the use of computer automation and industrial efficiency techniques. One of the earliest benefits of the Regenstrief EMR was improved access to patient information wherever and whenever clinical decisions were being made, independent of where the data were originally acquired. The Regenstrief Medical Record System (RMRS) has evolved over time and now functions as a citywide EHR system, allowing emergency room physicians to view a single virtual record for all patient care previously provided at any of 18 participating hospitals. Ambulances in Indianapolis also have laptops that can access the EHR in real time to provide up-to-date clinical information for diagnosis, treatment, and referral decisions about the patient (Regenstrief Institute 2012).

In addition to providing access to patient data for **clinical decision making** in the course of the care of the patient, the RMRS also provides a rich source of data for health services research. Clinical decision making is the process of utilizing information to formulate a diagnosis. RMRS has a database of 6 million patients, with 900 million online coded results, 20 million full reports including diagnostic studies, procedure results, operative notes, and discharge summaries, and 65 million radiology images (Regenstrief Institute 2012). This data is useful for research to support implementation of evidence-based practices. **Evidence-based medicine** is defined as use of the current best evidence in making clinical decisions about the care of individual patients by integrating individual clinical expertise with the best available clinical evidence from systematic research (Sackett 1996).

Major milestones in the evolution of the EHR in the 1980s include the implementation by the Veterans Health Administration (VHA) of an electronic health record system that is still in use today. Initially comprehensive patient scheduling software programs were launched. As the VHA system evolved through the 1970s and the 1980s, numerous agencies and organizations were involved in developing the scheduling system and encouraging an expansion to include support for clinical functions. The first program launched by VHA was the Decentralized Hospital Computer Program (DHCP) in 1981. The name of the system was changed when new groups, such as dentists, were added and their practice was not consistent with the name of the system. Other changes were made as different organizations became involved or new applications were added. Adopted in 1994, the system was named VistA (Veterans Health Information System and Technology Architecture) and is still in use today as an enterprise-wide information system. Nearly 160 integrated modules comprise the system for clinical care, financial functions, and infrastructure. The VistA system is open-source and readily available.

The 1990s saw the first Windows-based software for electronic health records. Software for **e-prescribing** enjoyed significant advances during this time. E-prescribing allows practitioners to use electronic devices to write and submit prescription orders directly to a participating pharmacy rather than faxing or providing the patient with a written prescription that must then be taken to the pharmacy. E-prescribing systems also incorporate reference software for practitioners' use as they consider the options of medications to be ordered. E-prescribing is also a requirement of the federal government's EHR Meaningful Use Incentive Program, which provides financial incentives for providers and hospitals for implementing health information technology (HIT).

The **Institute of Medicine (IOM)** has been a major force in the development of the EMR. The IOM is an independent, nonprofit organization that works outside of government to provide unbiased and authoritative advice to decision makers and the public. The IOM first presented a blueprint for the **computer-based patient record (CPR)** in 1991. The report defined the CPR as an electronic patient record that provides complete and accurate data, alerts, reminders, clinical decision support, links to medical knowledge, and other aids. The IOM proposed the adoption of CPR as the standard for all records related to patient care, and recommended the establishment of a public or private organization to focus on a national agenda and provide support for CPR research, development, and demonstration. They also proposed the promulgation of national standards for data and security, and laws and regulations to facilitate implementation of CPRs. A follow-up report in 1997 reported that the healthcare industry was lagging behind other industries in automating their data and called for the establishment of CPRs as the standard within 10 years (IOM 1997).

As a result of the gradual adoption over time of IT in the complex business of healthcare, health IT is not a single product, but rather a collection of hardware and software working within the healthcare organization or the healthcare delivery system. While there were published standards for the content of the paper medical record as defined by the Medicare Conditions of Participation and accrediting bodies such as the Joint Commission, the complex nature of healthcare and the lack of standardization have impeded the development and implementation of electronic medical records when compared to information systems development in the business and financial arenas. Data in the business and financial arenas are generally standardized and structured, but approximately 60 percent of healthcare documentation contains unstructured narrative text (Health Story Project 2012). Structured data are binary, computer-readable data, while unstructured data are nonbinary, human-readable information. For example, history and physical examinations, discharge summaries, nursing observations, physician progress notes, and consultation reports are generally handwritten or dictated and transcribed. In this unstructured narrative form, there are many ways to say the same thing, multiple terms with the same meanings, and acronyms that may represent multiple different phrases. For example, the medical term jaundice is synonymous with icterus. The acronym CVA is frequently used to refer to a cerebrovascular accident but just as commonly used to refer to costovertebral angle.

In 2001, the Institute of Medicine (IOM) noted that for most individuals "health information is typically dispersed in a collection of paper records which are not easy to retrieve, making it nearly impossible to manage illnesses, especially chronic conditions which require frequent monitoring and ongoing patient support" (IOM 2001, 15). The IOM called for a system in which knowledge is shared and information flows freely, where clinicians and patients communicate effectively and share information. The IOM emphasized the need for a commitment to the development of a national information infrastructure, with the expectation that such commitment could lead to the elimination of most handwritten clinical data by the end of the decade.

With mounting evidence supporting the premise that health IT can improve quality, safety, and cost effectiveness of care, it could be expected that the adoption rate would be high. However, a 2009 survey of all acute-care hospitals that are members of the American Hospital Association (AHA) demonstrated that this was not the case. On the basis of responses from 63 percent of the over 4,800 hospitals surveyed, only 1.5 percent of US hospitals had a comprehensive EHR in 2009. An additional 7.6 percent had a basic EHR in at least one clinical unit and 17 percent of hospitals had CPOE for medications. The survey also gathered data regarding barriers to the adoption of EHRs. Barriers cited included inadequate capital for purchases, unclear return on investment, maintenance costs, physician resistance, and inadequate IT staff (Jha 2009). Other reports indicate physician resistance can be attributed to the time it takes for them to learn the new system, the increased amount of time for them to document, and a perceived loss of connection with the patient as the physician attempts to document electronically while questioning and examining the patient.

The AHA study clearly demonstrated that cost was a major barrier to implementing health IT. Historically, the business case for health IT acquisition has not been as straightforward when compared to business planning for other types of technology. The benefits to be achieved with health IT often accrue to the payers, rather than the healthcare organizations that invest in the technology. For example, the availability of laboratory reports ordered by another provider and included in an EHR may avoid duplication of tests, but the savings for this avoided test would accrue to the payer and not the provider who made the investment in the EHR. Further, some of the benefits of health IT such as provider convenience, patient satisfaction, and improved communication are not easily quantified in evaluating the return on investment and building the business case for health IT. In 1991 the IOM first proposed that the costs of CPRs be shared among all users of the data (Dick 1991).

Despite the development of EHRs over three decades, research indicating improved quality of care, and the suggestions of the IOM, it was not until President George W. Bush noted in his 2004 State of the Union address "By computerizing health records, we can avoid dangerous medical mistakes, reduce costs, and improve care" that the issue of EHR came to the forefront for the American people and significant federal investment in health IT was initiated. President Bush created the **Office of the National Coordinator for Health Information Technology (ONC)** in 2004 with $50 million in funding, and doubled the investment for **health information technology (HIT)** to $100 million in 2005 (HIMSS 2004). The ONC's function is that of principal advisor to the Secretary of the Department of Health and Human Services on the development, application, and the use of HIT.

Between 2005 and 2009, there was gradual adoption of EHRs and the ONC developed and promulgated standards for health IT, but it was not until 2009 that the **American Recovery and Reinvestment Act (ARRA)** of 2009 provided a significant impetus to HIT through the allocation of $22.6 billion in funds to promote HIT. ARRA was an economic stimulus bill created to help the United States recover from the downturn of the economy with a total amount of $787 billion allocated to the recovery.

The **Health Information Technology for Economic and Clinical Health (HITECH) Act**, one part of ARRA, designated funding to modernize the healthcare system by promoting and expanding the adoption of HIT. HITECH provided $20 billion in Medicare and Medicaid incentive payments to physicians and hospitals for meaningful use of EHRs and $2.6 billion to support ONC initiatives. **Meaningful use** involves using the information from a certified EHR as a measure of quantity and quality of care. HITECH placed the payer (Medicare and Medicaid) into the business case for implementing health IT.

The HITECH funding and the ONC's coordinated nationwide effort to implement and standardize health IT resulted in a surge in health IT implementation in 2011 and 2012. As of the end of 2012, 42 percent of the primary care providers in the United States had signed up with the **Regional Extension Centers (RECs)** to participate in the Medicare and Medicaid Electronic Health Record (EHR) Incentive Programs. RECs were established by the ONC to assist primary care providers in quickly becoming adept and meaningful users of EHRs. RECs provide training and support services to assist doctors and other providers in adopting EHRs, share information and guidance to help with EHR implementation, and give technical assistance as needed. In December 2012, the Centers for Disease Control and Prevention's National Center for Health Statistics (NCHS) reported that the percentage of doctors adopting electronic health records increased from 48 percent in 2009 to 72 percent in 2012 (HHS 2012).

Check Your Understanding 2.1

Matching: Match the term with the appropriate description.

- **a.** Clinical decision making
- **b.** E-prescribing
- **c.** Evidence-based medicine
- **d.** Interface
- **e.** Interoperability

1. _____ Ability of systems to work together

2. _____ That which enables disparate systems to communicate with each other

3. _____ Facilitates transmission of medication orders from a physician to a pharmacist

4. _____ Utilizing information to formulate a diagnosis

5. _____ Relies on clinical expertise and the best research-based clinical evidence

---

⊙ Components

The electronic health record is not just software or a single computer system but is composed of multiple **integrated** applications. An integrated system is one that has been designed to bring together multiple information systems, and allows them to communicate in a timely and effective manner and work together as one system. There may be variations among systems regarding which ancillary services may be included. There may be differences in the means of the interfaces to access the ancillary systems, but all EHRs are designed to create an electronic record to bring together information from disparate systems that are in compliance with standards for the purpose of supporting quality of care, administrative functions, and research. As identified by the National Institutes for Health National Center for Research (NIH NCR) 2006 report on the Electronic Health Record, the key components of an EHR include systems for administrative functions, laboratory, radiology, pharmacology, and clinical documentation (NIH NCR 2006). Figure 2.1 depicts the integration of healthcare data from various systems for a single patient.

The component that is identified as administrative in nature includes those data that accurately identify the patient, such as the name and other demographics, and the registration, admissions, discharge, and transfer information, including such things as chief complaint and patient disposition. A vital administrative consideration is the unique patient identifier, which is at the core of an EHR and the means by which all information from the various components is linked to the patient. For confidentiality and security purposes the patient identifier is not known outside the organization.

In the majority of EHR systems, the laboratory systems remain as stand-alone systems that interface with the EHR. Lab systems routinely interface with

Figure 2.1 Electronic health record—concept overview

The EHR represents the integration of healthcare data from a participating collection of Systems for a single patient.

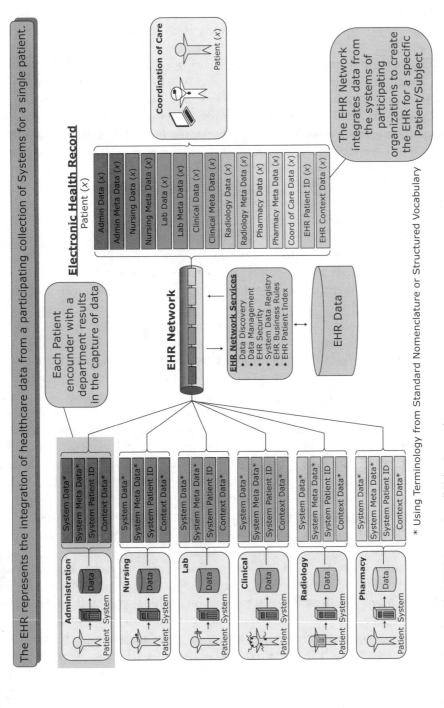

* Using Terminology from Standard Nomenclature or Structured Vocabulary

numerous laboratory instruments that process the lab specimens. A **laboratory information system (LIS)** may be a system that provides a hub to integrate laboratory information, including orders with results; there may be user access to the information. Other LIS functionality includes scheduling, billing, and other information needed by the lab; rarely is all of this information integrated with an EHR.

Radiology information systems (RIS) bring together patient radiology data with images. As seen with laboratory systems, RIS systems many times include patient tracking, scheduling, and reporting of results. Many systems are used with a **picture archiving and communication systems (PACS)**. PACS provide storage of electronic images and reports. While many hospitals have some sort of electronic system to support radiology, it does not mean that the system is necessarily integrated with the EHR.

As mentioned earlier in this chapter, computerized provider order entry (CPOE) systems were among the first applications deployed. Pharmacies are highly automated in other functions, including the use of robots to fill prescriptions. However, it is reported that the majority of pharmacy systems do not fully integrate with the EHR with many systems requiring the reentry of orders into the pharmacy system from the EHR, although this practice is improving.

Clinical documentation is the functionality of electronic capture of clinical notes. This would include patient assessments and clinical reports such as flow sheets and medication administration records. The clinical documentation that is entered into the patient record as text is not as easily automated due to the unstructured nature of the information. Unstructured clinical information would include notes written by the physicians and other practitioners who treat the patient, dictated and transcribed reports, and legal forms such as consents and advanced directives, to name a few. Information from medical devices may also be integrated into the information flow such as vital sign readings and intravenous pumps dosages and flow rates that can be sent directly to the patient record from the device where the data originated. With these components that provide the framework of the EHR systems, there are a number of other factors that must be considered in a discussion of the electronic health record. Many of these topics are related to regulations while others are identified as core functions and uses of the EHR that have been developed over time with the implementation and advancement of the systems.

In order to obtain HITECH funding, providers must implement an EHR that has been certified for meaningful use. Meaningful use is defined as the use of a certified EHR in a meaningful manner such as for e-prescribing; clinical decision support; maintenance of a problem list of current and active diagnoses; the exchange of health information; and the submission of quality or other measures. The Certification Commission for Health Information Technology (CCHIT) is one of the largest organizations authorized by the ONC to provide EHR certification. CCHIT is an independent not-for-profit organization that has been certifying EHRs since 2006. Other ONC authorized testing and certification entities include Surescripts, ICSA

Labs, SLI Global, InfoGuard Laboratories, Inc., and the Drummond Group, Inc. The certification process ensures that health IT products and systems are secure, can maintain data confidentiality, work with other systems to share information, and perform a set of well-defined functions (ONC 2013).

In 2003 a committee of the IOM identified a set of eight core care delivery functions that EHR systems should be capable of performing in order to promote greater safety, quality, and efficiency in healthcare delivery. Below are the eight functionalities with a brief description:

1. Health information and data—information for care providers to make clinical decisions about the care of the patient, including medical and nursing diagnoses, a medication list, allergies, demographics, clinical narratives, and laboratory test results.

2. Patient support—patient education has demonstrated significant effectiveness in improving control of chronic illnesses and computer-based patient education in particular has been found to be successful in primary care.

3. Order entry/management—can improve workflow processes by eliminating lost orders and ambiguities caused by illegible handwriting, generating related orders automatically, monitoring for duplicate orders, and reducing the time to fill orders.

4. Results management—managing results of all types (for example, laboratory test results, radiology procedure results reports) electronically.

5. Administrative processes and reporting—electronic scheduling admissions, procedures, and visits increase the efficiency of healthcare organizations, and provide better, timelier service to patients.

6. Reporting and population health—clinical data represented with a standardized terminology and in a machine-readable format would reduce the significant data collection burden at the provider level, as well as the associated costs, and would likely increase the accuracy of the data reported.

7. Decision support—computerized decision support systems for prescribing drugs, detection of adverse events and disease outbreaks, and computer reminders in such areas as vaccinations, breast cancer screening, colorectal screening, and cardiovascular risk reduction.

8. Electronic communication and connectivity—communication among healthcare team members and other care partners (for example, laboratory, radiology, pharmacy) and with patients (IOM 2003).

In addition to identifying the eight core functionalities for the EHR the IOM also identified primary and secondary uses of an EHR system as outlined in table 2.1.

The previously mentioned 2009 survey of AHA member hospitals on the level of implementation of EHRs also outlined four components of the EHR

Table 2.1 Primary and secondary uses of an EHR system

Primary Uses	Secondary Uses
Patient care delivery	Education
Patient care management	Regulation
Patient care support processes	Research
Financial and other administrative processes	Public health policy and homeland security
Patient self-management	Policy support

Source: IOM 1997.

that are useful as a framework for comparing levels of EHR adoption: clinical documentation, test and imaging results, computerized physician order entry, and decision support as core functionalities (Jha 2009). Ambulatory and inpatient EHRs have evolved differently over time and the specific components or functions also vary between ambulatory and inpatient EHRs. Ambulatory care is provided in a variety of locations by individual or groups of healthcare providers. Settings for ambulatory care may include physician offices, outpatient clinics, ambulatory surgery centers, and stand-alone laboratory and imaging facilities. In the ambulatory setting the patient generally moves themselves from setting to setting when receiving services from multiple providers. Inpatient care is generally provided in the hospital setting with many levels of providers and services concentrated within one setting.

Inpatient EHRs are generally comprised of multiple applications that are integrated and interoperable. Most ambulatory EHRs have been developed as complete systems that include practice management and clinical applications. Inpatient components may include financial and administrative applications, clinical systems, CPOE, **electronic medication administration records (EMARs)** (use of technology and bar coding to track medications from when ordered to when given to the patient), clinical data repositories, clinical decision support, document imaging, and PACS. Although inpatient and outpatient EHRs are different, there is a common set of functionalities that apply to both hospital and ambulatory EHRs as outlined below.

Electronic Functionalities

- Clinical documentation
  - Patient demographics
  - Physician notes
  - Nurse notes

- Problem lists
- Medication lists
- Discharge summaries
- Advance directives
- Results viewing
  - Laboratory reports
  - Radiology reports
  - Radiology images
  - Diagnostic test results
  - Diagnostic test images
  - Consultant reports
- Computerized physician order entry
  - Laboratory tests
  - Radiology tests
  - Medications
  - Consultation requests
  - Nursing orders
- Decision support
  - Clinical guidelines
  - Clinical reminders
  - Drug allergy alerts
  - Drug–drug interaction alerts
  - Drug–lab interaction alerts
  - Drug dosing support

Check Your Understanding 2.2

Matching: Match the term with the appropriate descriptions.
- a. E-prescribing
- b. Meaningful use
- c. Integrated
- d. EMAR
- e. Administrative

1. _____ System designed to bring together multiple information systems

2. _____ Use of a certified EHR for e-prescribing, health information exchange, and quality reporting

3. _____ Use of technology and bar coding to track patient medications

4. _____ Electronic transmission of prescriptions from the provider to the pharmacy

5. _____ Data that accurately identifies a patient

Ambulatory EHRs

Ambulatory EHRs were initially developed as **practice management systems (PMSs)** to support scheduling, financial, and billing activities. PMSs generally include patient registration, scheduling, eligibility verification, charge capture, electronic claims processing, billing, and collections. As ambulatory EHRs have evolved, they now include problem lists, medication lists, history and physical examinations, immunization records, patient progress and visit notes, clinical templates, electronic prescribing, medication management, health maintenance, disease management, outcomes reporting, clinical decision support, lab order entry, and results reporting.

Ambulatory EHRs may be characterized as complete or modular systems. In 2011, there were over 1,100 EHRs certified for meaningful use under the HITECH Act. Nearly two-thirds of the certified ambulatory EHRs were complete systems and one-third were modular systems. This changed dramatically from 2011 to 2012 as a result of new vendors moving into the marketplace and obtaining certification of their EHR products. By the end of 2012, there were 2,996 certified ambulatory EHRs; 50.9 percent complete systems and 49.1 percent modular components (ONC 2013).

Inpatient EHRs

As described earlier in this chapter, inpatient EHRs have evolved over time, beginning with business- and financial-based hospital information systems, followed by clinical information systems, and evolving to EHRs. Inpatient EHRs are generally comprised of a variety of source systems that feed data into the EHR.

Inpatient EHRs may also be classified as complete or modular. Of the inpatient EHRs certified by CCHIT in 2011, 75 percent were modular and only 25 percent were complete systems. At the end of 2012, the number of certified EHRs increased to 975: 29.1 percent complete systems and 70.1 percent modular systems (ONC 2013). Figure 2.2 illustrates all of the source systems and how they feed into the inpatient EHR.

The **Health Information and Management Systems Society (HIMSS)** EMR Adoption Model provides a framework for describing the components of an electronic medical record and measuring and reporting the stage of adoption by healthcare organizations (see figure 2.3). HIMSS is a cause-based not-for-profit organization exclusively focused on providing global leadership for the optimal use of IT and management systems for the betterment of healthcare. The HIMSS mission is to lead healthcare transformation through the effective use of HIT.

Table 2.2 depicts the level of adoption of health IT at the end of 2012.

The HITECH Act began to provide payment incentives for the implementation of EHRs by providers and healthcare organizations beginning in 2011 and these incentive payments will continue through 2016. However, beginning in 2016, providers who have not implemented an EHR will begin to be penalized through a reduction in Medicare payments. It is anticipated that the implementation and meaningful use of EHRs will continue to increase as more providers and healthcare organizations acquire EHRs and seek the incentive payments.

Figure 2.2   Source systems feeding data into the inpatient EHR

Source Systems

Administrative and Financial Applications

| R-ADT PMS | MPI | PFS | HIM | EDMS | QA | OC/RR |

Ancillary/Clinical Departmental Applications

Lab | Blood Bank | Radiology | Pacs | Inpatient Pharmacy | Others | Dietary

Specialty Clinical Systems

| Intensive Care | Perioperative/ Surgical | Cardiology | Labor and Delivery | Emergency Medicine | Long Term Care |

"Smart" Peripherals

| Monitoring Equipment | Robotics | Infusion Pumps | Dispensing Devices |

Core Clinical EHR Applications

Medication Management

| Results Management | POC Documentation | CPOE | BC-MAR | CDS | Reporting |

Supporting Infrastructure

- CDR - CDW - SAN - Interface Engine - Inference Engine -

Connectivity Systems

| LAN | Portals | CCR | CCD | PHR | WAN | Telehealth | HIE | NHIN |

Source: LaTour et al. 2013, 122.

Figure 2.3   HIMSS adoption model

- **Stage 0:** The organization has not installed all of the three key ancillary department systems (laboratory, pharmacy, and radiology).
- **Stage 1:** All three major ancillary clinical systems are installed (that is, pharmacy, laboratory, and radiology).
- **Stage 2:** Major ancillary clinical systems feed data to a **clinical data repository (CDR)** that provides physician access for reviewing all orders and results. The CDR is a centralized database focused on clinical information that usually contains a controlled medical vocabulary, and a **clinical decision support system (CDSS)** or engine for rudimentary drug or allergy conflict checking. A CDSS is a special subcategory of clinical information systems that is designed to help healthcare providers make knowledge-based clinical decisions such as those previously mentioned (AHIMA 2012, 85). Information from document imaging systems may be

(Continued)

Figure 2.3   HIMSS adoption model (*Continued*)

linked to the CDR at this stage. The hospital may be **health information exchange (HIE)**-capable at this stage and can share whatever information it has in the CDR with other patient care stakeholders. As used here, HIE refers to the actual exchange of health information between two parties who are using separate or different information systems.

- **Stage 3:** Nursing/clinical documentation (for example, vital signs, flow sheets, nursing notes, EMAR) is required and is implemented and integrated with the CDR for at least one inpatient service in the hospital; care plan charting is scored with extra points. The EMAR application is implemented. The first level of CDS is implemented to conduct error checking with order entry (that is, drug–drug, drug–food, drug–lab conflict checking normally found in the pharmacy information system). Medical image access from picture archive and communication systems (PACS) is available for access by physicians outside the Radiology department via the organization's intranet.

- **Stage 4:** CPOE for use by any clinician licensed to create orders is added to the nursing and CDR environment along with the second level of clinical decision support capabilities related to evidence-based medicine protocols. If one inpatient service area has implemented CPOE with physicians entering orders and completed the previous stages, then this stage has been achieved.

- **Stage 5:** The closed loop medication administration with bar coded unit dose medications environment is fully implemented. The EMAR and bar coding or other auto-identification technology, such as radio frequency identification (RFID), are implemented and integrated with CPOE and pharmacy to maximize point of care patient safety processes for medication administration. The "five rights" of medication administration are verified at the bedside with scanning of the bar code on the unit dose medication and the patient ID. (The five rights include right patient, route, medication, dose, and time.)

- **Stage 6:** Full physician documentation with structured templates and discrete data is implemented for at least one inpatient care service area (progress notes, consult notes, discharge summaries, or problem list and diagnosis list maintenance). Level 3 of clinical decision support provides guidance for all clinician activities related to protocols and outcomes in the form of variance and compliance alerts. A full complement of radiology PACS systems provides medical images to physicians via an intranet and displaces all film-based images. Cardiology PACS and document imaging are scored with extra points.

- **Stage 7:** The hospital no longer uses paper charts to deliver and manage patient care and has a mixture of discrete data, document images, and medical images within its EMR environment. Data warehousing is being used to analyze patterns of clinical data to improve quality of care and patient safety and care delivery efficiency. Clinical information can be readily shared via standardized electronic transactions (that is, a **continuity of care document (CCD)**) with all entities that are authorized to treat the patient or a health information exchange (that is, other nonassociated hospitals, ambulatory clinics, subacute environments, employers, payers, and patients in a data sharing environment). The hospital demonstrated summary data continuity for all hospital services (for example, inpatient, outpatient, ED, and with any owned or managed ambulatory clinics).

Source: Adapted from HIMSS 2013.

Table 2.2   Adoption level of health IT at the end of 2012

Stage	Cumulative Capabilities	2012Q4
Stage 7	Complete EMR; CCD transactions to share data; data warehousing; data continuity with ED, ambulatory, OP	1.9%
Stage 6	Physician documentation (structured templates), full CDSS (variance and compliance), full R-PACS	8.2%
Stage 5	Closed loop medication administration	14.0%
Stage 4	CPOE, clinical decision support (clinical protocols)	14.2%
Stage 3	Nursing/clinical documentation (flow sheets), CDSS (error checking), PACS available outside Radiology	38.3%
Stage 2	CDR, controlled medical vocabulary, CDS, may have document imaging; HIE capable	10.7%
Stage 1	Ancillaries—Lab, Radiology, Pharmacy—All installed	4.3%
Stage 0	All three ancillaries not installed	8.4%
		$N = 5458$

Source: Data from HIMSS Analytics® Database ©2012

Check Your Understanding 2.3

Instructions: Choose the best answer.

1. Which of the following information systems is not considered one of the three major ancillary systems?
   a. Laboratory information system
   b. Pharmacy information system
   c. Surgical information system
   d. Radiology information system

2. How much federal funding did the Health Information Technology for Economic and Clinical Health (HITECH) Act include for incentives to Medicare and Medicaid providers for adopting health information technology?
   a. $20 million
   b. $20 billion
   c. $2.6 billion
   d. $22.6 billion

3. Regional Extension Centers provide all but which of the following services for providers:
   a. Training
   b. Technical assistance
   c. Purchase of health information technology
   d. Information and guidance

4. "Clinical documentation" in the EHR includes all but which of the following:
   a. Patient demographics
   b. Diagnostic test images
   c. Discharge summaries
   d. Medication lists

5. What allows physicians and other providers the ability to directly enter medication, other orders, and medical instructions electronically?
   a. Pharmacy information system
   b. Electronic medication administration record
   c. Computerized physician order entry
   d. E-prescribing

⊙ Summary

The EHR evolution will continue as technology advances even more and the demand for healthcare data increases to support patient care, healthcare planning, and research. Systems will continue to be implemented in ambulatory and inpatient organizations with improved functionality. Health information exchange, the ability to exchange data across multiple entities, will continue to be a goal. As more information becomes available and usable due to advances in electronic health records, additional uses for the data will continue to surface. The EHR movement has evolved significantly in the past 40 years, but the potential is still significant with advances to come that we cannot even imagine at this time.

REFERENCES

AHIMA. 2012. *Pocket Glossary for Health Information Management and Technology*, 3rd ed. Chicago: AHIMA Press.

American Recovery and Reinvestment Act of 2009. Public Law 111–115.

Department of Health and Human Services. 2012. Press Release: More Doctors Adopting EHRs to Improve Patient Care and Safety. http://www.hhs.gov/news/press/2012pres/12/20121212b.html.

Dick, R.S., and E.B. Steen. 1991. *The Computer-Based Patient Record: An Essential Technology for Healthcare*. Washington, DC: National Academy Press.

Gungor, F. 2012. The History of Electronic Health Records Software. http://www.onesourcedoc.com/blog/bid/82838/The-History-of-Electronic-Health-Records-Software.

Health Story Project. 2012. http://www.healthstory.com/.

HIMSS. 2004. Top Line: President Bush Calls for EHRs for Most Americans in 10 Years; Creates New NHII Coordinator. *Health IT News*. http://www.himss.org/asp/ContentRedirector.asp?ContentId=47547&type=HIMSSNewsItem.

HIMSS. 2005. Interoperability Definition and Background. Approved by HIMSS Board of Directors. http://www.himss.org/content/files/interoperability_definition_background_060905.pdf.

HIMSS. 2013. U.S. EMR Adoption Model Trends. http://www.himssanalytics.org/docs/HA_EMRAM_Overview_ENG.pdf.

Institute of Medicine, Committee on Data Standards for Patient Safety. 2003. Key Capabilities of an Electronic Health Record System. Washington, DC: National Academy Press.

Institute of Medicine, Committee on Improving the Patient Record. 1997. The Computer-Based Patient Record: An Essential Technology for Health Care, Revised Edition. Washington, DC: National Academy Press.

Institute of Medicine, Committee on Quality of Health Care in America. 2001. Crossing the Quality Chasm: A New Health System for the 21st Century. Washington, DC: National Academy Press.

Jha, A., C. DesRoches, E. Campbell, K. Donelan, S. Rao, T. Ferris, A. Shields, S. Rosenbaum, and D. Blumenthal. 2009. Use of electronic health records in U.S. hospitals. *The New England Journal of Medicine*. 360:1628–1638.

LaTour, K., S. Eichenwald-Maki, and P. Oachs. 2013. *Health Information Management Concepts, Principles, and Practice*, 4th ed. Chicago: AHIMA.

Lippeveld, T., R. Sauerborn, and C. Bodart. 2000. Chapter 11 from *Health Systems Approach: A How To Manual*. Arlington: Management Sciences for Health.

McCullough, J. 2008. Adoption of hospital information systems. *Health Economics* 17:649–664.

National Institutes of Health, National Center for Research Services. 2006. Electronic Health Records Overview. http://www.himss.org/content/files/Code%20180%20MITRE%20Key%20Components%20of%20an%20EHR.pdf.

Office of the National Coordinator for Health Information Technology. 2013. http://www.healthit.gov/.

Regenstrief Institute. 2012. http://www.regenstrief.org.

Sackett, D. 1996. Evidence based medicine: What it is and what it isn't. *British Medical Journal* 312:71–72. http://www.bmj.com/content/312/7023/71.

Chapter 3

Information Infrastructure

By Diane Dolezel and Susan H. Fenton

Learning Objectives

- Understand the goals of a distributed system
- List and give examples of distributed systems
- Recognize the differences between two- and three-tiered network architectures
- Discuss the purpose of middleware
- Define collaborative computing
- Understand the design models of distributed systems
- Describe the development process of a distributed system
- Discuss the basic principles of cloud computing
- Describe the five basic characteristics of a cloud computing system
- List and give examples of the three major cloud computing service models

KEY TERMS

Architectural models
Broad network access
Centralized
Client-server
Cloud computing
Community cloud
Concurrent processes
Cost of ownership
Database management system
   (DBMS)

Decentralized
Dependability
Distributed systems
Fault tolerance
File server
Firewall
Future-proofing
Hybrid cloud
Information infrastructure
Infrastructure as a service (IaaS)

Local area network (LAN)	Resource sharing
Measured service	Scalability
Middleware	Security
Mobile computing	Software as a service (SaaS)
Mobility	Terminal emulation software
Network	Terminal-to-host
On-demand self-service	Three-tiered architecture
Openness	Topology
Physical models	Transparency
Platform as a service (PaaS)	Two-tiered model
Public cloud	Virtual private network (VPN)
Private cloud	Wide area network (WAN)
Rapid elasticity	Wireless network
Resource pooling	World Wide Web (WWW)

⊙ Introduction

Healthcare information professionals are increasingly finding a need for **information infrastructure**, specifically processing, tools, and technologies to support the creation, use, transport, and storage of information (Pironti 2006). This infrastructure will allow them to work faster, more efficiently, and more economically when managing healthcare data and information. There is also an increasing need to share expensive resources and to collaborate with others via networked systems and the applications that run in these environments. This can be accomplished by the use of collaborative computing. In the best of all possible scenarios, this would occur seamlessly without the user having to know any of the details, such as the location or types of the machines or applications functioning in the networked health information (HI) system environment, which is the idea behind cloud computing.

This chapter introduces the topic of distributed systems and their development relative to the healthcare informatics industry. The role of distributed systems in facilitating collaborative computer communication is explored and their design and development is addressed. The advantages and disadvantages of these systems are highlighted. Next, the technologies used to design and develop distributed information systems in healthcare are discussed. Finally, the evolution of information infrastructure is explored via the emerging technology of cloud computing and mobile computing as it relates to the future direction of networked computing.

⊙ Distributed Systems

Computer system networks can be classified as either **centralized** or **decentralized**. A **network** is a type of information technology that connects different computers and computer systems so they can share information (AHIMA, 2012, 286). A centralized system is one in which the systems processing functions occur on a single computer. Conversely, in a decentralized system the processing functions are split or distributed, among one or more machines in the network system. In most cases, all of the machines in the system are doing a portion of the overall work independently. In every case these distributed machines work together toward a common goal.

In a centralized system there is one component, such as a software program, shared by all users, all resources are accessible, and the system is homogenous. That is, all machines in the system are built with the same technology, and software runs as a single process with a single point of control and failure. A centralized system is therefore working or it is not. If the system is a relational database, then the users can all share the data at the same time. There is no need for an interface because there is only one system.

In a **distributed system** there are multiple autonomous components that are not shared by all users and the software runs concurrently on different processors with multiple points of control and failure. A distributed system is a decentralized system. It is defined as a collection of independent computers connected through a network and managed by system software that enables the computers to coordinate their activities and to share system resources such that the users perceive the system as a single, integrated system (Steen 2009). Other machines may use the machines in this system so there is a need for interfaces between them and for request management.

Sophisticated software checks the load of machines on the network and assigns the workload to machines in the system to better balance out the load. These machines can be geographically close and connected by a local area network (LAN). Or they could be geographically distant and communicating over a **wide area network (WAN)**, which could in fact be several LANs connected by a phone system or satellite. A WAN is a computer network that connects devices across a large geographical area (AHIMA, 2012, 434). For example, the Internet is a WAN. In any case, regardless of the connections, the goal of a distributed system is to make the system appear to the users as one computer.

Figure 3.1 illustrates the typical architecture in a distributed system configuration. Notice that there are three machines in this configuration. Each machine has its own operating system (OS) and all the machines are connected via a network. The distributed applications run across all machines and access the **middleware**, that is software and hardware services that form a bridge between applications (Abdelhak et al. 2012, 272), in order to provide seamless application access to the users on Machine A (with Local OS1), Machine B (with Local OS2), and Machine C (with Local OS3). Thus the user on say, Machine B, may actually be running an application in Local OS3, but this is transparent to the end user.

Notice this definition implies that in a distributed system the data, computation, and users are all dispersed. Users communicate via a web-interfaced application to multiple computers containing separate data stores in order to perform healthcare data processing. Examples of distributed systems include the **World Wide Web (WWW)**, a global network of networks offering services to users with web browsers (AHIMA, 2012, 437), an automatic teller machine (ATM), a LAN,

Figure 3.1   Distributed system

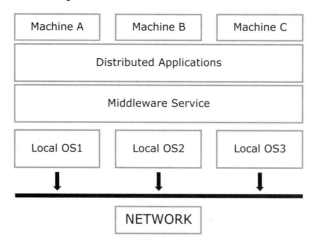

a database management system (DBMS) and an electronic health record (EHR) system.

The goals of a distributed system are

- ⊙ Resource sharing
- ⊙ Openness
- ⊙ Concurrency
- ⊙ Scalability
- ⊙ Fault tolerance
- ⊙ Transparency

Resource sharing means being able to use the hardware, software, or data anywhere in the system (Emmerich 1997). This is often implemented with a client-server architecture that allows the client PC and the server to interact. In this scenario, described in detail later, the server acts as the resource manager allowing the client to access hardware (that is, a file server) or data anywhere in the system.

Openness means flexibility to extend and improve the existing system with minimal impact. System openness is achieved by interfaces and interoperability between systems, which can be difficult in a heterogeneous environment. It could mean adding new interfaces or modifying existing servers or interfaces. Additionally, the data representations in the multiple vendors' interfaces must be managed transparently for openness to occur. An open system supports interoperability between the systems in the distributed network.

Concurrent processes run simultaneously and access shared resources such as databases. Concurrent processes in transactions require special handling so that changes made by one process are not lost. For example, suppose two processes are working concurrently to update a bank account balance level. It should be the case that the addition of money is applied simultaneously with the withdrawal of funds so that the account is not overdrawn. Similarly, in a concurrent database all the changes should be processed and applied accurately so that reporting from that system preserves data consistency.

In the case of a distributed database, the data is stored on two or more machines and the **database management system (DBMS)**, installed locally on each machine, is designed to keep track of data locations and coordinate data modifications. For example, a healthcare organization might consist of an acute-care hospital, an outpatient surgery center, and multiple remote clinics. Each facility has its own local applications and databases. All of the facilities are connected through a network that allows data sharing.

Scalability means the ability to support growth while maintaining the same level of service. The growth may occur for many reasons such as additional users, machines, and databases or expansion to another state or continent. In any case, users should not see a reduction of performance or reduced processing speed when the expansion occurs. Furthermore, scaling up should only require adding more processors, not redesigning the system. Note that while scalability should encompass adding more users and processes, even servers have an upper limit to the number of users that they can support, so this only works to a point.

Fault tolerant systems are highly available and remain in operation even when hardware, software, or network failures occur. This is usually achieved by having redundant systems and a good recovery plan. A redundant system could be a copy of the production server that is kept offline but updated frequently in case it needs to be switched out with the production server. Additionally, in a distributed system there is no single point of failure because resources, like data, are located across different servers, instead of centrally. Thus, if one server fails the others should be able to continue without the users being aware of any disruption.

Transparency means the end user sees the distributed system as a single machine. This is often achieved with the addition of middleware. An example of this would be using the Internet to do online shopping. The user does not need to know how the order gets into the remote system or gets processed. Transparency makes the resources available, distributes them transparently, and provides openness and scalability while hiding network failures. Distribution transparency means the user does not have to know how the data is represented, where it is stored, or if the data has been replicated, moved, or updated to be more consistent. This can be difficult to achieve if the users are on different continents and there are some network failures that can't be made transparent. Finally, it is difficult to be sure that system data was preserved in the event of a server failure. Transparency could include using web-based software to query a database in another state. The details of processing the request for data need not be known to the user nor does the location of the database matter.

Finally, distributed systems depend on middleware to facilitate communication between multiple heterogeneous machines. A distributed system has the goal of appearing as a single system multiprocessor system to the users. In an ideal world, we could just have a distributed OS implemented by a cluster of machines connected by high performance networks. In reality, this architecture is rarely seen. Instead, the machines in a distributed system are from various vendors, with different OSs and software installations. Middleware is the glue that allows messages to pass between the machines in the system.

Evolution of Distributed Systems

Distributed systems were not the model for systems processing in the past. In fact in the 1960s, when computer use began to be popular in healthcare, computer processing was largely centralized. Programmers sat at machines, called terminals, which were physically connected to large mainframe host systems. The terminals were used for data entry but had almost no processing power, so all the work was done on the host machine. The need for faster and better processing to support data processing brought about the modification of terminals to have added processing capabilities. This allowed some of the system workload to be shifted to the terminals and was the beginning of the client-server architecture model. Several architectures that describe the configurations, relationships, and structures of the components in a computer system will be examined next.

Two-Tiered Systems

The client-server architecture model is a **two-tiered model** composed of several client computers that are used to capture and process the data. The servers in this configuration are powerful machines that have application software installed on them and in turn store the data captured by client machines. The clients could be notebooks, desktops, tablets, smart phones, or other computers in the network. There may be multiple servers in the network; and each of them works to process requests from the less powerful clients (Abdelhak et al. 2012, 272).

When a client machine sends a request to the server for a service, the host handles the client's requests, processes the data or performs the requested service, and then returns the results of that processing to the client. For example, the client can be a laptop computer that sends a request to the mainframe for data and the mainframe would package the requested data and send a network message back to the client containing that information. The diagram in figure 3.2 depicts the basic client-server two-tier architecture with a database server and the clients, the computer laptops, sending their data requests across a LAN.

A **local area network (LAN)** is a network that connects various devices together via communications within a small geographic area such as a single organization (Abdelhak et al. 2012, 270). The users on a LAN can share printers, scheduling software, scanners, and files and can communicate by using network communication protocols. A single LAN has a limit as to how many PCs can be on the LAN. For example, a billing system at a physician's office might be on a LAN with 10 computers connected to a server. All the PCs on the network can share resources like printers and data files. And each of them can also execute software programs residing on their machines (such as Microsoft Word).

The Ethernet is the most widely used LAN network and it is a standard defined by the Institute of Electrical and Electronics Engineers (IEEE) as IEEE 802.3. The messages on an Ethernet are handled by all computers until they reach their final

Figure 3.2   Two-tiered system

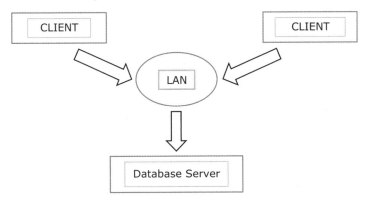

destination. The advantage of Ethernet communication is the high speed of data transmission, up to 100 megabytes bits per second (Mbps). However, if one part of the network fails, the entire network has problems since some of the computers are not available to handle the messages.

Three-Tiered Architecture

The **three-tiered architecture** expands on the two-tier system with the addition of an application server that contains the software applications and the business rules. Another difference is that clients in this architecture are called "thin clients" because most of the processing is done on the server, and the client has very little software installed on it. The business rules on the application server are logical rules that are used for processing the data and as such they are determined by the business. For example, a business rule might be "Display lab values only if not in normal range" (Abdelhak et al. 2012, 272).

There are several advantages to a three-tiered architecture. First, the business rules can be easily modified with minimal impact on the system since they are located on a separate server. Second, the system is scalable, that is, clients and applications can easily be added. And finally, the technology of the machines in the system is flexible, which means that servers can easily be replaced with a different vendor's system with minimal impact on the system.

In the diagram of the three-tiered system in figure 3.3 below, the flow of data starts with the client application sending a request across the LAN to the application server. The application server processes the request and sends its own request for data across the network to the database server. When the database server returns the requested data to the application server it is sent back to the client. Thus the application server is acting as middleware by functioning as a bridge for data communication and data management between the client applications and the database server.

Figure 3.3 Three-tiered system

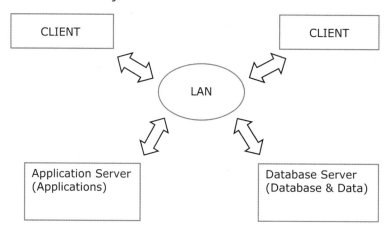

Web Services Architecture

A final computer structure called web services architecture (WSA) is needed for distributed computing in order to better integrate web-based healthcare applications with Internet protocols. It provides an environment that facilitates sharing of data behind a firewall across multiple systems using heterogeneous machines with different OSs (LaTour et al. 2012, 249). This would be used for all web-enabled client PCs in a facility to communicate with the EHRs and then again by the EHRs when they send and receive data from the various source systems.

To understand WSA one must first consider the nature of a web service. A web service is a software system that supports machine-to-machine communication. It is part of an XML-based message architecture system available over the Internet or an intranet, independent of OSs or programming languages. In this system a client browser sends a request, in the form of a message, to a web server. The message is then transported from the web browser client to the web server using Hyper Text Transfer Protocol (HTTP). The web server receives the message and passes it to a business objects component, which in turn contacts the database containing the requested data (W3C Working Group 2004).

Because the WSA is not tied to any particular OS or language, it can be implemented utilizing several open protocols or standards (TCP/IP, HTTP, Java, and XML) with a variety of software applications in various languages running on disparate platforms to exchange data over the Internet. For example, many standard web services currently use these components: Simple Object Access Protocol (SOAP), Universal Description, Discovery and Integration (UDDI), and Web Services Description Language (WSDL).

The layers for WSA architecture implementation are Discovery, Description, Messaging, and Networking (W3C Working Group 2004). The Discovery layer is where the requestor PC sends a message to the web service requesting a description of the service provider's interfaces. The reply from the web service provider would contain a set of documents, called a service description, which includes interface descriptions, information about what messages the requestor client can expect to receive, descriptions of the types of the responses that the client might send back to the server, and a description of the service's semantics. For example, WSDL is a commonly used standard language.

Next, the Messaging layer describes the XML-based message format that will be transported from the web service. Specifically it will outline what is in a request for service and what will be sent in the message. Generally, SOAP is the protocol used for the XML message.

The Networking layer is where the basic functions of networking are handled. These could include error processing, sending and receiving messages, contacting hosts, and routing messages. Figure 3.4 summarizes this model.

Collaborative Computing

Collaboration means working together to achieve a common goal. Common goals can be achieved by collaborative computing, which allows users to harness the power of Internet-based collaborative software to work simultaneously on documents and presentations, attend web meetings, plan using project management, or create content in other media like wikis.

Examples of collaborative software include Microsoft Office, Microsoft NetMeeting, Lotus Notes, online calendars, project management software, videoconferencing (such as Adobe Connect), and instant messaging, among others. On the social front collaborative software could be used for gaming, online dating, or social community sites like Facebook, LinkedIn, and Twitter. It could even include wikis when used for blogging, chatting, and surveys or creating social websites. Basically, collaborative computing occurs anywhere that individuals come together to work toward a common goal.

Figure 3.4   Web services architecture layers

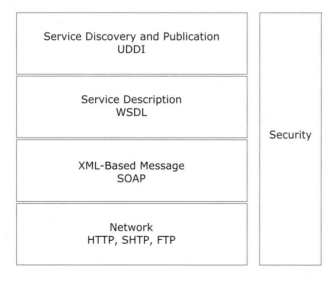

Figure 3.5   Collaborative computing

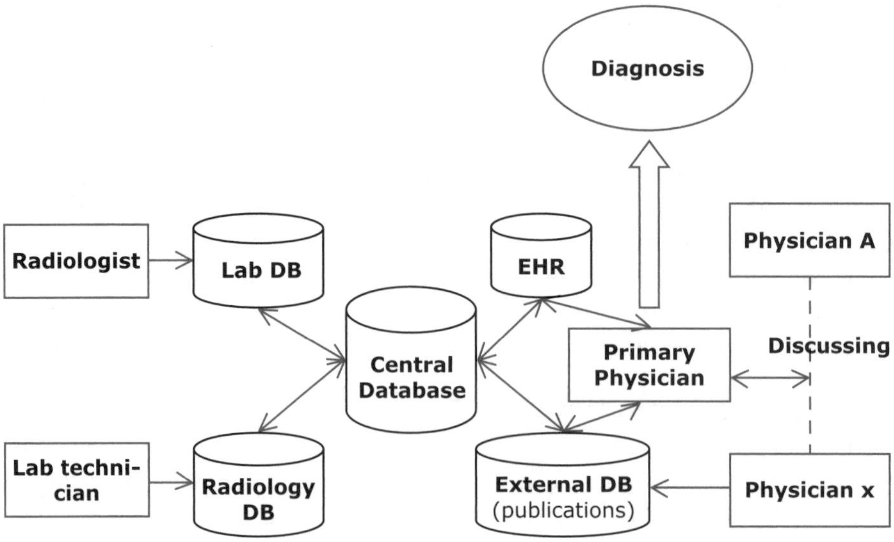

Medical work in general, in hospitals in particular, is highly collaborative due to the specialized nature of the medical treatment (Bardram and Christensen 2007). Collaborative computing is likely to be one of the solutions to the challenges in healthcare. For instance, a physician is trying to find a diagnosis of a patient. Traditionally, the physician can dictate the notes to a nurse to prepare the health record. During the radiology conference, the physician studies x-ray images with a radiologist. At the morning conference, the physician discusses proper medication with colleagues while browsing medicine catalogs. Later, the lab releases a blood sample result, and the physician must study it with a colleague while referencing recent publications. With collaborative computing it might be possible for many of these interactions to take place with minimal interference in the workflow. The physician might insert their own notes into the record, while using instant messaging to communicate with the nurse prior to rounds. The search for a medication and the implications of a laboratory result might take place within the EHR knowledgebase, with different practitioners communicating using internal instant messaging or e-mail (see figure 3.5).

Check Your Understanding 3.1

Instructions: Choose the best answer.

1. The flexibility to extend and improve a system with minimal impact refers to what characteristic of a distributed system?
   a. Openness
   b. Concurrency
   c. Fault tolerance
   d. Resource sharing

2. A distributed system that is seen by the end user as a single machine is said to be
   a. Shared
   b. Centralized
   c. Transparent
   d. Single processor

3. Which of the following refers to the ability to support the addition of users, machines, and databases without reduction in performance?
   a. Expansion
   b. Stability
   c. Concurrency
   d. Scalability

4. Which are examples of distributed systems?
   a. Single computer system
   b. Database management system
   c. Electronic health record
   d. A and B
   e. B and C

5. Redundant systems and a good recovery plan can help achieve
   a. Scalability
   b. Load balancing
   c. Fault tolerance
   d. Concurrency

⊙ Design and Development

A fully functioning information infrastructure for healthcare systems requires careful, considered, and informed design and development. Many factors must be considered beginning with user needs, the physical environment, the technology available, industry regulations, internal constraints, and any external threats. There are usually two different types of models, physical and architectural (logical), which are used to fully describe the information infrastructure for an organization.

Physical Models

Physical models capture the hardware composition of a system in terms of the computer and other devices. The physical infrastructure generally refers to the computers (workstations, servers, and so on) and connection media used for a network. The model is a pictorial representation of the arrangement of the different pieces and connection points (Wager et al. 2009, 206–207). A network consists of two or more computers linked by a communication line. There are many types of computers, including servers and user interface devices such as personal computers, laptops, tablet computers, and smart phones, among others. The communication media used in a network includes cables and noncabled media such as microwaves and radio waves, more commonly known as Wi-Fi, short for Wireless Fidelity.

The selection of servers, along with their configuration and capabilities, is very technical and usually the responsibility of the chief technology officer (CTO), chief information officer (CIO), or director of information systems. Generally, these same people are responsible for either the selection of user interface devices (computers, tablets, smart phones, and such) or setting standards for the user interface devices that may be purchased by others in the organization. Hopefully, these decisions will be made based upon the needs of the organization and users of the system. For example, an inadequate number of computers in an emergency room could lead to extreme user frustration or even a failure to document all of the care delivered.

The cabled communication media chosen for the physical infrastructure and model are categorized according to their varying transmission speeds. The categorizations range from 1 to 7, with speeds ranging respectively from 1 Mbps (megabytes per second) to 10 Gbps (gigabytes per second). Common types of cabling (or conducted media) include twisted pair, coaxial, and fiber-optic. Coaxial cable is typically used only for cable television, with twisted pair and fiber-optic preferred for other uses. Twisted pair can transmit a variety of speeds, though usually only over short distances. Fiber-optic can be used to transmit over longer distances; however it is more expensive (Wager et al. 2009, 208).

Noncabled communication media are usually termed wireless. When a network is created using noncabled communication methods to connect the computers and other resources it is known as a **wireless network**. They take the form of microwaves, including those used for satellite transmissions; other radio waves including the standards 802.11(a-n) used for Wi-Fi networks; cellular telephone technology; and the Bluetooth standard (Wager et al. 2009, 209). These wireless standards all have different specifications for speed of transmission, as well as supported distance between the sending device and receiving device.

There are additional devices that enable networked communication. Generally, these consist of hubs, bridges, routers, gateways, and switches. Much like a transportation hub such as a major rail station, a network hub brings together the data from a network. A bridge can be used to connect networks using the same communication protocol, while the more sophisticated router can play a role in directing the network traffic. Gateways connect networks using different communication protocols, while switches route data to their destination and may also be a gateway or router.

Physical models are typically described in terms of a **topology**. The topology is the network's physical layout. Types of cabled network topologies include point-to-point, star, bus, tree, or ring. The advantages and disadvantages are summarized in table 3.1. The last topology in the table is a mesh topology, which is largely confined to wireless networks, due to the exorbitant costs if a mesh network were to be attempted with cable.

In addition to the physical parts of a network, there are two software components that are integral parts of networking: **firewalls** and **virtual private networks (VPNs)**. The purpose of a firewall is to monitor and control all communication in to and out of an intranet. A firewall is implemented by a set of processes that act

Table 3.1   Network topologies pros and cons

Network Topology	Advantages	Disadvantages
Point-to-Point	• Speed	• Limited to two devices
Star	• Easy installation and device connection • Can connect and remove devices without disruption • Problems are easily identified	• Requires more cable than bus topology • Failure of a hub, switch, or concentrator disables nodes • More expensive than bus topology
Bus	• Easy device connection • Uses less cable than other topologies	• One break disables network • Terminators required at both ends of the backbone • Problems are hard to identify
Tree	• Point-to-point wiring for certain segments • Vendor neutral	• Length of a segment is limited by type of cable used • If backbone breaks an entire segment fails • More difficult to configure and wire
Ring	• Can support better performance than a star topology • Provides for orderly data transmission	• High performance under low loads • Expensive to implement • Any fault can cause network failure
Mesh	• Extensive redundancy with multiple connections • "Self-configuring" when new nodes are added • "Self-healing" to continue operations even when some nodes fail • More nodes increases speed	• Still in development, with no standards • Wireless is inherently unreliable • They are not completely seamless; moving nodes may result in failure

(Adapted in part from Florida Center for Instructional Technology 2013)

as a gateway to a network applying the organizational security policy. Firewalls in healthcare organizations usually keep hackers and other external threats from the Internet outside of the internal network; however, firewalls can also keep sensitive data such as individually identifiable patient HI from leaving the organization. See figure 3.6 for an illustration of a firewall.

Figure 3.6   Firewall

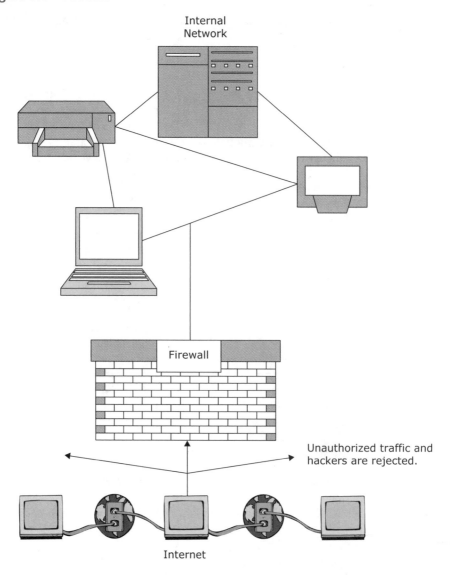

Sometimes there is a need to communicate across wide networks, which includes sending data via the Internet. Virtual private networks (VPNs) extend the firewall protection boundary beyond the local intranet by the use of cryptographically protected secure channels at the Internet Protocol (IP) level. A VPN is a private network that uses a public network (usually the Internet) to connect remote sites or users together privately.

Networks are often described in terms of the methods they use to distribute information. The most common distribution methods are **terminal-to-host**, **file server**, and **client-server**. With terminal-to-host, the application and any data stay on a host computer with the user connecting either via a "dumb" terminal or using

terminal emulation software on a personal computer to connect as if the user is on a dumb terminal. Sometimes this arrangement is also termed a thin client, with most of the actual processing taking place on a central computer (Wager et al. 2009, 210). A file server system runs entirely on the end user's workstation and transfers entire files, while the client-server method has multiple servers dedicated to different functions with workstations running the application and retrieving data from a server as needed. Client-server is the most used method, whereby some information and applications will sit on a local client; however, information or data can be pulled from a server (Wager et al. 2009, 210). A very common example of client-server is the use of e-mail, especially Microsoft Outlook, where Outlook runs on the local computer but pulls e-mail and other information from a server.

The physical model and distribution systems of a network are very important. While they do not determine the entire functionality, they can limit what can be done with a given system. It is very important to involve users as well as technical experts to ensure the choices made support the organizational needs.

Architectural Models

Distributed information systems are difficult to develop due to their complex and decentralized nature (Kart et al. 2007), basic safety (and security) requirements (Lamport 2001), as well as the need to achieve consistently high performance across a wide range of deployment settings (Mao et al. 2008). Healthcare, along with many other industries, faces these challenges, so a broad array of information modeling methods has been developed. These methods are often termed information **architectural models** as they provide a framework or structure for the flow of data and information within systems. This section will provide a brief review of different modeling approaches including Enterprise Knowledge Development (EKD), Service-Oriented Architecture (SOA), and Business Process Simulation (BPS). Each of these has its own methods, techniques, and tools, which are used to analyze, plan, design, and possibly change businesses (Stirna and Persson 2008, 85).

Before we begin exploring the different approaches and frameworks, it is important to understand that there are "languages" associated with information modeling. The most common are the Unified Modeling Language (UML), Extended or Enhanced Entity Relationship (EER), and Object-Role Modeling (ORM) (Halpin et al. 2008, 18). UML is a product of the Object Modeling Group, Inc., an international standards organization for the computer industry. With the use of various tools utilizing UML an organization can "specify, visualize, and document models of software systems, including their structure and design" (Object Modeling Group, Inc., 2013). The EER system began as entity relationship diagramming. It has been the subject of much research and is now widely used in various forms (Thalheim, 2011). Figure 3.7 is an illustration of a very simple EER representing potential values for the entity provider. Thus, EER is very useful for those who process data better visually. ORM is sometimes called fact-oriented modeling. It uses graphical and textual languages to model and query information, as well as a procedural language for designing conceptual models (Halpin 2009). Both EER and ORM have been incorporated into different tools to make their use easier.

Figure 3.7   Simple extended entity relationship (EER) diagram

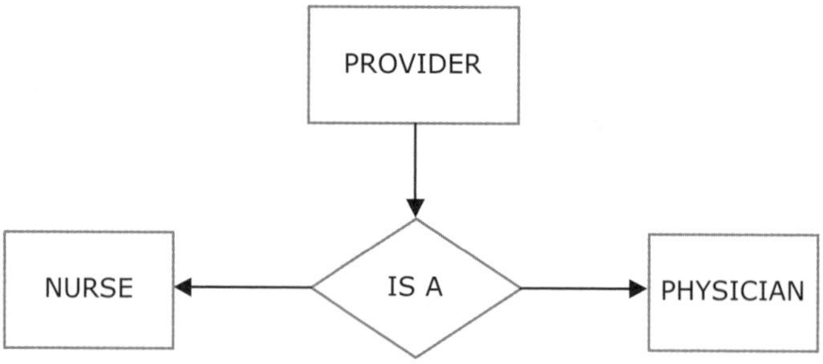

The selection of one of these tools is usually dependent upon organizational history or which tools key information systems personnel have used previously.

The EKD method evolved in Europe as a language for modeling business and information processes (Stirna and Persson 2008, 69). The overall model has six submodels that focus on different aspects of an organization: Goals Model (GM), Business Rules Model (BRM), Concepts Model (CM), Business Process Model (BPM), Actors and Resources Model (ARM), and Technical Components and Requirements Model (TCRM). The names are fairly self-explanatory with the exception of the CM, which is the ontology or domain of the organization for which the model is being created (Stirna and Persson 2008, 69–70). For example, the ontology for healthcare would be very different from the ontology for financial services.

The goal of the SOA approach is to build information systems that enable business to reuse existing assets effectively, create new assets, and support changes that will occur in the business and its needs (Hurwitz et al. 2009, 7). SOA is relatively new, having only arisen after 2003. However, it has proven to be quite popular and is used in many organizations, including healthcare organizations. That said, SOA is not an immediate silver bullet. Utilizing SOA in an organization is a journey, often without a definitive end. SOA consists of components, that is, building blocks, for which specifications define the storage of data, interactions of users, the communication of programs, as well as other functions (Hurwitz et al. 2009, 43–45). SOA is envisioned as a hierarchy, with the Application Front End as the top level. API, which stands for Application Programming Interface, can be thought of as the methods by which an SOA asset can be accessed. Within the Application are found the second level of Services, which are specific tasks or functions (Erickson and Siau 2008). For example, an SOA Service in healthcare might be titled "Patient Lookup." Using the same Service to accomplish this function throughout a healthcare organization and its software would ensure consistency and efficiency for users. Within Services are found the Contract, Interface, and Implementation (Erickson and Siau 2008). The Contract includes metadata such as who owns the service and how it is brokered; while the Interface connects the Service with the data or business logic, with the Implementation specifying which Contract and

Interface are to be used for each Service (Erickson and Siau 2008). Organizations will benefit from implementing SOA with the emphasis on standards and the reuse of software components.

The final information systems development process to be explored here is BPS. BPS is defined as "designing a model of a real system and conducting experiments with this model for the purpose either of understanding the behavior of the system or of evaluating various strategies (within the limits imposed by a criterion or set of criteria) for the operation of the system" (Elliman et al. 2008, 242). Proponents of BPS support its use throughout the entire development process, most notably to account for the impact of human dynamics with information systems. BPS can help information system developers understand current system operations, identify bottlenecks, evaluate various alternatives, and assess quantitative results on all of the above (Elliman et al. 2008, 251). BPS requires the active involvement of technical experts as well as business users to ensure the simulations created are accurate.

Check Your Understanding 3.2

Instructions: Choose the best answer.

1. This network design is more expensive than a hub; however, it is easier to install. It is a _____ network.
   a. Star
   b. Mesh
   c. Tree
   d. Bus

2. What is a private network that uses a public network (usually the Internet) to connect remote sites or users together privately?
   a. Extranet
   b. FTP
   c. VPN
   d. SFTP

3. What is the information distribution system that is the most widely employed in information systems?
   a. Internet
   b. Client-server
   c. Peer-to-peer
   d. Network

4. Which of the following is not a goal of Service-Oriented Architecture?
   a. Build information systems that enable business to reuse existing assets effectively
   b. Support changes that will occur in the business and its needs
   c. Create new assets
   d. Ensure services are delivered effectively

5. Architectural models are used for information systems to
   a. Provide a framework or structure for the flow of data and information within systems
   b. Determine the hardware necessary for the system
   c. Help technicians isolate problems in the system
   d. Assess quantitative results of evaluation data

Cloud Computing

One area of interest in distributed information systems is the emerging technology called **cloud computing**. One definition of cloud computing "is the dynamic delivery of information technology resources and capabilities as a service over the Internet" (Sarna 2010, 2). The National Institute for Standards and Technology (NIST) defines cloud computing as "a model for enabling ubiquitous, convenient, on-demand network access to a shared pool of configurable computing resources (e.g., networks, servers, storage, applications, and services) that can be rapidly provisioned and released with minimal management effort or service provider interaction" (Mell 2011). See figure 3.8 for an illustration of cloud computing. Several advantages make cloud computing very attractive including the ability to access and use resources as they are needed without having to pay for them if they are idle and distributed computing in a distant or even several locations, which provides some redundancy for business continuity purposes (Sarna 2010, 2).

The concept of cloud computing is popular. Most businesses are in the process of determining whether or not they wish to move some, or all, of their information infrastructure to the cloud. In an effort to standardize what can qualify as cloud computing and what does not, NIST established five essential characteristics that define a cloud. They are as follows:

1. **On-demand self-service**—Anyone with the appropriate permissions can make use of the resources without additional intervention.

2. **Broad network access**—Any capabilities available over the network can be accessed by a wide variety of interface devices (laptops, smart phones, and so on) using standard mechanisms.

3. **Resource pooling**—The cloud computing provider resources serve multiple consumers, usually independent of location, though these can be specified by the consumer.

4. **Rapid elasticity**—Service is provided on demand, meaning that more can quickly be provided when needed and reduced just as fast, so the consumer only pays for what they need and use.

5. **Measured service**—Use of resources in the cloud can be monitored, controlled, and reported, allowing for better management (Mell 2011).

NIST goes on to define three major cloud computing service models:

1. **Software as a service (SaaS)**—The highest level of cloud computing service models, SaaS enables access to the cloud computing provider's

applications via a variety of devices, usually through an interface such as a web browser. The only part of the SaaS that might not be standardized is any consumer-specific application configuration settings.

2. **Platform as a service (PaaS)**—At this intermediate level of capability consumers create or acquire applications using programming languages and tools supported by the cloud computing service provider. While the consumer does not control the underlying infrastructure they do exercise more control over the applications.

3. **Infrastructure as a service (IaaS)**—This is the most minimal level of cloud computing where the infrastructure is provided, but the consumer controls the OS, storage, and applications. The consumer may also have control over networking components such as the firewall (Mell 2011).

Depending upon the particular application an organization may choose to use cloud computing services at all three levels, having responsibility and direct control for only the applications deemed most important or critical. Regardless of the service model, the deployment of the cloud may be distributed to organizations using one of these four models:

1. **Private cloud**—The cloud is accessible to only one customer and can be operated by the organization, a third party, or a combination of the two, at the customer's location or offsite. Healthcare organizations, especially larger ones, may choose this option due to the need for patient information security or if sensitive research is being conducted.

2. **Community cloud**—This cloud is supported for use by a "community" of users who share some trait, such as security needs, in common. One or more of the community may own and operate the cloud, or it may be operated by a third party or a combination of the two. A healthcare example of a community cloud might be the data infrastructure needed for an accountable care organization or that required by a HI exchange.

Figure 3.8   Cloud computing

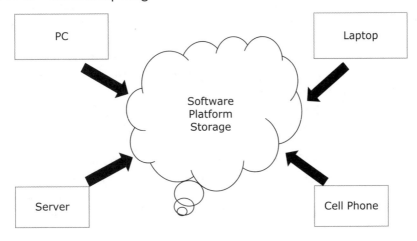

3. **Public cloud**—This cloud is open to the general public and owned by an academic institution, the government, or some other organization for the benefit of the public. As previously, the owner or a third party or some combination thereof can operate it, at any location.

4. **Hybrid cloud**—This consists of two totally separate cloud infrastructures (private, community, or public) that are unique, but share standardized or proprietary technology facilitating data and application portability (Mell 2011).

Everything discussed to this point lays the foundation of cloud computing so potential consumers can understand their options, as well as what cloud service vendors are offering. In essence, this is the beginning of standards related to cloud computing. The following are benefits of cloud computing:

⊙ Scalability—the ability to use multiple servers and increase or decrease usage very quickly

⊙ Preconfigured OS images—including both Linux and Windows-based servers

⊙ Virtual servers or physical servers—can be sized according to need with between one to four cores and one to four processors in a fault-tolerant RAID (redundant array of independent disks) configuration

⊙ Dedicated IP addresses—for cloud servers

⊙ Communication—extremely fast and without charge between services in the same cloud

⊙ Replication and distribution—for continuity or access over different geographical regions

⊙ Persistence—optional if a virtual server is used and it is shut down (Sarna 2010, 19)

One use of the cloud in healthcare is in the form of web-based EHRs. Providers access their cloud-based EHR applications via the Internet. This means that the hospitals and other facilities do not have to buy servers and storage. The provider may either purchase access to an EHR application or may be able to access the application for free. One researcher conducted a case study on a cloud-based EHR that can be used for free with the standard advertising found in many free information services, or for a fee, without the advertising. This EHR also sells deidentified data as a part of the revenue stream, while maintaining their offerings in their own private cloud in order to comply with the privacy and security regulations in the Health Insurance Portability and Accountability Act (HIPAA) (Sarna 2010, 275–280). It is important to note several caveats not called out in this case study. Healthcare providers using this "free" EHR would need to understand how the vendor may or may not be in compliance with separate privacy and security laws in the provider's location. For example, some states have stricter security requirements or restrict the sale of even deidentified data. It is the responsibility of the provider to comply with laws that apply to them. Additionally, the provider would need to ensure they will have access to the data should it be needed for legal purposes. In the case of pediatric records this can be a very long time, up to 20 or 21 years in the case of newborn records. Given that these services have existed for less than a decade, this assurance of availability may be difficult.

Thus, when exploring cloud computing for a healthcare organization several considerations must be investigated:

1. **Cost of ownership**—Using cloud computing can be more cost effective than maintaining a server onsite. Additional savings may be realized by reducing the number of employees and contractors needed for server maintenance, legacy system conversions, and upgrades.

2. **Dependability**—Cloud computing providers are dependable. They are up and running 24 hours a day, 7 days a week every day of the year, which ensures access to much needed items such as business applications, financial data, and help desk personnel. These providers also provide backup solutions, which relieve the facility of this chore and ensure business continuity in the case of a natural disaster such as a tornado, fire, or flood. Conversely since the cloud is Internet-based, any disturbance that causes loss of Internet access will impact the system by disrupting connectivity. To keep the business running redundant wireless hot points, leased lines, and fiber optics are recommended. Loss of Internet can come from malicious attacks by hackers or other sources. The cloud providers assist in this area by providing firewalls, which are protective boundaries between an intranet and the Internet that prevent unauthorized access from outside by filtering all incoming messages.

3. **Scalability**—Cloud systems can grow with the demands of the facility, which provides scalability for the business. This can be very important to companies that rely on web-based billing or sales for revenue. For example, if the size of the healthcare billing processing grows by 10 percent, due to the addition of additional outpatient services, then the cloud architecture would seamlessly provide additional computing power, storage, networking, and so on. Compare this to the amount of time, money, and meetings that would be required to plan a similar addition to resources if the healthcare facility had to add the resources themselves (that is, additional servers and PCs, extra networking, more software, personnel to maintain the additional resources).

4. **Mobility**—Data streaming from the clouds allows for greater mobility because the Internet is accessible from multiple mobile devices, such as smart phones and tablets, PDAs, virtual desktops, or traditional laptops or PCs. For example, the CIO could work on his MS Excel report from home on his iPad by accessing data from the hospital's EHR system (appropriately encrypted, of course). When completed the report could be put into MS PowerPoint slides and presented through the cloud by using Internet meeting software.

5. **Future-proofing**—Computer hardware, software, and networking solutions begin their move toward obsolescence almost as soon as they are implemented,

which can be costly. Cloud computing moves the cost of updating certain parts of the technology from the customer to the cloud provider, a substantial benefit given the rapid pace of the growth of Internet and other technologies.

6. **Security**—The security of the cloud application is paramount for healthcare providers to be able to ensure the privacy of individually identifiable healthcare data. Cloud computing service companies working with providers and others would be subject to all aspects of the HIPAA Privacy and Security Rules (Bellamy 2011).

Given that cloud computing, especially in the healthcare industry, is still very new, there are aspects that remain untested or still in development. These include issues very important to healthcare such as easy access to encrypted data (required for HIPAA compliance), as well as discoverability for legal purposes (Anthes 2010). For example, there is little legal precedent if the cloud provider is located within the United States, but the data center is in a different country or if the data is subpoenaed from the cloud provider instead of the healthcare provider (Anthes 2010). The bottom line for cloud computing in healthcare is the same as for all new technologies used in healthcare—users need to thoroughly investigate the pros and cons, seeking to protect patients and the organization, while maximizing productivity and efficiency.

Mobile Computing

Mobile computing, sometimes called mHealth, is quickly emerging as a technology infrastructure challenge for healthcare organizations. Mobile computing includes all types of computing accomplished on a device which can be moved, usually held in the hand of the user. Mobile devices of today have as much, if not more computing power, than desktop computers of the past. They offer practically unlimited access for busy clinicians and staff. However, they come with a separate set of concerns, which must be managed to maintain effective, efficient, and secure operations.

Initial issues to be addressed include the type and ownership of the devices. Whether the system is compatible with Apple's iOS, Android, or RIM's Blackberry systems (or all three) is a technical, infrastructure decision, which may be constrained by the EHR or other systems already installed. Related to the decision of which platforms or OSs to support is the ownership of the device. This decision can be very difficult, especially when users are vocal and do not always understand the complexity of the situation. The technical requirements for each platform come with their own challenges and organizations must be able to manage all of them effectively, while complying with myriad regulations. Users will often want to use their personal devices, often called "bring your own device" (BYOD). This is certainly easier for the user; however, using a personal device for accessing individually identifiable HI requires the device to meet very specific encryption standards. The healthcare organization is responsible for ensuring that any access to individually identifiable HI via any method is legal and secure. There are companies ready and waiting to help secure the data on mobile devices.

As with all tools, this functionality comes with a price. It is ultimately up to senior management to establish the level of acceptable risk versus the cost to protect the organization and its information assets.

Another decision point is the access to be supported. The organization must decide whether to only allow application access, such as with the EHR, or whether to include more expanded communication methods such as e-mail or text messaging, which are more difficult to manage. Additionally, the organization must determine whether to support mobile access for all employees or to limit it to physicians or some other combination of user types. Everyone always wants access; however, the support needs grow as access expands. As with the platform and device ownership decisions, the access decision must be carefully considered.

Mobile computing is in its infancy. Development and growth in this market is exponential with the advent of radio-frequency identification (RFID) for tracking assets, maybe even patients; real-time locator systems (RTLS); and portable wireless devices such as glucose monitors and blood pressure monitors. Healthcare organizations and health informatics professionals will have to engage in lifelong learning to provide their users, including patients, with the very latest technological tools in a protected environment.

Check Your Understanding 3.3

Instructions: Choose the best answer.

1. Which delivers Internet-based data as a service where users do not need to know the infrastructure or physical location of the hardware or software?
   a. Electronic health records
   b. Cloud computing
   c. Database management systems
   d. Personal data assistants

2. Which of the following describes the cloud service models where users interact with the service provider's applications from a web browser or client application without the customer having to buy the server or software license?
   a. Software as a service
   b. Platform as a service
   c. Infrastructure as a service
   d. Measured service

3. A cloud service that is distributed with an infrastructure physically located on premises owned by the cloud provider and freely accessible to everyone is called a
   a. Private cloud
   b. Community cloud
   c. Public cloud
   d. Hybrid cloud

4. Use of cloud computing may allow a facility to reduce the number of employees and contractors needed for server maintenance. This benefit helps reduce
   a. Mobility
   b. Cost of ownership
   c. Scalability
   d. Dependability

5. Decisions regarding mobile computing should be made after
   a. New technology emerges
   b. IT personnel tests the product
   c. When users demand it
   d. Following a thorough risk analysis

◉ Summary

It would be almost impossible to overstate the importance of the effective design and development of information systems, especially in the information-intensive healthcare industry. The choice of models, languages, and methods, as well as quality control for all of these, will impact the final results. The emergence of new technologies in the form of cloud computing, smart phones, and tablets will continue to challenge organizations and their IT staff. Organizations that are not large enough to have knowledgeable, full-time staff should choose their consultant advisors very carefully. Implementing information systems without the appropriate attention to the infrastructure can result in expensive mistakes, breaches of confidential information, and failed operations.

REFERENCES

Abdelhak, M., S. Grostick, and M.A. Hanken. 2012. *Health Information Management of a Strategic Resource*, 4th ed. St. Louis: Saunders.

Anderson, H. 2011. EHRs and Cloud Computing. http://www.healthcareinfosecurity.com/articles.php?art_id=3482&pg=1.

Anthes, G. 2010. Security in the cloud. *Communications of the ACM*. 53(11):16–18. doi:10.1145/1839676.1839683.

Bardram, J. and H. Christensen. 2007. Pervasive computing support for hospitals: An overview of the activity-based computing project. *Pervasive Computing, IEEE*. 6(1):44–51.

Bellamy, S., 2011. Is Cloud Computing for You? Five Points to Consider. Computer World. http://www.computerworld.com/s/article/9222249/Is_Cloud_Computing_for_You_Five_Points_to_Consider?taxonomyId=158&pageNumber=1.

Davis, Z. 2011. Network Operating System. PCmag.com.

Dean, T. 2009. Network operating systems. *Network+ Guide to Networks*. 421(483).

Elliman, T., T. Hatzakis, and A. Serrano. 2008. Business Process Simulation: An Alternative Modelling Technique for the Information System Development Process. In *Innovations in Information Systems Modeling: Methods and Best Practices (Advances in Database Research)*, 1st ed. Edited by Halpin, T., J. Krogstie, and E. Proper, 240–253. Information Science Reference. Hershey: IGI Global.

Emmerich, W. 1997. Distributed Systems Principles. http://www.cs.ucl.ac.uk/staff/ucacwxe/lectures/ds98-99/dsee3.pdf.

Erickson, J. and K. Siau. 2008. Service Oriented Architecture: A Research Review from the Software and Applications Perspective. In *Innovations in Information Systems Modeling: Methods and Best Practices (Advances in Database Research)*, 1st ed. Edited by Halpin, T., J. Krogstie, and E. Proper, 190–203. Information Science Reference. Hershey: IGI Global.

Florida Center for Instructional Technology. 2013. *An Educator's Guide to School Networks.* University of South Florida. http://fcit.usf.edu/network/.

Glandon, L., D. Smaltz, and D. Slovensky. 2010. *Information Systems for Healthcare Management.* Chicago: Health Administration Press.

Gruman, G. 2008. What Cloud Computing Really Means. InfoWorld. http://www.infoworld.com/d/cloud-computing/what-cloud-computing-really-means-031.

Halpin, T. 2009. Object-Role Modeling. In *Encyclopedia of Database Systems*, Edited by Liu, L. and M. Tamer Ozsu. New York: Springer.

Halpin, T., J. Krogstie, and E. Proper, eds. 2008. *Innovations in Information Systems Modeling: Methods and Best Practices (Advances in Database Research)*, 1st ed. IGI Global. Hershey: Information Science Reference.

Hugos, M. and D. Hulitzky. 2011. *Business in the Cloud.* Hoboken: Wiley.

Hurwitz, J., R. Bloor, M. Kaufman, and F. Halper. 2009. *Service Oriented Architecture (SOA) For Dummies*, 2nd ed. Hoboken: Wiley.

Kart, F., G. Miao, L.E. Moser, and P.M. Melliar-Smith. 2007. A Distributed e-Health System Based on the Service Oriented Architecture. Salt Lake City: IEEE International Conference on Services Computing.

Keidar, I. 2008. Distributed computing column 34 – Distributed computing in the clouds. *ACM SIGACT News* 39(4):53–54. doi:10.1145/1466390.1466402.

Lamport, L. 2001. Paxos made simple. *ACM SIGACT News* 32(2):18–25.

LaTour, K.M. and S. Eichenwald-Maki. 2013. *Health Information Management Concepts, Principles, and Practice*, 4th ed. Chicago: AHIMA.

Mao, Y., F. Junqueira, and K. Marzullo. 2008. Mencius: Building Efficient Replicated State Machines for WANs. OSDI '08 Proceedings of the 8th USENIX conference on Operating Systems design and implementation. Berkeley, CA. 369–384.

Mell, P. and T. Grance. 2011. The NIST Definition of Cloud Computing. National Institute of Standards. http://www.nist.gov/itl/csd/cloud-102511.cfm.

Object Modeling Group, Inc. 1997. Introduction to OMG UML. http://www.omg.org/gettingstarted/what_is_uml.htm.

Pironti, J. 2006 (May). Key Elements of a Threat and Vulnerability Management Program. *Information Systems Audit and Control Association Member Journal.* http://www.isaca.org/Journal/Past-Issues/2006/Volume-3/Pages/Key-Elements-of-a-Threat-and-Vulnerability-Management-Program1.aspx.

Sarna, D.E.Y. 2010. *Implementing and Developing Cloud Computing Applications,* 1st ed. New York: Auerbach Publications.

Schmidt, D. 2008. Software technologies for developing distributed systems: Objects and beyond. *Computer Society of India Communications,* Special Issue on OO Technologies. Edited by Jana, D., 30–37.

Simon, P. 2010. *The Next Wave of Technologies.* Hoboken: Wiley & Sons.

Steen, M. 2009 (Oct 25). Distributed System Paradigms. http://www.cs.vu.nl/~steen/courses/ds-slides/notes.01.pdf.

Stirna, J. and A. Persson. 2008. EKD: An Enterprise Modeling Approach to Support Creativity and Quality in Information Systems and Business Development. In *Innovations in Information Systems Modeling: Methods and Best Practices (Advances in Database Research),* 1st ed. Edited by Halpin, T., J. Krogstie, and E. Proper, 68–88. Hershey: Information Science Reference. Hershey: IGI Global.

Thalheim, B. 2011. The Enhanced Entity-Relationship Model. In *Handbook of Conceptual Modeling,* Edited by Embley, D.W. and B. Thalheim, 165–206. Berlin Heidelberg: Springer. http://link.springer.com.libproxy.txstate.edu/chapter/10.1007/978-3-642-15865-0_6.

Wager, K.A., F.W. Lee, and J.P. Glaser. 2009. *Healthcare Information Systems: A Practical Approach for Health Management,* 2nd ed. San Francisco: Jossey-Bass.

Watfa, M. 2012. *E-healthcare Systems and Wireless Communications: Current and Future Challenges.* Hershey: IGI Global.

W3C Working Group. 2004 (February). Group Note 11: Web Services Architecture. www.w3.org/TR/2004/NOTE-ws-arch-20040211/.

Chapter

4

Understanding Databases

By Susan White

Learning Objectives

- Understand flat file versus relational databases
- Learn basic SQL commands to select data for reporting and analysis
- Define the components of a data dictionary
- Learn the role of data modeling in database maintenance and design

KEY TERMS

Cardinality
Clinical data warehouse
Column-delimited data
Comma-separated values (CSV)
Data dictionary
Data flow diagram
Data model
Data table
Database
Database management system (DBMS)
Decision support databases
Diagram 0
Entity-relationship diagram (ERD)

Field
Flat file
Foreign key
Join
Method
Normalization
Object-oriented databases
Ontology
Primary key
Record
Relational databases
Select query
Structured Query Language (SQL)

⊙ Introduction

Healthcare is a data-rich business. On the business side of healthcare, claims are generated and submitted for payment. Payment transactions are then sent back to the provider. On the clinical side of healthcare, countless diagnostic tests are performed and the results of those tests are provided back to practitioners and providers. The introduction of the electronic health record (EHR) and sophisticated electronic medical record systems increased the amount of data available in the healthcare setting exponentially. The Centers for Medicare and Medicaid Services' (CMS) meaningful use criteria, value-based purchasing programs, and the formation of Accountable Care Organizations (ACOs) and other payment reform policies are driving the need for providers to use the data produced during the delivery of care to help improve the efficiency and effectiveness of the healthcare system. If these goals are to be met, then the data must be organized in a way that allows analysis and reports to be produced accurately and in real time. Databases give structure to the raw data and facilitate the manipulation of data to achieve these goals.

⊙ Database Terminology

Prior to studying the various types of databases and DBMSs, it is important to have a common set of terminology to describe the various components of a database. Databases may be envisioned as a collection of data tables. The most common form of a data table found in practice is a tab or worksheet within a spreadsheet.

Data tables include **records** or rows and **fields** or columns. For example, table 4.1 represents a table of patients and their associated appointments. The fields in this table represent data elements describing attributes of the appointment (provider, date, and time). A collection of fields that are related are placed in the same record. The records in this table represent the data describing the patient's appointment. Records in a data table may represent patient demographic information, attributes of a service provided to a patient, or even a diagnostic or procedural code (such as ICD-9) and its definition.

Table 4.1   Patients and their appointments

PatientID	ProviderID	AppointmentDate	AppointmentTime
ABD239	SMI123	1/23/2012	9:00 a.m.
DIR235	SMI123	1/23/2012	9:30 a.m.
JKF764	SMI123	1/23/2012	10:00 a.m.

Sets of records include a common set of fields and those related to the same business purpose or focus are collected together into a data table. Common data tables found in healthcare include

- Patient demographics
- Physician specialty and licensure
- Charge description master
- Patient services

A collection of data tables is called a **database**. Databases can have a variety of structures and may be created and maintained using a **database management system (DBMS)**. A DBMS provides a method for adding or deleting data and also supports methods to extract data for reporting.

Types of Databases

To decide on the type of database that is most appropriate to store data, the user must answer some key questions:

- How many records will the database contain (currently and in the foreseeable future)?
- How do the variables relate to each other?
- What database tools are available for use?
- How will the data be pulled or queried from the database?

The answers to these questions will drive the database type. There typically is not a right or wrong answer in database design. If the database is robust enough to hold all of the information required and extracting information is straightforward, then it should be considered a good quality design. The two most common types of databases used in practice are flat files or data tables and relational databases.

Flat Files

If the data structure is relatively simple, then a **flat file** or spreadsheet may be the right type of database. A flat file is a text file, usually delimited by a comma or tab, with one record found on each row. It has only one table of data. For instance, if a

Table 4.2   Flat file

Employee	Monday	Tuesday	Wednesday	Thursday	Friday	Weekly Total
Anne	4	9	6	6	5	30
Nicholas	6	10	7	3	6	32
Zach	4	7	9	8	4	32

practice manager wished to track the number of records coded by each employee, then the flat file displayed in table 4.2 is sufficient.

This structure allows the manager to see who is the most or least productive and may be expanded by adding additional columns to track more days. A series of flat files or individual spreadsheets may be used to track other information about the employees such as credentials or continuing education (CEU) credits. If the number of additional attributes is small, then they may be added to the records displayed in table 4.2. If there is a large number of additional attributes, they may be stored in a second flat file.

Flat file databases may be stored in a number of formats. Traditional spreadsheet tabs, such as those found in Microsoft Excel, are the most common format found in business applications. Flat files may also be stored in text files as columns of data or with the fields delimited by a character. Table 4.3 shows an example of **column-delimited data** and table 4.4 shows the same data stored in a comma-delimited or **comma-separated value (CSV)** file. Column-delimited data must be accompanied by documentation that lists the order and position of the variables so that the data may be interpreted properly.

CSV files may include the variable names in the first row. If not, then they too require documentation to identify the variables in each position.

Flat data tables have an intuitive two-dimensional format of rows and columns. The number of rows and columns is limited only by the software tool used to store and analyze the data. If a spreadsheet program is used to store the data, then formulas may be embedded into the table structure and are stored as part of the data table. A flat data table may be sorted or filtered to select particular values of the variables.

Table 4.3   Column-delimited data

Employee	Monday	Tuesday	Wednesday	Thursday	Friday	Weekly Total
Anne	4	9	6	6	5	30
Nicholas	6	10	7	3	6	32
Zach	4	7	9	8	4	32

Table 4.4   Comma-separated values

Employee, Monday, Tuesday, Wednesday, Thursday, Friday, Weekly Total
Anne,4,9,6,6,5,30
Nicholas,6,10,7,3,6,32
Zach,4,7,9,8,4,32

The two primary limitations of storing data in flat tables are first that the design does not allow relationships between variables in separate tables. This limits the ability to cross-check values for data integrity to those variables stored in the same table. For instance, if the charge description master (CDM) includes current procedural terminology (CPT) codes, the validation of the CPT code could only be accomplished by relating the CDM in one table to the CPT code table using the CPT code. The second limitation is that the same data element may need to be stored in multiple tables to allow for useful reporting. Data redundancy is not a good practice in database design and can cause serious data integrity issues when a variable is updated in one table, but not the others in which it is stored. If the tables used to store the various data elements need to be combined or must be validated against each other to ensure data integrity, then a relational database is a better choice.

Relational Databases

Relational databases were first conceptualized by Edgar F. Codd. Codd proposed that data should be stored in a way that allowed users to query and analyze data without having to restructure it (Codd 1970, 377). As an example, suppose a data analyst wished to create a report of the number of patients served by zip code and clinical department. The data reside in two tables. One holds the patient demographic information. The second holds the information about the patient's visit, including the clinical department. If the database is stored in flat files, then the clinical department must be added to the first file or the zip code must be added to the second file. If the database is relational, then the two tables may be joined or linked using the patient identifier as a common data element.

In a relational database, data with a common purpose, concept, or source are arranged into tables. The relationship between the tables is displayed in an **entity-relationship diagram (ERD)**. Figure 4.1 displays a simple ERD relating a patient information table to a table containing the dates of service for each visit for all patients. This ERD shows that the patient information and visit tables are related by the PatientID variable.

Figure 4.1   Entity relationship diagram

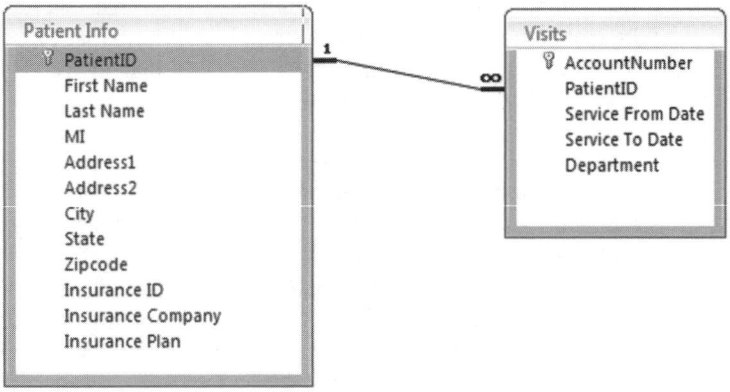

Relational databases are structured in a way that helps ensure data integrity. Notice that in figure 4.1, one variable in each table has an icon of a key next to it. These are the primary key in each of the tables. The **primary key** uniquely identifies the row in the database. PatientID uniquely identifies a row in the patient information table and AccountNumber uniquely identifies the row in the visits table. Properly defining the primary key field in a table prevents adding of duplicate values of that field in the tables. A **foreign key** is a variable in one table that is a primary key in another table. In this example, PatientID is a foreign key in the visits table.

The line extending in figure 4.1 from the PatientID variable in the patient information table to the PatientID variable in the visits table indicates that these two tables are related through the PatientID. Notice that the line has a 1 at the PatientInfo end and the infinity sign (∞) at the visits table end. These symbols represent the **cardinality** of the relationship between the two tables. Cardinality for each table refers to the number of elements in each table. Table 4.5 presents three types of relationship cardinality in relational databases:

1. One-to-one: Each row in one table relates to one and only one row in the other.

2. One-to-many: Each row in one table may relate to many rows in a second table; each row in the second table relates to only one row in the first table.

3. Many-to-many: Each row in one table may relate to many rows in a second table; each row in the second table may relate to many rows in the first table.

Table 4.5　Cardinality

Cardinality	Table A	Table B	Explanation
One-to-one (1:1)	Patient ID Discharge status code	Discharge status code Definition	Each patient has only one discharge status code; each discharge status code has only one definition.
One-to-many (1:N or 1:∞)	Account number Patient name	Account number Diagnosis code sequence ICD-10-CM diagnosis code	Each account may have many associated diagnosis codes.
Many-to-many (N:N or ∞:∞)	Account number Bill type Bill date	Account number Bill type Bill date Payment amount	Each account may have multiple bill types and bill dates. Each bill type and bill date may have multiple payments.

Carefully defining the variables in each table and the primary key fields for each table is the first step in ensuring data integrity. Data redundancy or duplication should be avoided in a relational database. The practice of **normalization** of a database prevents duplication of data elements and ensures the data all conform to a standard. There are three forms of normalization:

1. First Normal Form
   a. Eliminate repeating groups in individual tables
   b. Create a separate table for each set of related data
   c. Identify each set of related data with a primary key

2. Second Normal Form
   a. Create separate tables for sets of values that apply to multiple records
   b. Relate these tables with a foreign key

3. Third Normal Form

   a. Eliminate fields that do not depend on the key (Microsoft 2007).

Case Study: Normalizing Data Tables

In this case study, the flat data table included in table 4.6 will be converted to a relational database with a normalized form. When data is normalized, the data in one flat file may result in a number of tables.

The first normal form requires that the repeating groups are eliminated, separate tables are created for each set of related data, and each resulting table has a primary key. In table 4.6, the variables may be segmented into patient information (table 4.7) and service information (table 4.8).

The services table may be further broken down into a revenue code definition table, services by account number, and a CDM table. These are displayed in tables 4.8a, 4.8b, and 4.8c.

The final step in first-order normalization is to identify the primary key fields in each table. The primary key for the visits table is account number. The primary key in table 4.8a is a combination of the account number and the CDM item. The primary key in table 4.8b is the CDM item and, finally, the primary key in table 4.8c is the revenue code.

By eliminating repeating rows, the tables now actually conform to the second normalized form. Recall that the second normalized form requires that separate tables be created for sets of values that apply to multiple records and that the tables are related with a foreign key.

The ERD displayed in figure 4.2 shows the relationships between the normalized tables. Notice that the field names were converted to single words by inserting an underscore between the words in the original variable names. It is best practice to use single-word variable or field names and table names to simplify the syntax for writing queries and reports.

Table 4.6   Normalized data

MRN	Account Number	Date of Service	CDM Item	Revenue Code	Revenue Code Definition	HCPCS Code	Units	Charge
123ABC	1	011011	L01	0300	LABORATORY OR LAB	36415	1	$ 55.75
123ABC	1	011011	L02	0300	LABORATORY OR LAB	84066	1	$ 51.50
123ABC	1	011011	L03	0301	LAB/CHEMISTRY	84153	1	$ 92.25
123ABC	1	011011	C01	0331	CHEMOTHER/INJ	96402	1	$ 168.50
123ABC	1	011011	D01	0636	DRUGS/DETAIL CODE	J9217	1	$ 507.77
987ZYX	2	010411	D02	0250	PHARMACY		6	$ 306.04
987ZYX	2	010411	S01	0270	MED-SUR SUPPLIES		1	$ 11.25
987ZYX	2	010411	S02	0270	MED-SUR SUPPLIES	A6257	1	$ 0.42
987ZYX	2	010411	L04	0305	LAB/HEMATOLOGY	85025	1	$ 107.00
987ZYX	2	010411	C02	0335	CHEMOTHERP-IV	96413	1	$ 495.00
987ZYX	2	010411	E13	0510	CLINIC	99213	1	$ 136.50
987ZYX	2	010411	D03	0636	DRUGS/DETAIL CODE	J2405	8	$ 50.65
987ZYX	2	010411	D04	0636	DRUGS/DETAIL CODE	J9305	100	$ 10,714.56
987ZYX	3	020611	S03	0270	MED-SUR SUPPLIES		1	$ 11.25
987ZYX	3	020611	S02	0270	MED-SUR SUPPLIES	A6257	1	$ 0.42
987ZYX	3	020611	E13	0510	CLINIC	99213	1	$ 136.50

Table 4.7 Patient information

Patient_ID	Account_Number	Service_Date
123ABC	1	01/10/2011
987ZYX	2	01/04/2011
987ZYX	3	02/06/2011

Table 4.8 Service information

Services						
Account number	CDM Item	Revenue Code	Revenue Code Definition	HCPCS Code	Units	Charge
1	L01	0300	LABORATORY OR LAB	36415	1	$ 55.75
1	L02	0300	LABORATORY OR LAB	84066	1	$ 51.50
1	L03	0301	LAB/ CHEMISTRY	84153	1	$ 92.25
1	C01	0331	CHEMOTHER/ INJ	96402	1	$ 168.50
1	D01	0636	DRUGS/DETAIL CODE	J9217	1	$ 507.77
2	D02	0250	PHARMACY		6	$ 306.04
2	S01	0270	MED-SUR SUPPLIES		1	$ 11.25
2	S02	0270	MED-SUR SUPPLIES	A6257	1	$ 0.42
2	L04	0305	LAB/HEMATO LOGY	85025	1	$ 107.00
2	C02	0335	CHEMOTHERP-IV	96413	1	$ 495.00
2	E13	0510	CLINIC	99213	1	$ 136.50
2	D03	0636	DRUGS/DETAIL CODE	J2405	8	$ 50.65

(Continued)

Table 4.8   Service information (*Continued*)

Account number	CDM Item	Revenue Code	Revenue Code Definition	HCPCS Code	Units	Charge
			Services			
2	D04	0636	DRUGS/DETAIL CODE	J9305	100	$ 10,714.56
3	S03	0270	MED-SUR SUPPLIES		1	$ 11.25
3	S02	0270	MED-SUR SUPPLIES	A6257	1	$ 0.42
3	E13	0510	CLINIC	99213	1	$ 136.50

Table 4.8a   Services

Account number	CDM Item	Units
	Services	
1	L01	1
1	L02	1
1	L03	1
1	C01	1
1	D01	1
2	D02	6
2	S01	1
2	S02	1
2	L04	1
2	C02	1
2	E13	1
2	D03	8
2	D04	100

Services		
Account number	**CDM Item**	**Units**
3	S03	1
3	S02	1
3	E13	1

Table 4.8b Charge description master

Table 4.8c Revenue codes

Charge Description Master				
CDM Item	**Revenue Code**	**HCPCS Code**	**Unit Charge**	
C01	0331	96402	$	168.50
C02	0335	96413	$	495.00
D01	0636	J9217	$	507.77
D02	0250		$	51.01
D03	0636	J 2405	$	6.33
D04	0636	J 9305	$	107.15
E13	0510	99213	$	136.50
L01	0300	36415	$	55.75
L02	0300	84066	$	51.50
L03	0301	84153	$	92.25
L04	0305	85025	$	107.00
S01	0270		$	11.25
S02	0270	A6257	$	0.42
S03	0270		$	11.25

Revenue Codes	
Revenue Code	**Revenue Code Definition**
0250	PHARMACY
0270	MED-SUR SUPPLIES
0300	LABORATORY OR LAB
0301	LAB/CHEMISTRY
0305	LAB/HEMATOLOGY
0331	CHEMOTHER/INJ
0335	CHEMOTHERP-IV
0510	CLINIC
0636	DRUGS/DETAIL CODE

Figure 4.2   Relationships between normalized tables

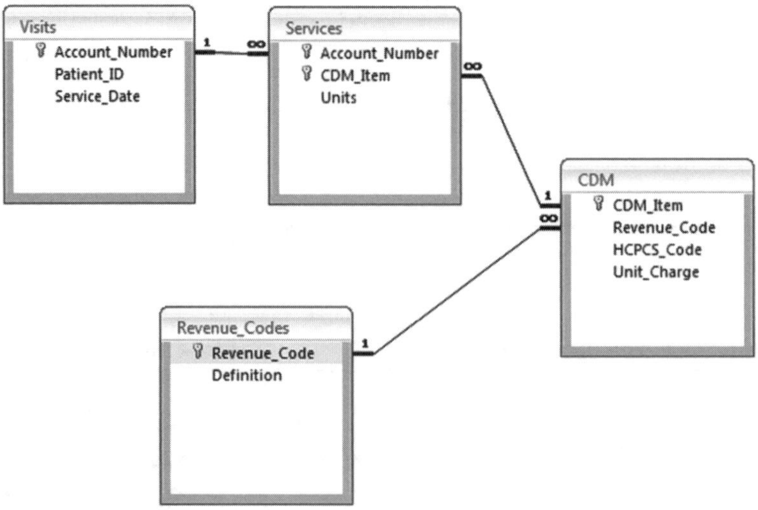

Used with permission from Microsoft.

The final step in normalization is to check the third normalized form. To conform to the third normalized form, all fields that do not depend on a key (primary or foreign) must be eliminated. The tables in figure 4.2 do not include any fields that do not depend on the key fields and therefore the tables are completely normalized.

Object-Oriented Databases

Object-oriented databases are designed to handle data types beyond text and numbers. Flat file and relational databases were developed to store data that fits into rows and columns. Object-oriented databases may be used to store images or videos. In healthcare, object-oriented databases may be used to store images from an MRI or x-ray, or even an audio file capturing the heartbeat heard during a prenatal ultrasound. The building blocks of an object-oriented database are the objects, as opposed to the tables in a relational database system

An object-oriented database stores two types of information about the object. The first element is the data itself (audio clip, image, video file, and such). The second element stored describes how to use the data and is called the **method**. Object-oriented databases are currently not used widely in practice, but the expansion of EHRs will require the storage of many objects beyond the simple rows and columns of numbers and text that may be stored in relational databases.

Database Management Software

To access and manipulate a database, it must reside in a software tool. The choice of database software depends on the type of database, the size of the database, and the complexity of the relationships between the database elements. Relational databases are found most often in practice. The most common relational database software applications include Microsoft Access, Oracle, and Microsoft SQL Server.

Microsoft Access is typically run from a workstation and is appropriate for smaller department-specific applications. It is also useful for prototyping larger enterprise-wide database systems. Once the number of users expands and Access can no longer efficiently accommodate the database, the database may require a more sophisticated software application. Microsoft offers a wizard that allows users to convert an Access database to a SQL Server database (Microsoft 2011).

Check Your Understanding 4.1

Instructions: Choose the best answer.

1. A data table
   a. Cannot be empty
   b. Is made up of rows and columns
   c. Holds alphanumeric data
   d. May only store one type of data

2. DBMS is an acronym for
   a. Database manipulation standards
   b. Database management standards
   c. Database management system
   d. Database manipulation system

3. A flat file database is a
   a. Database that only has simple data tables
   b. Database with only one table
   c. Database that contains records with a large number of fields
   d. Database manipulation system

4. A primary key
   a. Uniquely identifies a record
   b. Contains only numeric values
   c. May be repeated across rows
   d. Represents the relationship between two fields

5. Microsoft Access in an example of:
   a. Relational database management software
   b. A spreadsheet program
   c. A program to manage flat data files
   d. A querying language

⊙ Data Dictionary

A **data dictionary** is a tool that provides metadata or information about data. Metadata is defined as data about data. For example, the data element of First Name might include metadata such as the field length, that it is an alphanumeric field, and that the field is required. A key focus of a data dictionary is to support and adopt more consistent use of data elements and terminology to improve the use of data in reporting. A data dictionary promotes clearer understanding; helps users find information; promotes more efficient use and reuse of information; and promotes better data management (Bronnert 2011, 5).

A data dictionary should document the following attributes (or metadata) for the fields in a data table at a minimum:

- Field name
- Table name
- Description of the field
- Data type (numeric or text, field length)
- Data frequency (required field or not)
- Primary or foreign key
- Valid values
- Data source
- Field creation date
- Field termination date
- Update frequency

The data dictionary in table 4.9 documents the contents of the CDM table found in the normalization example. The details included in this table allow a user with little or no knowledge of the contents of the table to understand the fields present and their various roles.

⊙ Structured Query Language (SQL)

Structured Query Language (SQL) is the programming language that is used to manipulate data in a relational database. SQL is sometimes pronounced "sequel." SQL fulfills many roles in a DBMS:

- SQL is an interactive query language. Users type SQL commands into an interactive SQL program to retrieve data and display it on the screen, providing a convenient, easy-to-use tool for ad hoc database queries.
- SQL is a database programming language. Programmers embed SQL commands into their application programs to access the data in a database. Both user-written programs and database utility programs (such as report writers and data entry tools) use this technique for database access.
- SQL is a database administration language. The database administrator responsible for managing a minicomputer or mainframe database uses SQL to define the database structure and control access to the stored data.
- SQL is a client/server language. Personal computer programs use SQL to communicate over a network with database servers that store shared data. This client/server architecture has become very popular for enterprise-class applications.

Table 4.9 Data dictionary

Field Name	Table	Description	Data Type	Field Length	Data Frequency	Key?	Valid Values	Data Source	Field Creation Date	Field Termination Date	Update Frequency
CDM Item	CDM	CDM item code	Text	20	Required	Primary	Alpha-numeric	Finance	01/01/1900		N/A
Revenue Code	CDM	UB-04 revenue code	Text	4	Required	Foreign	Valid revenue code	HIM	01/01/1900		Annual
HCPCS Code	CDM	CPT/ HCPCS Level II	Text	5		Foreign	Valid HCPCS	HIM	01/01/1900		Annual
Unit Charge	CDM	Charge per unit	Currency	10	Required		>= $0.00	Finance	01/01/1900		Annual

⊙ SQL is an Internet data access language. Internet web servers that interact with corporate data and Internet application servers all use SQL as a standard language for accessing corporate databases.

⊙ SQL is a distributed database language. Distributed DBMSs use SQL to help distribute data across many connected computer systems. The DBMS software on each system uses SQL to communicate with the other systems, sending requests for data access.

⊙ SQL is a database gateway language. In a computer network with a mix of different DBMS products, SQL is often used in a gateway that allows one brand of DBMS to communicate with another brand (Groff 2010, 6).

The role of SQL as an interactive query language is described in more detail in the following section. The other roles of SQL are beyond the scope of this text, but health information management (HIM) professionals should be aware that SQL is far more than just a tool used to extract data from a relational database.

SQL commands that may be used to retrieve data follow a basic structure that allows nonprogrammers to understand and write queries. For example, a SQL command to collect all of the visits for a particular patient in the visits table found in Table 4.7 is

SELECT * FROM visits WHERE patient_id = '987ZYX'

The results of the query are the two records displayed in Table 4.10.

This is called a **select query**. The purpose of a select query is to pull records that meet a certain criteria from a particular table or combination of tables. The words SELECT, FROM, and WHERE are capitalized in the query because they represent key words or instructions in the SQL command.

In this case, the two visit records for patient 987ZYX were selected from the three records found in the visits table. The query may be modified to present the records in a particular order. For instance, the records in the previous example may be sorted by descending service date by revising the query to include an ORDER BY statement:

SELECT Visits.Account_Number, Visits.Patient_ID, Visits.Service_Date

FROM Visits

WHERE Visits.Patient_ID="987ZYX"

ORDER BY Visits.Service_Date DESC;

The ORDER BY clause states that the results of the query should be sorted by descending service date. The results of this query are presented in table 4.11.

Table 4.10   Select query

Account_Number	Patient_ID	Service_Date
2	987ZYX	01/04/2011
3	987ZYX	02/06/2011

Table 4.11   Select query example results

Account_Number	Patient_ID	Service_Date
3	987ZYX	02/06/2011
2	987ZYX	01/04/2011

A select query may be used to combine data from two or more tables by defining a **join**. For example, a SQL query to select all of the patients that received the medical supply with the CDM item code S02 would require the services table be joined to the visits table. The relationship between these tables is found in the ERD displayed in Figure 4.2. The tables must be combined or joined based on the Account_Number field. When more than one table is included in a query, the fields are referenced by both the table and field name concatenated together and delimited by a period. For example, when referring to the field Account_Number in the visits table, the user would reference the field as Visits.Account_Number. The following select query will find the patients who received CDM item S02:

> SELECT Visits.Account_Number, Visits.Patient_ID, Visits.Service_Date, Services.CDM_Item,
>
> Services.Units
>
> FROM Visits INNER JOIN Services ON Visits.Account_Number = Services.Account_Number
>
> WHERE Services.CDM_Item="S02";

In this query, the SELECT statement includes the fields that are desired; the FROM statement includes the two tables (Visits and Services) as well as how those two tables should be related (Account_Number). Finally, the WHERE statement indicates that only rows where the CDM_Item is equal to S02 in the Services table. The results of this query are presented in table 4.12.

A SQL command may also be used to summarize data. In the above example, a count of the number of visits for each patient may be generated with the following query:

> SELECT Visits.Patient_ID, Count(Visits.Service_Date) AS CountOfService_Date
>
> FROM Visits
>
> GROUP BY Visits.Patient_ID;

This query includes the familiar SELECT and FROM keywords, but notice that there is now a GROUP BY statement. When a query is used to summarize data the summary statistic and the field that designates the group to be summarized must be designated. In the example, the SELECT statement includes a command that creates a count of the number of service dates (Count(Visits,Service_Date)) and stores that result in a new field called CountOfService_Date. The GROUP BY portion of the query states that the counts should be presented by Patient_ID. The result of this query is presented in table 4.13.

Table 4.12   Join query example results

Account_Number	Patient_ID	Service_Date	CDM_Item	Units
2	987ZYX	1/4/2011	S02	1
3	987ZYX	2/6/2011	S02	1

Table 4.13   Count of service dates

Patient_ID	CountOfService_Date
123ABC	1
987ZYX	2

Check Your Understanding 4.2

Instructions: Choose the best answer.

1. SQL is an acronym for
   a. Sequential Query Language
   b. Structured Query Language
   c. Selective Question Language
   d. Sequential Question Language

2. SQL is used to manipulate
   a. Data in a relational database
   b. Data in a flat file database
   c. A data warehouse
   d. Unstructured data

3. Which of the following SQL statements will select all columns and rows from the table visits?
   a. SELECT patient_id FROM visits
   b. SELECT * FROM visits WHERE service_date = #1/1/2010#
   c. SELECT * FROM visits
   d. SELECT account, count(patient_id) FROM visits

4. Which of the following is included in a data dictionary?
   a. Field length
   b. Data type
   c. Field description
   d. All of the above

5. The field reference cpt.code in a SQL query refers to
   a. The database named cpt.code
   b. The field code in the table named cpt
   c. The field cpt in the table named code
   d. The table named code found in the database named cpt

⊙ Data Modeling

A **data model** is a representation of the data to be stored in a database and the relationships between the tables and data fields. Prior to the design of the database, the business process to be supported by the database must be modeled. This may be accomplished through the use of process and data flow diagrams. The components of a database, discussed previously in this chapter, are designed and assembled in a way that supports the business process requirements. Data modeling may be carried out using either an object-oriented or entity-relationship approach. The entity-relationship approach will be outlined here.

There are two important outputs to the data modeling process. The first output is the ERD, a graphical representation of the tables in the database and their relationships. The second output is the data dictionary. Both of these documents were discussed earlier in this chapter. The data model serves as the basis for the database structure and design as documented by the ERD and data dictionary.

The process of data modeling includes three steps: the conceptual model, the logical model, and the physical data model. The conceptual model includes a mapping of the business requirements for the database using nontechnical terms that end users can understand. A database that does not meet the need of the end users is of no value, so they must be involved in the design process at the earliest stage. The conceptual data model is independent of the type of database that will ultimately be used to store the data. The conceptual data model may be mapped using a context-level **data flow diagram**, which maps out the database's boundary and scope. Figure 4.3 shows a context-level data flow diagram for the claims database example used earlier in this chapter. Notice that the diagram does not include any field or table information. It simply displays the general categories of data and their roles in the business process. The details regarding the actual database structure are fleshed out in the logical modeling step.

Figure 4.3   Context-level data flow diagram

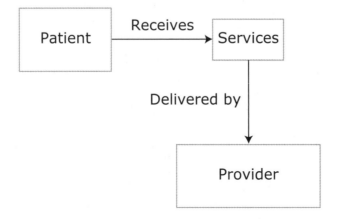

The logical model is the next step in database modeling. During this phase the tables start to take shape. The fields are not defined, but the basic contents of the tables and how they relate are defined. In our claims data example, the tables are

- Patient information
- Visit for each patient
- Services provided to patient
- Charge for services

The relationships between the tables may be mapped out in a **Diagram 0** data flow diagram. A Diagram 0 data flow diagram expands on the context diagram and adds details regarding the tables and their relationships. Figure 4.4 displays a Diagram 0 for the claims database example.

The final step in the database modeling process is to determine the physical model. This includes mapping out the tables, keys, and relationships using an ERD as well as determining the DBMS and hardware to house the database. The ERD for this example is displayed in figure 4.2. At this point in the modeling process a database type may be selected. Since this database requires multiple tables that may need to be linked together for reporting purposes, a relational database is the best choice for this business process. There are a number of DBMSs that support relational database structures. Some examples include

- Microsoft Access
- Microsoft SQL Server
- Informix
- Oracle
- MySQL

Figure 4.4   Diagram 0

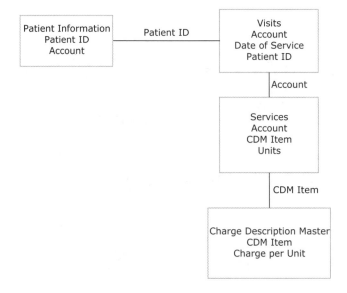

The choice of specific DBMS software should be based on the size and scope of the database as well as the budget for the project. Microsoft Access is an excellent choice for small departmental databases, but is not suited for enterprise-wide databases with many users because the administration of user access at various levels is not possible. Oracle is an extremely robust DBMS and can accommodate very complex models with many users. Oracle licenses tend to be significantly more expensive than Microsoft Access. For this reason, departmental-level databases are often maintained in Microsoft Access. There are some open-source DBMSs that are free to the public, but may not have the support network that some of the commercial products have.

The physical model also includes a specification of the computer hardware that will be used to house the database. The amount of storage or disk space required for the database should be determined prior to selecting any hardware platform. Estimating the space required for the database currently and for the foreseeable future will help determine the appropriate hardware and software to select for implementation of the database.

Check Your Understanding 4.3

Instructions: Choose the best answer.

1. Which phase of data modeling includes a description of the business process?
   a. Physical model
   b. Logical model
   c. Conceptual model
   d. None of the above

2. Which phase of data modeling describes the relationship between the data tables?
   a. Physical model
   b. Logical model
   c. Conceptual model
   d. None of the above

3. Which phase of data modeling includes the selection of the database type?
   a. Physical model
   b. Logical model
   c. Conceptual model
   d. None of the above

4. An entity-relationship diagram describes all of the following except
   a. Tables in the database
   b. Relationship between the tables
   c. Key fields
   d. DBMS software

5. Which of the following is not a database management software package?
   a. Microsoft Access
   b. Oracle
   c. MySQL
   d. Microsoft Excel

⊙ Clinical Data Warehouses

Clinical databases are found throughout healthcare operations. The example in this chapter was a very simple database designed to hold information about the services provided to a patient. Clinical databases may be found in various departments throughout a healthcare facility including

- ⊙ Patient accounting
- ⊙ Clinical departments
- ⊙ Pharmacy
- ⊙ Clinical trials
- ⊙ Marketing
- ⊙ Quality measurement

Combining these data sources into a **clinical data warehouse** is an effective method of making the data accessible to a wider audience of users. A clinical data warehouse must be designed in a way that maintains sufficient detail so that the data is useful for research and analytic purposes and related in a way that supports real-time access to the data by users. Data warehouses are snapshots of a variety of databases found throughout a company that are combined for the purpose of reporting and analysis. The data warehouse does not include the "live" or transaction data that are used for business operations, but instead are populated by periodic downloads from the live database. The frequency of refreshing the clinical data warehouse depends on the volatility of the underlying data (how often it changes) and the need for timely reporting.

The Stanford School of Medicine has an extensive clinical data warehouse called STRIDE (Stanford Translational Research Integrated Database Environment) that stores data that supports clinical and translational research (Stanford Center for Clinical Informatics 2012). STRIDE includes data from both hospitals affiliated with Stanford. The hospitals use different billing systems and yet the warehouse is designed to combine the datasets across the facilities. In January 2013, the STRIDE warehouse included

- ⊙ 1.85 million pediatric and adult patients with clinical and demographic data (1994 to present)
- ⊙ 21.5 million Clinical Encounters (1994 to present)

- 40 million ICD-9 coded inpatient and outpatient diagnoses (1994 to present)
- 25 million ICD-9 and CPT-coded inpatient and outpatient clinical procedures (1994 to present)
- 3.1 million radiology reports (2005 to present)
- 1.3 million surgical pathology reports (1995 to present)
- 21 million transcribed clinical documents (2005 to present)
- 145 million laboratory test numeric results (2000 to present)
- 14 million inpatient pharmacy orders (2006 to present)
- 99,000 dates of death drawn from hospital and Social Security Administration records

Clinical data warehouses like Stanford's STRIDE are becoming widespread as the technology to support the storage and access of huge volumes of data.

Decision support databases are a common example of a clinical data warehouse. These databases are found in many healthcare entities and may include claims data, financial data, and quality data combined in one database to support both internal and external reporting. One of the unique challenges in combining clinical data is that any release of that data may be subject to HIPAA regulations if it includes any of the protected health information fields such as dates or Social Security numbers. Any efforts to combine data into a clinical data warehouse should include the involvement of a compliance officer or other professional with knowledge of the rules and regulations surrounding deidentification of data and the release of identifiable data.

Much of the time and effort invested in compiling a clinical data warehouse is used to clean and combine the data. Although clinical data is singularly focused on healthcare and patient information, the coding systems may or may not be consistent. For instance, pharmacy databases may include the National Drug Code (NDC) or may only include an inventory or CDM code that only has meaning inside a particular facility or system of facilities. The mapping between code sets and standardization of coding systems is an age-old issue in healthcare data. Many thought that the HIPAA regulations specifying only one coding system for each purpose would solve this problem. The concept of common **ontology** or system of categories as a method of combining data that may be categorized by clinical classification systems such as ICD and CPT codes as well as those categorized by clinical nomenclatures such as Systematized Nomenclature Of Medicine Clinical Terms (SNOMED) has emerged. An effective ontology is "a theory of those higher-level categories which structure the biomedical domain, the representation of which needs to be both unified and coherent if it is to serve as the basis for terminologies and coding systems that have the requisite degree and type of interoperability" (Smith and Ceusters 2007). A properly designed ontology may allow the automated combining of data from many sources. Such a system would speed the design and delivery of new clinical data warehouses.

⊙ Summary

Understanding the basic structure and guidelines for database design is a critical skill for health information and informatics professionals. Healthcare has a wealth of data that must be organized in a way that allows accurate and efficient processing and reporting. The type of database selected for a business process should be based on the level of complexity of the relationships between the data.

Many database concepts are applicable across the spectrum of database types. The design of the database through the stages of data modeling is as necessary when designing a flat file to hold data with a relatively simple structure as it is when designing an object-oriented database that holds multimedia files as well as numeric and text format data. Data dictionaries are also useful for all database types. Without documentation to inform the user of the format, type, and definitions of data elements the data may not be used for reporting. The basic SQL commands covered in this chapter are transferable across a variety of DBMSs for relational databases. There are slight syntax differences between the various database software products, but the basic structure and key words are transferable across products.

REFERENCES

Bronnert, J., J. Clark, L. Hyde, J. Solberg, S. White, and M. Wolin. 2011. *Health Data Analysis Toolkit*. Chicago: AHIMA.

Codd, E.F. 1970. A relational model of data for large shared data banks (P. Baxendate, ed.). *Communications of the ACM*. 13(6):377–387.

Groff, J., P. Weinberg, and A. Oppel. 2010. *SQL: The Complete Reference*, 3rd ed. New York: McGraw-Hill/Osborne.

Microsoft. 2007. Description of the Database Normalization Basics. Microsoft Support. http://support.microsoft.com/kb/283878.

Microsoft. 2011. How to Convert an Access Database to SQL Server. Microsoft Support. http://support.microsoft.com/kb/237980.

Smith, B. and W. Ceusters. 2007. Ontology as the Core Discipline of Biomedical Informatics: Legacies of the Past and Recommendations for the Future Direction of Research. In *Computing, Philosophy, and Cognitive Science—The Nexus and the Liminal*. Edited by G.D. Crnkovic and S. Stuart, 104–122. Cambridge: Cambridge Scholars Press.

Stanford Center for Clinical Informatics. 2013. Clinical Data Warehouse Projects— SCCI Stanford Medicine. Stanford Center for Clinical Informatics. https://clinicalinformatics.stanford.edu/projects/cdw.html.

5

Data and Information

By Susan H. Fenton

Learning Objectives

- Describe the types of data, as well as the relationship between data and information
- Explain how health information standards are developed and why they are important
- Define data mapping and the various types of data maps
- Compare different needs for and methods of data collection
- Apply data quality principles and practices
- Utilize effective policies, processes, and techniques for data analysis
- Design appropriate data presentations

KEY TERMS

Ad hoc standards
American National Standards Institute (ANSI)
Categorical data
Classification system
Certification
Certification Commission for Health Information Technology (CCHIT)
Characteristics of data quality
Code set

Concept
Concept identification
Consensus standards
Continuous data
Crosstabs
Data cleaning
Data dictionary
Data governance
Data mapping
Data Quality Management Model
Data standards

Data-interchange standard
Data set standard
De facto standards
Descriptive statistics
Discrete data
Equivalence
Expressivity
Forward map
Frequency
Government mandate
Health Information Technology for
    Economic and Clinical Health
    (HITECH) Act
Health Insurance Portability and
    Accountability Act (HIPAA)
    of 1996
Health IT Standards Committee
Health IT Policy Committee
Imputation
International Organization for
    Standardization (ISO)
Interval data
Narrative-text string

National Institute of Standards and
    Technology (NIST)
Natural language processing (NLP)
Negation
Nominal data
ONC-Authorized Testing and
    Certification Bodies
Ordinal data
Post-hoc text processing
Ratio data
Reverse map
Semantic interoperability
Source
Standards development organizations
    (SDOs)
Structured data
Target
Temporal
Terminology
Transaction set
Transaction standard
Unstructured data
Vital statistics

⊙ Introduction

Data and information are the resources that fuel the healthcare industry. Getting the right data or information to the right person at the right time is essential for the delivery of high-quality care as well as the financial well-being of healthcare provider organizations. Data can be entered into electronic health records (EHRs) to be used for clinical care, disease management, or disease prevention. They are also found in large data sets or data warehouses where clinicians, researchers, payers, and others access the data for a variety of purposes.

It is imperative that health informaticists understand the basics of data, the relevant data standards, issues involved with data collection, how to ensure the quality of the data, as well as concerns related to the analysis and presentation of data.

⊙ The Basics of Data

Data are the dates, numbers, images, symbols, letters, and words that represent basic facts and observations about people, processes, measurements, and conditions (AHIMA 2012). The terms datum or data can be used as a singular noun to refer to specific bits of information. Data is always used as the plural noun in reference to many bits of information. Examples of singular data include the patient's address, a single laboratory result, one blood pressure reading, the charge for one day in the hospital, and so on. Examples of plural data can include the entire set of entries for a single patient in the EHR or data sets such as the National Center for Health Statistics' (NCHS), National Hospital Discharge Data Set (NHDDS), or all of the Centers for Medicare and Medicaid Services (CMS) claims data (see figure 5.1).

There are many different types of data in healthcare. There are numerical data and alphabetical data. In some instances such as an address, the data are alphanumeric. Data can be categorical (discrete) or continuous. It is important for the health informaticist to understand data types in order to utilize the data appropriately.

Categorical or **discrete data** are data elements that represent mutually exclusive categories or labels. These categories or labels can be further broken down into **nominal** and **ordinal data**. **Nominal data** are those data where the categories are simply names. For example, a data element often collected for healthcare consumers is gender. A person can be male, female, or, in some cases, gender may be unknown or other. At any given point in time, a person can have only one gender. In contrast, **ordinal data** are data where the names or labels have an order to them with meaning attached. For example, a patient may be diagnosed with cancer, which is often represented as Stage I, Stage II, Stage III, or Stage IV. These are mutually exclusive categories; however, there is an order to the labels, with Stage IV cancer being more advanced than Stage I cancer.

Continuous data are numerical data where there is an equal interval between the data points. There are two types of continuous data, **ratio** and

Figure 5.1 Examples of singular and plural data

Singular Data Examples
Patient Address: 123 Any Street, City, ST 10000
Hemoglobin Level: 12.6 grams per deciliter
Blood Pressure: 120/80 mm Hg
Room Charge: $650 per day

Plural Data Examples
National Center for Health Statistics' National Hospital
Discharge Data Set, http://www.cdc.gov/nchs/nhds.htm
Centers for Medicare and Medicaid Services Medicare Provider Analysis and Review File (MEDPAR), https://www.cms.gov/LimitedDataSets/02_MEDPARLDSHospitalNational.aspTopOfPage

interval data. In addition to the equal intervals between data points, ratio data have a true zero (0) point. An example of ratio data in healthcare would be "patient weight." No human can weigh less than 0 pounds or ounces so this data element would be ratio. Interval data do not have a true zero and can have negative numbers. An example of interval data is temperature, which can be negative or positive.

Data Related to Information

While data are important, it is often difficult to utilize them effectively even for a single patient unless they are processed into information. So, how does the health informaticist get from individual data elements to information that can be used effectively and efficiently?

Foremost is an understanding of the original purpose for which the data is used or collected. For example, data that are collected for clinical purposes may be, and often are very different from data that are collected for reimbursement or research purposes. Clinical data are often very detailed, for instance, vital signs can be collected every 15 minutes in the intensive care unit (ICU), while the reimbursement data for the same patient will only include the more general diagnostic code. It is important to consider whether there are mandated or generally accepted **data standards** for the data. Standards may be related to the data set, such as the data elements specified for the Uniform Hospital Discharge Data Set, or the allowable data values, such as a selection list being provided for the address data element of State. Standards such as the allowable data elements within a data set, the definitions of the different data elements, or the allowable data values, which constrain the data that can be entered into a field, ensure that the data is as accurate as possible.

An additional consideration is the data collection method that was utilized. There are many different methods of data collection, such as keyboard, voice recognition, and automated methods, where data are transferred directly from digital thermometers, scales, blood pressure cuffs, and so on. The quality of the data must be assessed. It is difficult to produce good quality information when the data itself is of poor quality. It is also vital to understand the analysis that the data are intended to undergo or the analysis that was used to develop or produce the information. Finally, it is important to present the data so that it can be easily understood. Figure 5.2 presents total cholesterol levels for a patient in two different forms, tabular and graphical. It is generally easier to detect the rise of this patient's cholesterol levels using the graphical representation. Figure 5.3 presents these issues in the form of questions health informaticists can pose while they are working with data.

These and other concerns are important to address in order to ensure the data and information used in healthcare can be relied upon for all of the varied purposes. This chapter will examine these different aspects of data that are important to the production of information.

Figure 5.2   Examples of data presentation
PATIENT X Cholesterol (normal is less than 200)

Date	Cholesterol Level
January 2011	153
February 2011	168
March 2011	160
April 2011	174
May 2011	168
June 2011	181

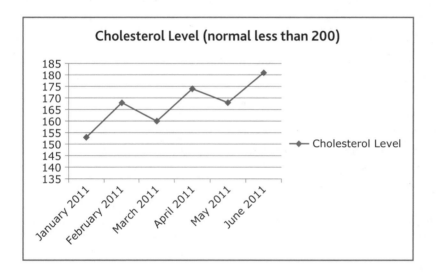

Figure 5.3   Understanding data and information

Questions to Ask about the Data or Information

1. For which purpose or use was the data originally collected?
2. Are there any data standards related to the data?
3. How was the data collected?
4. What is the quality of the data?
5. How will the data be analyzed to produce information?
6. How can the data or information be presented so that it is meaningful to users?

Check Your Understanding 5.1

Instructions: Match the terms with the appropriate descriptions.

- **a.** Nominal
- **b.** Ordinal
- **c.** Ratio
- **d.** Interval

1. _____ These data do not have a true zero and the distance between the data points is consistent.

2. _____ These data separate records into mutually exclusive categories in a meaningful order.

3. _____ These data have a true zero and the distance between the data points is consistent.

4. _____ These data separate records into mutually exclusive, named, categories with no order.

Instructions: Choose the best answer.

5. This type of data typically has many measurements.
   - **a.** Ordinal
   - **b.** Continuous
   - **c.** Discrete
   - **d.** Nominal

6. This is the most important consideration regarding data collection.
   - **a.** Standards
   - **b.** Quality
   - **c.** Purpose
   - **d.** Method

⊙ Data Standards

Standards permeate our lives even though we are rarely conscious of it. In fact, we often only become attuned to the need for standards when they do not exist. Consider our ability to travel across the country in our automobiles. We could not do this if there were no standards for the width of cars and trucks or highways. Standards bring order and understanding to situations where too much variety will result in confusion or an inability to achieve certain goals (Hammond and Cimino 2001, 214). This section will explore the healthcare data standards development process, as well as discuss the different types of standards needed to support health information for the healthcare industry.

Standards Development

One of the challenges encountered when working with healthcare data standards is understanding the process by which the standards are developed. However, it is not uncommon for informaticists to be asked to assist in the development of standards or policies and practices related to standards implementation and use. The four basic methods of standards development follow:

- ⊙ **Ad hoc standards** are those that are established by a group of stakeholders without a formal adoption process.
- ⊙ **De facto standards** have evolved over time to become universally used without a government or other mandate.
- ⊙ Standards that are specified or established by the government for certain purposes are a **government mandate**.
- ⊙ **Consensus standards** are those that are developed through a formal process of comment and feedback by interested stakeholders (Hammond and Cimino 2001, 215–216).

These four methods of standards development are not mutually exclusive. For example, there are many standards that were developed using the consensus method which are now either de facto or governmentally mandated standards. Table 5.1 outlines the different methods and provides an example of each type of standard.

Table 5.1   Standards development methods

Standard Development Method	Definition	Example
Ad hoc	Agreed upon by a group of stakeholders with no formal adoption process.	The Logical Observation Identifiers, Names, and Codes (LOINC) and Digital Imaging and Communications in Medicine (DICOM) standards were developed using the ad hoc method by groups of interested experts.
De facto	A standard that evolves over time due to widespread, nonmandated adoption.	The Microsoft Windows operating system is a de facto standard due to its widespread adoption.
Government mandate	The government either develops the standards or specifies a certain standard be used for a purpose.	The code sets mandated by the government under the Health Insurance Portability and Accountability Act provisions are an example of governmentally mandated standards.
Consensus	Standards developed when stakeholders come together to reach formal agreement on the specifications.	Health Level 7 standards, developed by the HL7 organization and its members, are an example of consensus standards.

Whichever of these development methods is used, there are steps required for standards development. There are many different **standards development organizations (SDOs)** involved in creating and maintaining healthcare standards. The internationally recognized standards development body is the **International Organization for Standardization (ISO)**. The United States representative to the ISO is the **American National Standards Institute (ANSI)**. In order to promulgate a recognized standard, SDOs must be accredited by ANSI and, if applicable, the ISO. The ISO outlines a six-step standards development process.

1. Proposal—This is the stage in the process where there is a recognized need for a new standard. The stakeholders involved often vote or otherwise agree to the need for a new standard.

2. Preparatory—In this stage, a group of experts develops a draft of the proposed standard.

3. Committee—The original draft is reviewed and revised by the full committee of stakeholders until consensus is reached regarding the new standard.

4. Enquiry—The proposed standard is circulated throughout the entire organization for review and approval as a final draft standard.

5. Approval—The final draft standard is voted on again. At this stage, no substantive changes are allowed.

6. Publication—The standard is published with only minor editorial changes made if needed (ISO 2013).

Each standards development organization has its own process. For example, the Health Level Seven (HL7) organization outlines its standards development processes in its Governance and Operations Manual. The manual is very detailed, including guidance for the development of workgroups, as well as information gathering, balloting procedures for standards, and much more information (HL7 2013). Standards that are developed within a single organization may often undergo a much less formal process.

United States Health Information Technology Standards

The Health Information Technology for Economic and Clinical Health (HITECH) Act enacted as part of the American Recovery and Reinvestment Act (ARRA) of 2009 established the **Health IT Standards Committee**, an official federal advisory committee (US Government 2009). The Health IT Standards Committee is "charged with making recommendations to the National Coordinator for Health IT on standards, implementation specifications, and certification criteria for the electronic exchange and use of health information" (HHS 2013).

Representatives on the Health IT Standards Committee come from across the healthcare industry and bring a variety of stakeholder viewpoints to the standards designation process. The Health IT Standards Committee has divided their work into different categories including Clinical Operations, Clinical Quality, Privacy and Security, and Implementation, among others (HHS 2012). The HIT Standards Committee assesses the policy recommendations of the

Health IT Policy Committee, another federal advisory committee established under HITECH, and determines whether standards, implementation guidance or other assistance is needed for the healthcare industry (HHS 2012). Past, present, and future recommendations of the Health IT Standards Committee include standards for EHR certification for CMS's EHR meaningful use incentive program, as well as recommendations related to privacy and security, digital certificates, and so on (HHS 2012).

Prior to the HITECH Act, the majority of governmentally mandated health information technology standards were specified as a part of the **Health Insurance Portability and Accountability Act (HIPAA) of 1996**. These standards included the Privacy Rule, the Security Rule, Transaction and Code Sets, as well as a provision for a National Provider Identifier (US Government 1996). Aside from the obvious focus on privacy and security, the HIPAA standards were largely administrative in nature, supporting the efficient processing of claims to insurance companies and government payers for reimbursement. The increasing use of governmentally mandated standards serves to bring added complexity to healthcare data, while at the same time ensuring it is interchangeable and comparable.

Data Set Standards

One of the oldest types of data standards found in healthcare is the **data set standard**. An early example of the use of data set standards can be found in the London Bills of Mortality (Graunt 1665). Data set standards have historically been established to assist in the tracking and understanding of important events such as births, deaths, hospital discharges, and so on. In the United States, we consider events such as birth and death to be important enough that the data are designated as **vital statistics**.

Prior to computers, healthcare data set standards were established, usually by the government, to collect various types of data. These data set standards established the data elements or data variables to be collected and defined each data element. Medical or other records were carefully examined by clerical personnel. The data was abstracted and entered onto forms and mailed to the controlling governmental agency or entered into computer terminals and transmitted via dedicated lines. It is difficult to overstate the importance of these data sets as they often served as the foundation for public health management and other healthcare research.

Data set standards have evolved along with the information systems supporting them. Due to increased computerization, the time and money involved in establishing a new data set standard can be reduced. An example of a relatively recent data set standard established because of increased availability of information systems is the ImmTrac immunization tracking registry in Texas (Texas Department of State Health Services 2010). This data set standard specifies required demographic and immunization fields, as well as preferred demographic, immunization, and provider fields (Texas Department of State Health Services 2010). Although the United States survived for many years without an immunization registry, the availability of this tool enables better management of health, healthcare, and even national defense in the face of emerging pathogens such as H1N1 or biological weapons such as anthrax.

Data set standards are foundational to healthcare information standards. They continue to evolve, now being used for quality management as with the Health Plan Employer Data and Information Set (HEDIS) (LaTour et al. 2013) and for the continuity of patient care as with the Continuity of Care Document (CCD) (ASTM Standard 2005). The need to collect and use explicitly defined data elements will not abate in the near future. Health informaticists should explore the different data sets standards that can meet a variety of healthcare information needs.

Classification, Code Set, and Terminology Standards

It is all very well and good to have data set standards that specify and define the data elements that are collected regarding certain events. This is necessary, but not always sufficient, to utilize the data and information effectively. Some data elements have such a large number of potential values that those values demand a standard themselves.

Among John Graunt's many accomplishments was that he analyzed the causes recorded for the deaths in the London Bills of Mortality, crude as they might be (WHO 2011). This set the stage for what is now the widespread use of code sets, classification systems, and clinical terminologies. Code set is the term used by the Department of Health and Human Services (HHS) in the seminal health information law, the HIPAA of 1996. HHS defines **code set** as "any set of codes used to encode data elements, such as tables of terms, medical concepts, medical diagnostic codes, or medical procedure codes. A code set includes the codes and the descriptors of the codes" (HHS 1996). A **classification system** is defined as "a system that arranges or organizes like or related entities for easy retrieval" (AHIMA 2012, 77). A **terminology** is defined as "a set of terms representing the system of concepts of a particular subject field" (AHIMA 2012, 408). A code set and classification system are many times synonymous. A terminology is often much more detailed than a classification system. This is because a terminology is intended to represent the details, while a classification system or code set is usually utilized to divide concepts into categories.

It is vital to have either mandated or de facto standards, whether it be a terminology or a classification system, for representing different concepts in healthcare. Both the human users and the computer processors need standards for enhanced understanding. What is a concept? At its most simple, a **concept** is an idea or "unique unit of knowledge or thought created by a unique combination of characteristics" (AHIMA 2012, 95). Concepts are not the same as words or terms. Consider, for example, the word "cold." This simple four-letter word can have many different meanings. The patient can report having a "cold." The patient can state that they feel "cold." It can be "cold" outside. If a code set, classification system, or terminology only focused on the term, the usage of any identifiers related to "cold" would soon become very confusing.

As the health information industry develops and researchers learn more about representing the complex world that is healthcare, it has become clear that it would be beneficial to have guidelines for classification and terminology standards. The most important guideline is to clearly articulate and focus the purpose of a classification or terminology (Cimino 1998). This is not always as easy as it might seem. For example, the stated purpose for the International Classification of Diseases (ICD) is public health reporting and tracking. In the United States, ICD-10 is currently used for mortality reporting, while for morbidity reporting ICD-9-CM is now used and ICD-10-CM will be used beginning in 2014. However, in 1979, ICD-9-CM was adopted for use as a reimbursement classification system, with special guidelines and rules related to the reimbursement purpose (Zeisset 2010). The result has been the use of ICD-9-CM to support reimbursement rather than pure public health reporting. This is not, in and of itself, wrong. However, this mixing of purpose will, by definition, change the evolution and eventual content of the ICD-9-CM classification system. Thus, purpose of the classification system or clinical terminology is paramount and should always remain a central consideration for health informaticists.

Data Mapping

Data mapping is defined by ISO as "the process of associating concepts or terms from one coding system to concepts or terms in another coding system and defining their equivalence in accordance with a documented rationale and a given purpose" (AHIMA 2011b). For the purposes of mapping, the term "coding system" is used very broadly to include classification, terminology, and other data representation systems. Mapping is necessary as the healthcare information systems and their use evolves in order to link disparate systems and data sets. This section will introduce basic mapping concepts for health informaticists.

As with coding, classification, and terminology systems, the creation of a map must begin with a clearly defined purpose for the map. Maps can be created for reimbursement, clinical care, or other purposes. It is important to note that the map created for reimbursement will be different from the clinical map, even if using the same coding or data sets. Any data map will include a source and a target. The **source** is the code or data set from which the map originates. The **target** is the code or data set in which one is attempting to find a code or data representation with an equivalent meaning. **Forward maps** are those that map from an older source code or data set to a newer target code or data set. A **reverse map** goes from a newer source code or data set to an older target code or data set. Maps must be specified as to their source, target, and direction for an understanding of the map.

The relationship in maps are often determined and defined by the purpose of the map. An example of types of map relationships could include

- One-to-one—The source entry has an exactly matching target entry.
- One-to-many—The source entry has many potential target entry matches.
- No match—The source entry has no matches in the target system.

The level of equivalence can indicate the relationship between two code or data sets. **Equivalence** in a map is determined by the distribution of map relationships for a given map. For example, a map containing 50 percent one-to-one maps would have a higher level of equivalence than one containing 20 percent one-to-one maps (AHIMA 2011b).

Transaction Standards

Health information **transaction standards** are also often called **data-interchange standards**. These standards establish the means by which a sender transmits or communicates data or information to a receiver. The data required to complete a specified communication is termed a **transaction set** (Hammond and Cimino 2001, 220). These standards set out the technical format for the communication so the sender knows which data needs to be included in which format and the receiver knows which data to expect and in which format.

There are many different types of transaction standards, including X12 5010, National Council for Prescription Drug Programs (NCPDP), and the HL7 messaging standards, among others. The Accredited Standards Committee (ASC) X12 5010 standard is used by providers and insurance companies for claims processing. The NCPDP is used for e-prescribing. HL7 has a variety of standards, including their messaging standards, supporting the interchange of data between software applications and, ultimately, providers. Users should note that, though the transaction standards ensure both communicating parties understand the message type and the format, these standards do not interpret the content, nor do they constrain the use of the data on the receiving end. They are a transport mechanism only.

EHR Standards and Certification

All of the standards previously discussed are not sufficient to ensure adequate, standard, usable EHRs. HL7 has an EHR functional model, in addition to the messaging standards already discussed. The EHR functional model has been adopted as the foundation of EHR standards. However, with no motivation or incentive to adopt standards, vendors or developers may ignore them or only adopt them in part. The health information industry took action.

Thus, in 2004, the **Certification Commission for Health Information Technology (CCHIT)** was established. CCHIT is an industry-wide initiative engaging a diverse group of stakeholders in a voluntary, consensus-based process that began certifying EHRs in 2006 (CCHIT 2011). **Certification** is an evaluation performed to establish the extent to which a particular computer system, network design, or application implementation meets a prespecified set of requirements (AHIMA 2012, 66). This proved to be a very valuable point of information for EHR purchasers, who could now determine which EHRs met the specified standards, which are always publicly available.

In 2009, the certification of EHRs was codified in legislation and made a requirement for hospitals and physicians receiving payment by the CMS (US Congress 2009). The regulations implementing this section of the **Health Information Technology for Economic and Clinical Health (HITECH) Act** are extensive and incorporate many of the previously discussed standards while incorporating additional technical standards from the **National Institute of Standards and Technology (NIST)** (HHS 2010). It is important to note that the standards and certification of the Office of the National Coordinator for Health Information Technology (ONC) are not all-encompassing and focus on the ability of a software product to enable a provider to demonstrate meaningful use of the product and qualify for payment incentives. In addition to the standards for EHR software, the legislation required the ONC to create an accreditation program to establish **ONC-Authorized Testing and Certification Bodies** (ATCBs) (HHS 2011). ATCBs are empowered to perform complete EHR or EHR module testing and certification. They utilize conformance testing requirements, test cases, and test tools developed by the National Institute for Standards and Technology (NIST) to determine whether the software complies with the EHR Incentive Program requirements for establishing meaningful use of an EHR. At the time this section was written, the number of EHR certification organizations had grown from one to six (HHS 2011). The ultimate goal of EHR certification to specified standards is **semantic interoperability**, that is, the ability to exchange data and information with its original meaning intact and understood by all receivers.

Check Your Understanding 5.2

Instructions: Match the terms with the appropriate descriptions.
Standards Development Matching

    a. Ad hoc
    b. Consensus
    c. Government mandate
    d. De facto

1. _____ Standards that are established by a group of stakeholders without a formal adoption process.

2. _____ Standards that have evolved over time to become universally used without a government or other mandate.

3. _____ Standards that are specified or established by the government for certain purposes.

4. _____ Standards that are developed through a formal process of comment and feedback by interested stakeholders.

Types of Standards

    a. Data set standards
    b. Classification standards
    c. Transaction standards
    d. EHR standards

5. _____ These are developed with the intent of ensuring adequate, standard, usable application software.

6. _____ Systems that arrange or organize like or related entities.

7. _____ These establish the means by which a sender transmits or communicates data or information to a receiver.

8. _____ These establish the data elements or data variables to be collected and define each data element.

⊙ Data Collection

The collection of healthcare data oftentimes must conform to the standards already described. Data can be entered by users via keyboard, handwriting, speech recognition, or direct feed from machines. However, data collection must also be carefully planned, keeping in mind the expected uses of the data and the needs and workflow of the users. Generally, data entry can be classified as either structured or unstructured. Figure 5.4 outlines questions that should be answered by organizations planning their EHR data collection efforts. Ultimately, the choices are usually between structured data entry, unstructured data entry, or a carefully considered combination of the two methods.

Structured Data Entry

The structured entry of healthcare data involves the use of templates and on-screen forms with the possible entry fields and the potential entries in those fields controlled, defined, and limited. **Structured data** can have many benefits including completeness, quality (Johnson et al. 2008), and accessibility of the data for a variety of purposes (van Mulligen et al. 1998). Structured data is often entirely appropriate and highly recommended for data entry when the options are limited or are required to conform to a specific standard. For example, the collection of race and ethnicity data is specified by the US government (US Census Bureau 2003). While this could be a free-text field, the need to report data in conformance with the government standard has led most informaticists to limit the entries in the race and ethnicity fields. Structured data is often also highly desired for uses such as clinical decision support or quality measure reporting where false positives or false negatives could place either patients or organizations at risk (van Mulligen et al. 1998).

Figure 5.4   Data collection considerations

- Why is the organization entering these data? Is it for patient care? To secure payment? To comply with a regulation?
- What data need to be entered? Is there a standard for the data?
- Who will enter the data? Will it be clinicians, nurses, ancillary staff, clerks, or a combination?
- What will be the most efficient method of data entry for each type of user?
- Under what circumstances will users enter data? Will they be rushed, or will they have adequate time? What will be the setting (admissions, emergency room, intensive care, or the patient's home)?
- What use does the organization expect to make of the data? Will they be used for patient care, reimbursement, quality improvement, or research?

Source: Fenton 2006

Structured data is not without its negative aspects. Some studies have suggested that structured data entry can slow down users decreasing their productivity (Rosenbloom et al. 2011; Ash et al. 2007). In addition, structured data entry tools can be incomplete for user needs as well as inflexible when new or unexpected demands arise (Rosenbloom et al. 2011). Finally, structured data entry templates can be developed that insert a more complete narrative with a particular selection; however, the majority of structured data entry systems appear to be found in niche settings and specific clinical domains (Rosenbloom et al. 2011).

Unstructured Data Entry

Unstructured data entry is the use of free text or narrative data in the health record. In the paper record, a large amount of the data, especially the day-to-day progress notes, were unstructured. The clinician determines the level of detail entered and often the formatting used for the data entered in unstructured data entry. This enables the clinician to include the nuances and details that might otherwise be missed with the use of structured data entry. This is called **expressivity**, which is defined as "how well a note conveys the patient's and provider's impressions, reasoning, and thought process; level of concern; and uncertainty to those subsequently reviewing the note." (Rosenbloom et al. 2011).

The main drawback to unstructured data entry centers on the general inability to determine the completeness of the data (Fenton 2006) during the data entry process. Until methods can be developed that can assess the requirements for unstructured data relative to the document it is being used for (the type of patient, the setting of care, and such) this will remain a serious challenge when handling unstructured data.

Another challenge with unstructured data usage is the ongoing and increasing need to use the data in ways that require it to be structured. Health informaticists and linguists have been researching different methods of **post-hoc text processing**, which is using algorithms after data is entered. Some of the different methods that have been studied include searching for narrative-text strings or string patterns; concept identification or indexing; and combining concept indexing with negation or temporal algorithms to approach quite complex and sophisticated **natural language processing (NLP)** (Rosenbloom et al. 2011). NLP is a technology that converts human language (structured or unstructured) into data that can be translated then manipulated by computer systems (AHIMA 2012, 283). **Narrative-text string** or string pattern searches are similar to the "find" functionality used every day in software such as Microsoft Word or Adobe Reader. **Concept identification** methods map the text to standardized concepts using clinical terminologies with high levels of recall and precision (Rosenbloom et al. 2011). **Negation** and **temporal** issues are two that have proven to be obstacles for widespread use of NLP in the real-time clinical domain. Negation involves the ability of the processor to detect the differences between "no chest pain," meaning it is absent, and "chest pain," meaning it is present. Temporal means the computer can detect any time frames included when the concept is identified. For example, "past history of cancer" is very different from simply "cancer." NLP approaches vary by developer and software. Advances in the last four to five years have been significant with expanded use, though anecdotal reports from clinical users are that NLP software can still pose challenges.

Whether an organization chooses structured or unstructured data entry depends upon the purpose of the data entry and the eventual uses of the data. Data entry acceptable for administrative purposes may not be adequate for clinical processes. Organizations must carefully investigate data entry when considering an EHR. Ultimately, each organization will need to make its own carefully considered decision when selecting data entry methods for its EHR (Fenton 2006).

Check Your Understanding 5.3

Instructions: Indicate which type of data entry (s = structured; u = unstructured) applies to the pros and cons.

Pros

1. _____ The data will have detail and nuance.
2. _____ The data are easily used for analysis and reporting.
3. _____ It is easy to determine if these data are complete.
4. _____ These data usually reflect more of the clinician's thought processes.

Cons

5. _____ It usually takes more time to enter data using this method.
6. _____ It is more difficult to use this data for reporting or clinical decision support algorithms.
7. _____ This type of data entry tends to be very inflexible.
8. _____ It is difficult to determine the completeness of this data.

⊙ Data Management

Data are an asset to an organization similar to the personnel, buildings, or other resources. As such, data require attention and maintenance to ensure the data are capable of supporting organizational needs and goals. The management of data is as important to a healthcare organization as the management of its buildings, capital equipment, and information technology infrastructure.

Data Governance

Data governance is an emerging practice in the healthcare industry. Definitions for data governance are that it is "the exercise of decision-making and authority for data-related matters" (The Data Governance Institute 2013), or that it "is about establishing a culture where quality data is achieved, maintained, valued and used to drive the business" (Fisher 2009). Regardless of which definition one subscribes to, it is clear that any industry as reliant upon data as healthcare needs a plan for managing this asset.

Data Governance Process

As with most important healthcare processes, data governance is not a one-time effort, nor should it be "fast-tracked." It is important to take a considered approach, as the decisions made for data governance will have a long-term impact upon the organization. A suggested process follows:

1. Discover—Identify the databases or datasets or applications that store data; the relationships between the different datasets; the meaning of the data to the organization; and who has responsibility for the data. This step requires the business users to be involved.

2. Design—Consolidation and coordination of organizational data and the environment focusing on consistency of any governing rules; consistency of the organizational data model; and consistency of the business processes. This step requires the involvement of the business users.

3. Enable—This step takes a considerable amount of time and effort, as this is when the new data governance standards are applied to each data source, business process, and application. It is recommended that the standards be deployed to the entire network, rather than embedded in each source, process, or application. Although this includes business users much of the responsibility falls on IT staff.

4. Maintain—A robust monitoring and reporting system is required to ensure that the data remains fit-for-purpose for the organization. The monitoring requires involvement from both business users and IT. The monitoring should be as automated as possible, with reporting to the responsible parties who then have the authority to make changes resulting in optimal standards and processes. Any changes must be documented so the data can be thoroughly understood when it is used.

5. Archive or Retire—It is important to ensure that the data that are no longer needed are retired in a methodical, considered fashion. This may involve complying with the legal requirements for maintaining the data, as well as understanding the different uses of the data within the organization (Fisher 2009, 146–161).

Data governance and stewardship are relatively new aspects of data management in healthcare organizations. Although the processes can be difficult and time-consuming they are essential to any organization wishing to maximize the use of their valuable data assets.

Data Quality

Assessing and understanding the quality of healthcare data is an extremely important and often overlooked aspect of managing data and information in healthcare provider settings. Ensuring that the data and information are correct has implications for the quality of patient care, reimbursement, and research. In short, it is important for all of the reasons providers document in patient records to begin with. For example, something as simple as the wrong patient weight could result in an incorrect drug dosage calculation and medication administration error.

At least one study has been published supporting claims that using an EHR will result in more complete data than that found in a paper record (Tang et al. 1999). While this may be true, others have researched data quality in EHRs and found an average of 7.8 documentation entry errors per admission (Weir et al. 2003). Rather than get bogged down in the details of studies regarding data quality, this section will discuss various aspects of data quality and draw from more general computer information systems theory to suggest methods for assuring high-quality data and information for healthcare.

Characteristics of Data Quality

Data quality can seem an overwhelming topic. There are many ways for data to be of poor quality and, in fact, the quality of the data can sometimes resemble the quality of patient care—it can vary according to the consumer. "Data are of high quality if they are fit for their intended uses in operations, decision making, and planning. Data are fit for use if they are free of defects and possess desired features" (Redman 2001, 73). This emphasizes that the data consumer and the use of the data are essential to any determination of data quality. In 1998, the American Health Information Management Association (AHIMA) Data Quality Management Task Force developed a **Data Quality Management Model** (AHIMA 1998). The model is seen in figure 5.5 and covers the different processes of data handling during which data quality should be addressed. The data handling processes are

- Application—The purpose for which the data are collected
- Collection—The processes by which data elements are accumulated
- Warehousing—Processes and systems used to archive data and data journals
- Analysis—The process of translating data into information utilized for an application

Figure 5.5 Data quality management model

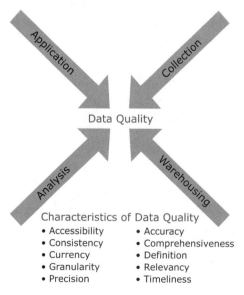

Characteristics of Data Quality
- Accessibility
- Consistency
- Currency
- Granularity
- Precision
- Accuracy
- Comprehensiveness
- Definition
- Relevancy
- Timeliness

Source: AHIMA 2012.

In addition, 10 **characteristics of data quality** were identified and defined. The definitions and examples are provided in table 5.2. The 1998 model was updated in 2012. Though the fundamentals remain the same, understanding of how they can most effectively be implemented in healthcare continue to evolve.

It is important to understand that these processes and characteristics do not exist in a vacuum. Just as everyone who has a driver's license has to meet certain

Table 5.2   AHIMA data quality characteristics, definitions, and examples

DATA QUALITY CHARACTERISTIC AND DEFINITION	HEALTHCARE EXAMPLE
Accuracy—The extent to which the data are free of identifiable errors.	The data element gender is completed for all patients and a random check of 500 records performed annually revealed only one demographic data element in conflict with the documentation.
Accessibility—Data items that are easily obtainable and legal to access with strong protections and controls built into the process.	All persons with access to the EHR have the ability to search the master patient index and the search function is designed such that the wrong patient is rarely accessed.
Comprehensiveness—All required data items are included; ensures that the entire scope of the data is collected with intentional limitations documented.	Providers may decide that recording external cause data is not useful. If so, their data dictionary for the diagnoses data elements would need to include this as an intentional limitation.
Consistency—The extent to which the healthcare data are reliable and the same across applications.	Within the EHR data such as allergies must be consistently displayed within different applications or screens to prevent confusion.
Currency—The extent to which data are up-to-date; a datum value is up-to-date if it is current for a specific point in time, and it is outdated if it was current at a preceding time but incorrect at a later time.	Patient age is generally current when the care is delivered. If age is not reentered the software needs to be have functionality to automatically update the age when appropriate.
Definition—The specific meaning of a healthcare-related data element.	Address as a data element label can mean the street address or it can mean the entire address to include city, state, and zip code.
Granularity—The level of detail at which the attributes and values of healthcare data are defined.	Adult weights are usually only recorded in pounds, possibly tenths of a pound. Newborn weights must be recorded in terms of ounces for accuracy.

(Continued)

Table 5.2 AHIMA data quality characteristics, definitions, and examples (*continued*)

DATA QUALITY CHARACTERISTIC AND DEFINITION	HEALTHCARE EXAMPLE
Precision—Data values should be strictly stated to support the purpose.	Diagnosis related group (DRG) values are carried out to four digits behind the decimal. It would be inaccurate to have the system only use two digits behind the decimal.
Relevance—The extent to which healthcare-related data are useful for the purposes for which they were collected.	Recording a primary diagnosis for hospital inpatients would be irrelevant because coding guidelines mandate collection of the principal diagnosis, which can be entirely different.
Timeliness—Concept of data quality that involves whether the data is up-to-date and available within a useful time frame; timeliness is determined by the manner and context in which the data are being used.	It would be inappropriate for blood pressure readings from ICU monitors to only be updated each hour.

Source: AHIMA, 2012

criteria, but not all drivers are not equally accomplished, all data that meet these criteria may still not be appropriate or adequate. This is why the process of assessing data quality is so significant. Failure to address the quality of the data may mean that the massive increase in data collected and available due to the increased use of computers in healthcare has only resulted in an increase in poor quality data and, hence, decision making.

The Data Quality Assessment and Management Process

The process of data quality assessment is similar to and, in some instances, uses the same methods as healthcare quality assessment and management. This section will outline generally accepted steps to quality assessment through the lens of quality management. It has been explicated using examples from the healthcare industry.

Who Are the Data Consumers?

Any health informaticist tasked with assessing or managing data quality must first understand who the data consumers are. This involves making a list of all of the internal and external data consumers. Likely internal data consumers for healthcare data managers include patients, clinicians, administrators, and researchers. External data consumers might include payers, public health agencies, and law enforcement agencies. Once a complete list has been compiled the consumer list must be prioritized. This is an essential step. It will be impossible for the data manager to meet all of the needs of all of the data consumers. However, by enumerating all of the data consumers, data managers will begin documenting the full depth and breadth of data use in their organization.

What Are the Needs of the Data Consumers?

This step in the process is usually very challenging. Most data consumers do not understand their needs well enough to articulate them effectively. So, what is the data manager to do? Rather than asking what the data consumer needs, the data manager should ask the consumer to describe how they use the data, the decisions that are made, the potential consequences of a wrong decision, and so on. As an example, consider the data use of clinical decision support. Even within this seemingly single data use task there are nuances. Allergic drug reactions as well as a preventive service reminders are each considered clinical decision support. However, allergic drug reactions are much more important because incorrect data could result in immediate, serious patient injury, even death. While preventive service reminders are certainly important, they rarely, if ever, rise to the level of immediate injury or death. The person working with the consumers to determine their needs must explore each data use thoroughly.

The data manager must take a controlled and careful approach to collecting data consumer needs. By now it should be obvious that the initial steps of implementing a data quality process will not be quick. However, the data manager should better understand the needs of the various consumers upon completion of the template or similar tool. In addition, the data manager will now have a complete list of data consumer needs to carry forward for consideration by senior management if necessary. It would be usual and expected for senior management to become involved in data consumer and data needs prioritization efforts. Table 5.3 is an example of a needs and requirements collection template that might be used.

Table 5.3   Data consumer needs assessment tool

CONSUMER:																					
CONSUMER NEEDS (Adapted from Redman 2001)						**PRODUCT FEATURE REQUIREMENTS**									**GAP ANALYSIS**							
Primary Needs	Secondary Needs	Tertiary Needs	Translated Needs	Source	Unit of Measure	Accuracy	Accessibility	Comprehensiveness	Consistency	Currency	Definition	Granularity	Precision	Relevancy	Timeliness	Accuracy	Accessibility	Comprehensiveness	Consistency	Currency	Definition

What Are the Required Features and Quality Characteristics?

After documenting the consumer needs, the functionality requirement associated with each quality characteristic needs to be identified. Building on the drug allergy reaction alert data use, each data quality characteristic will be examined in light of the functionality required. The following might be a partial list of the requirements:

⊙ Accuracy—The lists of drugs will need to utilize the current EHR data standard for pharmaceuticals. Allergies will need to be recorded as structured data or processed using an NLP algorithm after entry to be usable for drug allergy reaction processing.

⊙ Accessibility—The data entry methods for the allergies and drugs will be dependent upon the workflow of the organization and the abilities of the persons entering the data. This requires further study.

⊙ Comprehensiveness—Allergies are a required data element for the EHR. If the patient has no allergies the field should reflect "No allergies reported." If the clinician is not able to determine whether the patient has allergies the field should reflect "Unknown."

⊙ Consistency—Once recorded an allergy should become a permanent entry in the patient EHR, which is always incorporated into the information presented to the clinician.

Once the functionality requirements are identified across all of the characteristics, the data consumer should review them to ensure they meet consumer needs. Seeing the requirements specified in this fashion may result in the consumer identifying additional, important uses that will also need to be specified using these methods.

The end result of the requirements and quality characteristics specification involves a dual examination of both the stringency of the requirements and a prioritization of all requirements. The most stringent requirement may not be at the top of the prioritization list, but it is the highest level of functionality required.

How Well Do Our Current Information Products Meet the Needs and Requirements?

After identification of the most important needs and requirements, it is now time to determine how well any current information products perform. There are several steps for this process:

1. Ask the data consumers.

2. Measure the data where possible and appropriate.
   a. Select a business process or operation that uses the suspect data.
   b. Determine a desired sample size and selection method.
   c. Decide on the assessment criteria. In healthcare we would like to strive for 100 percent accuracy or correctness; however, there may be instances in nonclinical data where data are "seriously flawed" or "flawed but acceptable."
   d. Establish the estimated impact by asking the people who work with the end data. Does flawed data impact patient care? Does it impact

the ability to seek reimbursement? What are the impacts upon time, expenses, customer satisfaction, or other issues?

   e. Measure associated activities such as productivity and consumer satisfaction.

3. Include the results of the data measurement on the needs and requirements spreadsheet.

Where Are the Gaps and How Important Are They?

The data manager should now create a list of all of the gaps between the consumer needs and requirements and the current information products and performance identified in the previous steps. Once the gaps have been enumerated, the data manager can move forward with creating a priority list of areas or functionality needing attention. As always, this should not be done in a vacuum. The development of the list should be iterative, undergoing review by affected data consumers as well as senior management.

Check Your Understanding 5.4

Instructions: Match the terms with the appropriate descriptions.

   a. Accuracy
   b. Accessibility
   c. Comprehensiveness
   d. Consistency
   e. Currency
   f. Definition
   g. Granularity
   h. Precision
   i. Relevance
   j. Timeliness

1. _____ The data are at the appropriate level of detail for the uses of the data.

2. _____ Each data element must be defined with a clear meaning and allowable values.

3. _____ All data required for the specified purpose are included. Any intentional limitations are documented.

4. _____ The data must be meaningful for the purpose.

5. _____ Data values are appropriate for a given time frame and then become obsolete.

6. _____ The exactness of the data is related to purpose of the data.

7. _____ The data must be able to be accessed or used within a given time frame as determined by the purpose of the data.

8. _____ Data items should be easily obtainable, legal to collect, and protected as necessary.

9. _____ Data values are reliable across applications, time, or other parameters as needed.

10. _____ Data which are valid, that is, within the allowable values, and are the correct values, not in error.

Instructions: Indicate whether the following statements are true or false (T or F).

11. Data governance or stewardship is an optional function for data-rich healthcare organizations.

12. Business users of data can allow IT to be totally responsible for data governance activities.

13. Ongoing maintenance of the data governance processes is required to maximize use of the data asset.

⊙ Data Analysis

The increasing computerization of the healthcare industry has left many organizations awash in data. Effective data analysis plans, techniques, and processes are needed in order to turn the data into usable information.

Understanding the Data

The first, most essential step to analyzing any data is acquiring a thorough understanding of the data to be analyzed. This is best done by studying the **data dictionary**. The data dictionary is vital to understanding the data set. The data dictionary and minimum requirements are discussed in greater detail in Chapter 4.

The data dictionary may include information related to the originating source system, data owner, data entry date, and data termination date (AHIMA 2011a). In addition, the data dictionary should include any information regarding special processing utilized in the production of the data set. It is not uncommon for some data records to have missing values. Depending upon the type of analysis, the records with missing values may be eliminated or, using special statistical methods, the missing values may be provided using a process called **imputation**. Imputation methods must be described fully and imputed values clearly labeled.

One part of understanding the data that can easily be overlooked is an understanding of the data collection methods. Laboratory data that are loaded directly into a laboratory information system and then transferred to an EHR automatically are likely to be of better quality than data that were entered manually. This holds for all data. Each time the data are handled or touched by a human the opportunity or likelihood of error increases. However, this understanding of the data collection can also be more subtle. Consider the many claims databases that are used for research, quality measure development, and so on. While these are often the most easily accessed, they may not always be the best. Some hospitals code their inpatient records very completely, including all secondary diagnoses regardless of their impact upon reimbursement as well as all External Causes (E-codes) and Factors Influencing Health Status (V-codes). Other hospitals code only the Principal Diagnosis and the Secondary Diagnoses, which will impact the reimbursement. Often these different methods of data collection are made for very pragmatic reasons such as coder workforce shortages. However, a failure to understand these differences when using large data sets from multiple organizations could result in false conclusions being drawn regarding the causes of injuries or the presence or absence of certain health factors.

Cleaning the Data

The largest part of any data analysis project should begin with cleaning the data. **Data cleaning**, sometimes termed data scrubbing, involves examining the data thoroughly to detect wrong or inconsistent data. This is a necessary task even if the data are drawn from a data set that is managed with a data quality program. When data are subset or transferred between data applications, the opportunity exists for the introduction of data errors.

The first step in data cleaning is to load or label the data. This process may be largely automated or users may have to perform it themselves. Either way, the data analyst needs to validate the data elements in the data set against the data dictionary.

Once the data are loaded and labeled each data element needs to be examined. **Descriptive statistics**, also known as summary statistics, such as frequencies, mean, mode, range, and standard deviation, should be run for all continuous data elements. Table 5.4 is an example of descriptive statistical output for the continuous data element of age. Upon initial examination, the output seems fine,

Table 5.4   Descriptive statistics for a continuous variable

Age	
Mean	60.834375
Standard Error	3.851114233
Median	66.4
Mode	N/A
Standard Deviation	21.78519191
Sample Variance	474.5945867
Kurtosis	–1.25981969
Skewness	–0.38286422
Range	268
Minimum	23.3
Maximum	291.3
Sum	2146.7
Count	32

with a reasonable mean and median. However, continued examination of the output reveals a range of 268. Without looking at the minimum and maximum, the data analyst can tell that errors exist for this data element because 268 is not a valid entry for age. Either a negative age was entered for a patient or an incorrect, large entry was made for age. In this instance the minimum is 23.3, entirely reasonable, but the maximum is 291.3, not reasonable.

Correcting the continuous data element error first necessitates identifying the record(s) with the error. If available, it is always preferable to return to the source data to determine the correct value. If the source data are not available, the correct value may be imputed, as previously discussed, or the incorrect record may have to be eliminated from the analysis.

Categorical data require a different method of examination for data cleaning purposes. Frequencies should be run on all categorical data elements. Table 5.5 is an example of a **frequency** for a categorical data element. A frequency is the number of times that a particular observation or value occurs in a dataset. This type of output should prompt the data analyst to examine the data dictionary for the allowable values for this data element. Either the label for a valid entry was not captured correctly or there are a significant number of records with an invalid entry.

The relationships between the data elements may also prompt categorical data cleaning using **crosstabs**. Crosstabs serve to highlight any errors where there is an expected or explicit relationship between two data elements. Table 5.6 is an example of a crosstab analysis for two categorical data elements. The use of crosstabs for data cleaning is more ambiguous than the use of descriptive statistics or frequencies for single data elements. Often the data cleaning using crosstabs may not be done until the type of data analysis being attempted is known.

Correction of categorical data errors can be handled in a manner similar to continuous data errors. First the record with the error must be identified. However, unlike continuous errors where the only options are imputation or reviewing the

Table 5.5 Frequency exploration of categorical data

Discharge Disposition	Count	Percent	Cumulative Percent
Home	100	33.33%	
Nursing Home	50	16.67%	50.00%
Rehabilitation	50	16.67%	66.67%
Died	50	16.67%	83.34%
99	50	16.67%	100.00%
			(rounding)
TOTAL	300	100%	

Table 5.6   Crosstab of categorical data

Procedures by Gender	Male	Female	Total
Laparoscopy	200	350	550
Cardiac Catheterization	40	25	65
Arthroscopy	350	300	650
Hysterectomy	5	25	30
TOTAL	595	700	1295

source data, the correct categorical data can sometimes be deduced from other data element entries. For example, the records with the errors in table 5.6 could be examined to attempt to determine whether the procedure was incorrect or gender was incorrect. Other data that might provide a clue include preventative services such as a prostate exam or mammogram. The other options of imputation and reviewing the source data are also available.

If performing data analysis using an unknown or untested data set, data cleaning can sometimes take as much as 75 to 80 percent of the entire data analysis time. The most sophisticated analysis is useless if the data that went into it are not cleaned.

Analyzing the Data

The production of information and new knowledge is predicated on asking the right questions and knowing how to utilize a given data set. Specification of the question(s) is not necessarily as easy as might be expected, nor is use of a given data set to answer a question. The question or request can range from a specific report to an in-depth research study analysis. Whatever the question or request the first step is to ensure complete understanding (AHIMA 2011a). Suggested steps for data analysis specification include the following:

1. Determine the goals and objectives. Are you analyzing data at one point in time or trending it longitudinally or both? Is this a quality management or research study? The type of analysis planned will determine whether institutional review board (IRB) approval is needed.

2. What is the level of analysis for the study? Is it the organization, clinical specialty, patient? This will determine sampling methods and data elements needed for the analysis.

3. What are the limitations of the data? Some of these issues were discussed in the data cleaning section but bear repeating here since they can impact the conclusions drawn from the data.

4. What tools are available for the analysis? Is Microsoft Excel the only tool available or is statistical software such as SPSS, SAS, or Stata, or business intelligence software such as Cognos or Tableau available?

5. What are the analyses needed? Will data elements need to be calculated or derived? Will descriptive statistics, simple inferential statistical tests such as chi-square or correlation, or something more sophisticated such as Bayesian statistics or structural equation modeling be needed? Inferential statistics are those that help researchers draw conclusions regarding relationships between data elements.

6. How will the results be used? Is this a report for a journal manuscript or a presentation or some other presentation mode? (AHIMA 2011a).

Appendix A is a suggested outline for a Study Report and Request Form taken from the 2011 AHIMA Data Analysis Toolkit. Use of such a tool is highly recommended to ensure no important questions are overlooked.

Validating the Analysis

While the analysis is being conducted, and once it is believed to be complete, the analysis itself has to be validated. The types of examinations may include the following:

⊙ A review of any data elements added from the merging or matching of data sets that were not previously checked.

⊙ Data cleaning or review of any derived data elements that have not been checked previously.

⊙ Verification of the time frame of analysis used and any data elements that may have changed or are subject to change over time. An upgrade in EHR software may have resulted in acceptable value changes for certain fields at a given point in time. Diagnostic and procedural codes as well as payment mechanisms change according to a government schedule each year. Do the data cross the change dates?

⊙ Do the statistical results, descriptive or inferential, make sense? Do counts and percentages add up as they should? Can the results of the inferential analyses be interpreted or understood? Some of these answers may only be available from a statistician (AHIMA 2011a).

The overriding message from this section is to never "trust" the data analysis. It is always possible that the wrong data element was selected or that the wrong test was selected or some other seemingly simple error occurred.

Check Your Understanding 5.5

Instructions: Choose the best answer.

1. A data dictionary consists of
   a. The names, definitions, and attributes of data elements
   b. Synonyms for specific data variables
   c. All possible data elements in the healthcare industry
   d. Hints for using data elements

2. Once any records with data errors are identified the data analyst should
   a. Delete the records with the errors
   b. Perform imputation to determine the correct values
   c. Determine whether the source records are available in order to validate the data
   d. Attempt correcting the data from the other data in the record

Indicate whether each task is related to analysis (A) or validation (V).

3. _____ Counts and percentages are checked.

4. _____ The limitations of the data are known and accounted for.

5. _____ Derived data elements are examined thoroughly.

6. _____ The goals and objectives are explained and understood.

⊙ Data Presentation

Presenting the results of a data analysis effectively can be a challenge. The data output from an analysis may or may not be clear and easy to understand. Numbers are factual data. However, when displayed incorrectly, they can be deceiving. Incomplete or misrepresented data may leave the reader with unanswered questions (AHIMA 2011a). Whether presented with words, in tabular form, or in a graph or picture it is imperative the presentation be clear.

Tables

A table is an organized arrangement of data, usually in columns and rows. Many different types of quantitative data can be displayed in tables. For examples of tables see tables 5.1 through 5.6. Tables should be used with care because the inclusion of too much data in a table can increase rather than decrease confusion.

If the decision is made to use a table it is helpful to keep the following guidelines in mind:

⊙ The table should be a logical unit that is self-explanatory and stands on its own.

⊙ The source of the data in the table should be specified.

⊙ Headings for rows and columns should be understandable.

⊙ Blank cells should contain a zero or a dash.

⊙ Formatting for headings and cell contents should be consistent so that the eye is not confused (LaTour et al. 2013, 508).

In some instances, a table can be the basis for a chart or graph to display the data.

Charts and Graphs

One of the benefits of a highly computerized world is that it is now relatively easy to generate charts and graphs for data analysis results. Charts and graphs can be very useful for emphasizing important points and conveying information about a topic. Guiding principles for the creation of charts and graphs include

- Distortion—The representation of numbers or percentages should be proportional to the quantities represented.
- Proportion and scale—Graphs should emphasize the horizontal and be greater in length than height. A general rule is that the y-axis (height) be three-quarters the x-axis (length) of the graph.
- Abbreviations—Any abbreviations used should be spelled out for clarity.
- Color—Color should be used as appropriate to the use of the graph. If the chart is going to be printed will it be printed in black and white or color?
- Text—The font and use of capitalization needs to be considered carefully. The use of all capital letters can sometimes be difficult to read (LaTour et al. 2013, 510).

Ideal graphs will

- Show the data
- Induce the viewer to think about the substance rather than the methodology, graphic design, technology, or other things
- Avoid distorting what the data have to say
- Present many numbers in a small space
- Make large data sets coherent
- Encourage the eye to compare different pieces of data
- Reveal the data at several levels of detail
- Serve a reasonably clear purpose
- Closely integrated with the statistical and verbal descriptions of the data set (Tufte 2001)

There are many resources available to assist in determining the best type of graph or chart for data display including books, AHIMA Data Analysis Toolkit, YouTube videos, and tutorials from software makers.

Check Your Understanding 5.6

Instructions: Match the data display tool with its description.

    a. A horizontal or vertical arrangement of rectangular shapes that represents data from one or more groups or categories

    b. An orderly arrangement of values that displays data in rows and columns

    c. An arrangement of pieces in a circular shape that represents the component parts of a single group or variable

    d. One or more series of points connected by a line or lines to represent trends over time

1. ___ Table
2. ___ Bar chart
3. ___ Pie chart
4. ___ Line graph

⊙ Summary

Data and information have been key to the development of healthcare throughout the ages. The ability to communicate healthcare data and information efficiently and effectively is crucial for the global healthcare industry. The uses of data and information are only expected to grow and accelerate in the future. Without the widespread use of standards, semantic interoperability will be impossible to achieve. Data are an asset to an organization similar to the personnel, buildings, or other resources. As such, they require management, attention, and maintenance to ensure they are capable of supporting organizational needs and goals. However, the misuse of data and information can retard industry growth, injure patients, and imperil organizations.

Data analysis and reporting is incredibly detailed work that must be performed with great care. This field is expected to grow exponentially in the future as healthcare organizations seek to utilize their EHR and other data assets effectively and efficiently. The most important concept to keep in mind when considering the presentation of any data is that the user of the data presentation must be able to understand it with as little effort as possible. Presentations that require a great deal of time or analysis by the user are less likely to be effective or communicate the information intended. Health informaticists must make every effort to use and help others to use data and information effectively.

REFERENCES

AHIMA. 2011a. Health Data Analysis Toolkit. Chicago: AHIMA. http://library.ahima .org/xpedio/groups/public/documents/ahima/bok1_048618.pdf.

AHIMA. 2011b. Data mapping best practices. *Journal of AHIMA* 82(4):46–52.

AHIMA. 2012. *Pocket Glossary for Health Information Management and Technology*. 3rd ed. Chicago: AHIMA.

AHIMA Data Quality Management Task Force. 2012. Data Quality Management Model.

Ash, J.S., D.F. Sittig, E.M. Campbell, K.P. Guappone, and R.H. Dykstra. 2007. Some unintended consequences of clinical decision support systems. *Journal of the American Medical Informatics Association.* 14(4):415–423.

ASTM Standard. 2005. E2369 – 05e1 Standard Specification for Continuity of Care Record (CCR). American Society Testing and Materials. http://www.astm.org/ Standards/E2369.htm.

CCHIT. 2011. About Certification Commission for Health Information Technology. http://www.cchit.org/about.

Cimino, J. J. 1998. Desiderata for controlled medical vocabularies in the twenty-first century. *Methods of Information in Medicine* 37(4-5):394–403.

Department of Health and Human Services. 1996. Health Insurance Portability and Accountability Act. *Code of Federal Regulations.* http://edocket.access.gpo.gov/cfr_2007/octqtr/pdf/45cfr162.103.pdf.

Department of Health and Human Services. 2010. Health Information Technology: Initial Set of Standards, Implementation Specification and Certification Criteria for Electronic Health Record Technology. *Code of Federal Regulations.* Vol. 111-5. August 27. http://edocket.access.gpo.gov/2010/pdf/2010-17210.pdf.

Department of Health and Human Services. 2011. HealthIT.hhs.gov: ONC-Authorized Testing and Certification Bodies. *ONC-Authorized Testing and Certification Bodies.* http://healthit.hhs.gov/portal/server.pt?open=512&mode=2&objID=3120.

Department of Health and Human Services. Health IT Standards Committee. healthit.hhs.gov. http://healthit.hhs.gov/portal/server.pt/community/healthit_hhs_gov__health_it_standards_committee/1271.

Fenton, S.H. 2006. Structured or unstructured? Options for clinician data entry in the EHR." *Journal of AHIMA* 77(3):52.

Fisher, T. 2009. *The Data Asset.* Hoboken: Wiley.

Graunt, J. 1665.*Reflections on the Weekly [sic] Bills of Mortality for the Cities of London and Westminster, and the Places Adjacent but More Especially, So far as They Relate to the Plague and Other Mortal Diseasesthat We English-Men Are Most Subject Unto: With an Exact Account of the Greatest Plagues That Have Happened Since the Creation.* London: Printed for Samuel Speed.

Hammond, W., and J. Cimino, eds. 2001. "Standards in medical informatics." In *Medical Informatics Computer Applications in Health Care and Biomedicine,* 212–256. New York: Springer-Verlag.

Health Level Seven International. 2013. HL7 Governance and Operations Manual. HL7, January 7. http://www.hl7.org/documentcenter/public_temp_F525E34A-1C23-BA17-0C7C0AA8A8F7ABCD/membership/HL7_Governance_and_Operations_Manual.pdf.

International Organization for Standardization. 2013. ISO—Standards development processes—Stages of development of International Standards. http://www.iso.org/iso/standards_development/processes_and_procedures/stages_description.htm.

Johnson, S.B., S. Bakken, D. Dine, S. Hyun, E. Mendonça, F. Morrison, T. Bright, T. Van Vleck, J. Wrenn, and P. Stetson. 2008. An electronic health record based on structured narrative. *Journal of the American Medical Informatics Association* 15(1):54–64. doi:10.1197/jamia.M2131.

LaTour, K.M., S. Eichenwald-Maki, and P. Oachs. 2013. *Health Information Management: Concepts, Principles, and Practice,* 4th ed. Chicago, IL: AHIMA.

Rosenbloom, S.T., J.C. Denny, H. Xu, N. Lorenzi, W.W. Stead, and K.B. Johnson. 2011. Data from clinical notes: A perspective on the tension between structure and flexible documentation. *Journal of the American Medical Informatics Association* 18(2):181–186. doi:10.1136/jamia.2010.007237.

Tang, P.C., M.P. LaRosa, and S.M. Gorden. 1999. Use of computer-based records, completeness of documentation, and appropriateness of documented clinical decisions. *Journal of the American Medical Informatics Association* 6(3):245–251.

Texas Department of State Health Services. 2010. ImmTrac Electronic Data Reporting. http://www.dshs.state.tx.us/immunize/immtrac/data_reporting.shtm.

The Data Governance Institute. The Data Governance Institute Data Governance Framework. http://www.datagovernance.com/dgi_framework.pdf.

Tufte, E. 2001. *The Visual Display of Quantitative Information.* 2nd ed. Cheshire, CT: Graphics Press.

United States Congress. 2009. Health Information Technology for Economic and Clinical Health (HITECH) Act. *Code of Federal Regulations.* http://edocket.access.gpo.gov/2010/pdf/2010-17210.pdf.

United States Government. 1996. Health Insurance Portability and Accountability Act of 1996. *United States Code.* http://www.gpo.gov/fdsys/pkg/PLAW-104publ191/pdf/PLAW-104publ191.pdf.

United States Government. 2009. American Recovery and Reinvestment Act of 2009. http://frwebgate.access.gpo.gov/cgi-bin/getdoc.cgi?dbname=111_cong_bills&docid=f:h1enr.pdf.

US Census Bureau. 2003. Revisions to the Standards for the Classification of Federal Data on Race and Ethnicity. *Race Data.* January. http://www.census.gov/population/www/socdemo/race/Ombdir15.html.

van Mulligen, E. M., H. Stam, and A. M. van Ginneken. 1998. Clinical data entry. *Proceedings / AMIA ... Annual Symposium. AMIA Symposium:* 81–85.

Wager, K.A., F.W. Lee, and J.P. Glaser. 2009. *Health Care Information Systems.* 2nd ed. San Francisco: Wiley.

Weir, C.R., J.F. Hurdle, M.A. Felgar, J.M. Hoffman, B. Roth, and J.R. Nebeker. 2003. "Direct text entry in electronic progress notes. An evaluation of input errors." *Methods of Information in Medicine* 42(1):61–67. doi:10.1267/METH03010061.

World Health Organization. 2011. History of the Development of the ICD. WHO. http://www.who.int/classifications/icd/en/HistoryOfICD.pdf.

Zeisset, A. 2010. "International Classification of Diseases (ICD) and the U.S. Modifications." In *Healthcare Code Sets, Clinical Terminologies, and Classification Systems,* 2nd ed. edited by K. Giannangelo. Chicago, IL: AHIMA.

6

Implementing Healthcare Information Systems

By Kim Murphy-Abdouch and Susan H. Fenton

Learning Objectives

- Understand the need for and roles of leadership related to healthcare information systems implementation
- Create a strategic plan for healthcare systems implementation
- Describe the Systems Development Life Cycle related to EHR implementation
- List and describe the steps in an EHR implementation
- Explain the issues associated with the hybrid EHR
- Discuss the impact of usability on EHR utility

KEY TERMS

Accountable Care Organization (ACO)
American Recovery and Reinvestment Act (ARRA)
Application service provider (ASP)
Chief information officer
Computers-on-wheels (COWs)
Functionality
Health Information Technology for Economic and Clinical Health (HITECH)
Hybrid
International Organization for Standards (ISO)

Legacy data
Meaningful use
ONC-Authorized Testing and Certification Bodies (ATCBs)
Physician champion
Practicality
Reputation
Request for information (RFI)
Request for proposals (RFP)
Stakeholders
Usability

⊙ Introduction

The successful implementation of healthcare information systems (HISs) is becoming integral to the success of healthcare organizations of all types and sizes. HISs are extremely complex, support all aspects of healthcare delivery and are very susceptible to error when implemented poorly or utilized by untrained users. This chapter discusses the many aspects of HIS implementation, focusing on the extremely important human elements. Ultimately, it is vital to remember the purpose of the HIS or electronic health record (EHR) is "to handle the medical information necessary for patient care and improve the efficiency and accessibility of that information" (Corrao et al. 2010).

⊙ Leadership, Roles, and Strategic Planning

Key to successful implementation of an EHR is strong leadership from a variety of roles at different levels in the organization, as well as ensuring the HIS is aligned with the strategic goals of the organization. Lack of leadership from the top of the organization or from key roles in the organization could result in inadequate resources for or other fatal flaws in the implementation. Alignment with the organizational strategic plan is required to ensure system **stakeholders** (persons, roles, or organizational units with a vested interest) can use the EHR to accomplish their goals.

Leadership

Top leadership in healthcare organizations can vary from a single, primary owner in a solo practice to a large board of trustees in a nonprofit healthcare organization to a board of directors in for-profit corporations to state and federal officials of government-run healthcare organizations. Top leadership implements the strategic direction of the healthcare organization through five primary activities:

- ⊙ Select and work with the chief executive officer (CEO)
- ⊙ Establish the organization's mission, vision, and values
- ⊙ Approve strategies and budget to implement the mission
- ⊙ Maintain quality of care
- ⊙ Monitor results for compliance with the goals, laws, and regulations (Griffith and White 2010)

The extent of these activities or the ways in which they are manifested differs by organizational setting and size; however, the overall role of top leadership related to EHR implementation is to establish the strategic goals for the organization, identify initiatives that will be enabled by or benefit from an EHR, and provide resources to achieve those goals.

The governing body delegates responsibility for the daily operations of the healthcare organization to the senior management team through the CEO. Senior management support from the "C-suite," the chief financial officer (CFO), **chief**

information officer (CIO), chief nursing officer (CNO), chief medical officer (CMO), and chief medical information officer (CMIO) is also essential to the success of EHR initiatives.

A recent study of EHR implementation in an academic ambulatory setting identified six themes for EHR implementation best practices:

1. Effective communication
2. Successful system migration
3. Technical equipment, support, and training
4. Safeguards for patient privacy
5. A focus on improved efficiency
6. A sustainable business plan (Yoon-Flannery et al. 2008)

Effective communication must occur at and between all levels of the organization from top leadership all the way to the front lines as well as with the persons working behind the scenes. Communication can take many forms these days including meetings, newsletters, and even social media. Successful system migration might lead one to believe that an EHR must already be in place; however, a migration must occur even if the facility is almost entirely paper based or has implemented parts of an EHR previously. Technical equipment, support, and training encompasses not only computer servers, routers, wireless access points, and other infrastructure but also includes IT personnel such as network and database administrators, clinical "super-users" for algorithm construction and maintenance, as well as EHR trainers for both go-live, ongoing, and new employee training. Safeguards for patient privacy are paramount. No patient wants their identifiable data released and no healthcare provider wants to have to contact patients to let them know their data has been compromised. Support for the EHR should include business analysts to ensure the EHR is used with maximum effectiveness. This is one of the implementation themes because an EHR that impairs efficiency or results in lower patient care quality will result in extreme user frustration. Finally, each organization must approach the implementation of an EHR with a clear plan for the long-term financial viability and sustainability of the system and the organization. All of these elements must be considered in strategic planning for the EHR or an HIS.

In organizational strategic planning, the top leadership sets the organization's direction, defines key relationships with all stakeholders and positions the organization through its missions, values, services, and partnerships. To develop the strategic plan, top leadership engages senior management and key stakeholders to identify, prioritize, and implement strategic opportunities to achieve the long-term vision of the organization. Many strategic opportunities in healthcare are likely to require the implementation or enhancement of an EHR to achieve the organization's goals.

In high performing healthcare organizations, there is high employee satisfaction, strong earnings, and high quality of care (Griffith and White 2010). The EHR facilitates excellent care, but it is not essential, and high performing healthcare organizations have built a culture and operational infrastructure of excellence first, and moved later to automate the supporting patient record (Griffith and White 2010). This serves to support the contention that successful implementation of an EHR is more dependent upon the people and other factors than the latest and greatest technology.

Implementation of an EHR is a journey toward goals that are aided by technology. The organization must establish its goals and determine whether the path toward those goals can be assisted with the implementation of an EHR. Most healthcare organizations have some EHR components already in place. It is important to maintain the perspective that an EHR is one of many organizational assets that can be used to enable the healthcare organization's mission and services. Other factors such as knowledge of the regulatory environment and healthcare financing initiatives may also facilitate identification and achievement of strategic goals.

For example, one organizational goal may be to participate in the Medicare **Accountable Care Organization (ACO)** program. An ACO is an organization of healthcare providers accountable for the quality, cost, and overall care of Medicare beneficiaries who are assigned and enrolled in the traditional fee-for-service program (AHIMA 2012, 9). The goal is to achieve higher quality at lower costs with Medicare paying incentives to ACOs that meet quality measures and achieve cost savings. ACOs will require accurate, timely, and well-coordinated health records and effective information flow in order to achieve the quality and cost savings goals. It is possible to achieve the requisite information flow with paper records, but coordinating information across multiple providers and healthcare organizations will be greatly facilitated with an EHR. Consider the example of ordering a laboratory test for a patient in the ACO. To check with all other providers and organizations in the ACO to be sure that the test has not recently been completed would be very labor intensive without an EHR; multiple sites would have to be contacted by telephone, fax, or e-mail and there could be delays as the information was retrieved from the paper records. With an EHR, immediate access to lab results would be available to the provider at the time they determined that they needed the information in order to diagnose or treat the patient in a timely manner. In this example, it is not likely that the provider would delay ordering the test while all other providers in the ACO were contacted, and lack of timely access to an EHR would result in duplicate testing.

Another goal for a healthcare organization may be to become the community leader in quality measures. Collecting and reporting quality measures is facilitated by timely access to accurate and complete patient information so they can be reported to the Centers for Medicare and Medicaid Services (CMS), the Joint Commission, and other quality monitoring organizations. It is possible to report quality measures without an EHR, but electronic capture, analysis, and reporting will facilitate the timeliness and accuracy of the data.

Historically, the business case for the acquisition of an EHR has not been as straightforward as compared to business planning for other types of technology. Benefits of a full-fledged EHR often accrue to the payers, rather than the entities that invest in the technology. For example, the physician office must pay for the EHR and associated technology. However, if the patient requires fewer visits then the physician will ultimately lose money; however, the payer will enjoy higher profits. Additionally, some of the benefits of health IT such as provider convenience, patient satisfaction, and improved communication are not easily captured on the bottom line (Garrido et al. 2004). Strategic planning for health IT must consider both financial and nonfinancial benefits.

Recent federal initiatives are changing the business case. The Office of the National Coordinator for Health Information Technology (ONC) Federal Health Information Technology Strategic Plan for 2011 through 2015 noted that the lack of capital for small- and medium-sized providers has slowed acceptance of EHRs and widespread health information exchange (HIE). The ONC also noted that there was a lack of skilled health IT professionals to support providers as they transition from paper records to EHRs (ONC, DHHS 2011). These barriers are being addressed through the **Health Information Technology for Economic and Clinical Health (HITECH)** section of the **American Recovery and Reinvestment Act (ARRA)**, which provides funding for incentives, education, and training (US Congress 2009).

The ARRA-funded EHR incentive program has provided additional weight to the business cases for implementing a fully functioning EHR. In 2011, healthcare organizations and providers became eligible for incentive funding for implementing and using EHRs meaningfully and will begin to incur penalties for not doing so by 2016 (US Congress 2009). In general, the incentive funds will not fully cover the cost of implementing the EHR, but the additional funding opportunity needs to be considered in the EHR planning business case (Dimick 2011).

Overall, it is expected that most healthcare organizations and providers will seek to shift from paper-based patient records to EHRs. The paper records are often incomplete, illegible, and unavailable when and where they are needed. Within EHRs, the patient clinical information is integrated, complete, and stored electronically, so that it can be available to the patient and other authorized persons, anywhere, anytime. How this is achieved will vary greatly from organization to organization, but common roles in strategic planning can be identified and should be considered to help prepare the organization for this shift.

Strategic Planning Roles

The requirements for EHR strategic planning will vary by the size and type of healthcare organization. Planning for the small physician practice may be accomplished in a less formal manner than the methods required for a large healthcare facility or system. In any setting, it is imperative for top leadership to support the implementation of the EHR and for all key stakeholders to be involved in the planning process. Table 6.1 identifies leadership and stakeholder roles in the inpatient environment and in the small physician practice. This table may be used as a starting point to identify the leadership and stakeholders across the full spectrum of sizes and types of healthcare organizations.

Table 6.1   Strategic planning roles

Role	Inpatient Environment	Physician Practice
Leadership	Governing body (Board) Senior administrative leadership Senior clinical leadership	Physician
Internal stakeholders	Medical Staff Nursing Laboratory Radiology Pharmacy Respiratory Case management Other clinical departments Finance Information systems Health information management Patient access Patient financial services	Physicians Physician extenders Nursing Medical assistants Other caregivers Administrative support staff Scheduling Insurance verification Coding Billing
External stakeholders	Patients Payers Licensing and accrediting organizations Health information exchanges	Patients Payers Licensing and accrediting organizations Health information exchanges

Internal Stakeholders

The support of internal stakeholders, which includes clinicians—physicians, nurses, pharmacists, therapists, and others who use clinical information to care for patients, is critical to successfully implementing the EHR. They must be involved in the entire process in order to ensure the needs of the users are fully addressed, the most appropriate system is selected, and the implementation is successful.

Three levels of communication within and among internal stakeholders have been noted to be important to successful EHR implementation: between executive leadership and internal stakeholders, stakeholder to stakeholder, and among the executive leadership, stakeholders, and vendors (Yoon-Flannery et al. 2008). The importance of this communication and active listening between all parties cannot be overstated. There have been a number of unsuccessful implementations of computerized provider order entry (CPOE) reported that have been attributed in great part to communication issues. These include an implementation that was undertaken with the involvement of internal stakeholders, but when it was made mandatory to use CPOE, the physicians voted almost unanimously to suspend the CPOE system (Bass 2003), as well as the implementation of a hospital-wide EHR where leadership apparently did not involve internal stakeholders to the detriment of the implementation (Han et al. 2005). The CIO where CPOE had been mandated stated "you cannot communicate enough with physicians" (Bass 2003). While it is important to involve physicians due to their responsible role in patient care, it is also important to remember that all internal stakeholders perform vital functions and all types of stakeholders need to be involved in any EHR implementation.

External Stakeholders

External healthcare organization stakeholders include actual and potential patients, payers, HIE, as well as licensing and regulatory organizations. Involving patients is especially important if the healthcare organization is considering a patient portal to facilitate patient access to their personal health information within the healthcare organization's EHR. However, other external stakeholders should also be considered. For example, payers may begin requiring quality measures or other data from providers, while regulatory organizations can require specific technological standards. For example, specific standards must be used for effective HIE or for submitting Joint Commission core measures. Healthcare organizations must also ensure that systems selected will be able to effectively exchange information with all necessary external stakeholders such as other treatment providers or pharmacies.

Check Your Understanding 6.1

Instructions: Indicate whether the following statements are true or false (T or F).

1. The purpose of the EHR is to handle the medical information necessary for patient care and improve the efficiency and accessibility of the information.

2. Successful implementation of an EHR is more dependent upon the human factors than the most recent and advanced technology.

3. Input from internal stakeholders is not essential for a successful EHR implementation.

4. Top leadership for a healthcare organization implementing an EHR always includes a board of directors.

Instructions: Choose the best answer.

5. The leadership of a healthcare organization is responsible for all but which of the following primary activities:
   a. Establish the organization's mission, vision, and values
   b. Approve the strategies and budget to implement the mission
   c. Select the organization's EHR vendor
   d. Maintain quality of care

⊙ Systems Development Life Cycle

It can be very helpful to have a framework for considering the processes and stakeholders in the development and implementation of health IT. The systems development life cycle (SDLC) includes four primary phases: planning and analysis, design, implementation, and maintenance and evaluation (LaTour et al. 2013, 105). The framework is depicted in figure 6.1. It can be used as the framework for a wide range of initiatives, from small health IT projects to the transition to a complete EHR. Within a full-blown EHR implementation, many different SDLC processes may be occurring at the same time at various levels of the implementation. The entire SDLC process begins with the identification of a need and ends when the benefits of system no longer outweigh costs, at which point the life cycle would begin again.

Planning and Analysis

Implementing an EHR represents a significant investment in time and money for healthcare providers and organizations of all sizes and types. Selecting the right product requires an investment in advanced planning to guide the selection process. Once a strategic decision is made to explore the use of technology to solve a business need, the planning and analysis phase of the SDLC is initiated. It is in this phase of life cycle development that the organization first defines the goals and scope of the project, taking into account the unique needs and characteristics of the organization including the size, complexity, and scope of services provided. The focus in this phase is on defining the organization's business problem and the resources that may be needed to develop the project. The resources to be defined in this phase include people, time, and funds. The specific technology is not included here. It will be addressed in a later phase.

Figure 6.1 Systems development life cycle

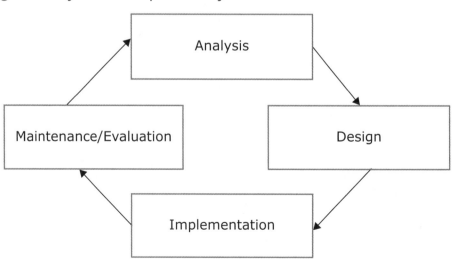

An in-depth assessment of the needs of the user and their functional requirements must be accomplished in this planning and analysis phase. The assessment should include widespread participation from all end-users of the technology to ensure that the key stakeholder's needs and gaps in present technology and processes are clearly defined. The current system(s) and the user's response to the system should be analyzed to identify opportunities for improvement.

Areas to be addressed in the assessment include

- Identification of the technology currently being used and how it is used
- Analysis of current work and data flow processes
- Efficiency assessment of current technology and workflow
- User proficiency in using the current technology
- Timeliness and availability of data and information
- User satisfaction with the current system and processes
- Patient satisfaction, if applicable
- How the use of technology is expected to
  - Increase efficiency
  - Enhance quality
  - Meet other goals of the users

It is possible that the planning and analysis phase may reveal that the business problem is actually caused by issues with the workflow, processes, procedures, or training, and that new technology may not be required or that the technology being used is obsolete. If a business need for a technology solution is identified, the planning and analysis phase is also the time to carefully consider whether it is technologically, financially, and operationally feasible to undertake the implementation of new technology to solve the business need.

The planning and analysis phase creates the blueprint for the project. This phase must take into account the unique characteristics of the organization to ensure that there is a strong foundation upon which to build the system and that the system is aligned with the healthcare organization's strategic goals.

Design

Once a determination is made that new systems or technologies are required, the design phase begins. In this phase, a project manager should be designated and a project steering committee of key stakeholders established to oversee and manage the project. The role of the steering committee is to plan, organize, coordinate, and manage the design and acquisition of the new technology. The role of the project manager is to lead the steering committee and keep the project on track.

The steering committee should be comprised of key stakeholders, including physicians, nurses, and other clinical disciplines and administrative personnel who will use the system. It is important that all groups who have an interest in the system be represented on the steering committee, including individuals who have expertise in information technology. Organizations that lack internal expertise in information management may choose to contract with an IT consultant to join the steering committee and assist throughout the life cycle of the project.

Define the System Goals

The goal of a systems implementation is very important to the ultimate design. Each organization will have goals aligned with its vision and mission. At the same time, goals can originate from external sources too. ONC is "charged with coordination of nationwide efforts to implement and use the most advanced health information technology and the electronic exchange of health information" (ONC, DHHS 2012a,b). To support these implementation and exchange efforts, CMS administers the EHR Incentive Program, which provides "incentive payments to eligible professionals, eligible hospitals and critical access hospitals (CAHs) as they adopt, implement, upgrade, or demonstrate meaningful use of certified EHR technology" (CMS 2012). Working together these two agencies promulgate a variety of regulations and guidelines, including EHR certification criteria and clinical quality measures for providers. The steering committee should consider these regulations and guidelines in defining the system goals. The goals should be clearly identified and measurably defined.

Examples of goal statements include

- Facilitate the exchange of information throughout the integrated delivery system by establishing a single EHR for the enterprise.
- Enable the physicians in a large multispecialty clinic to create and exchange information electronically from multiple locations, including the hospital, clinic offices, and at home using a wide variety of devices including smart phones and tablets.

These goal statements should be aligned with the strategic goals of the organization and should serve as measures of performance throughout the SDLC.

Define Project Objectives and Scope

The project objectives and scope should be clearly defined. Projects may range from a limited scope, such as managing an upgrade to an existing application, to the much larger project of leading a complete assessment of the organization's information management needs and implementation of an enterprise-wide EHR.

Determine and Prioritize the System Requirements

Once the goals have been developed and evaluated against the organization's strategic goals, the specific requirements should be identified and prioritized. As an example, the goal to enable the physicians to create and exchange information electronically from multiple locations will require specifically defining the information they need as well as the methods the will use to create and exchange information.

The foundation of requirements needs to begin with any defined regulatory requirements. Any additional requirements can be determined by interviewing individual users and by establishing focus groups. In many cases, the users are unable to clearly identify their specific requirements, so vendor demonstrations or exploratory site visits to similar organizations may be necessary to develop their system requirements. Defining and prioritizing the functional and technical requirements requires the clear identification of the current state workflow analysis and development of the future state workflow. The Agency for Healthcare Research and Quality (AHRQ) has a *Workflow Assessment for Health IT Toolkit* that includes educational presentations, research compilations, tools, and examples of how to use the tools available via the Internet (AHRQ 2012). Utilizing a framework such as the AHRQ tool can be very helpful for many organizations. This part of the process is of vital importance. Failure to assess workflow and requirements adequately can result in the purchase of software that will not meet user needs.

Screen the Marketplace for Potential Vendors

Once the project objectives and scope are defined, research should be conducted to identify potential vendors. The definitive resource for identifying an EHR solution or multiple solutions is the ONC Certified Health IT product list (ONC 2013). The ONC issues EHR certification criteria to ensure compliance with the CMS EHR Incentive Program, also known as **meaningful use** (MU).

To ensure EHR software is certified appropriately, the ONC has designated **ONC-Authorized Testing and Certification Bodies (ATCBs)**. ATCBs are empowered to perform complete EHR or EHR module testing and certification. ATCBs utilize conformance testing requirements, test cases, and test tools developed by the National Institute for Standards and Technology (NIST) to determine whether the software complies with the EHR Incentive Program requirements for establishing MU of an EHR (ONC, DHHS 2012a,b).

Other sources of information may include trade shows and conferences operated by groups such as the American Health Information Management Association (AHIMA), Health Information Management Systems Society (HIMSS), and the American Medical Informatics Association (AMIA). There is also an abundance of EHR vendor information available on the Internet. Vendor information may also be obtained by contacting similar healthcare facilities to determine the technology they utilize.

There are usually two types of EHR software to consider: best-fit and best-of-breed. Best-fit refers to a single EHR product that provides a comprehensive integrated solution. For example, a physician practice may wish to select the best fit from among EHR vendors that offer a practice management system and clinical documentation as one system. Best-of-breed refers to products selected from a variety of vendors. Best-of-breed allows the user to find products that most closely meet their needs and preferences. However, best-of-breed products may not be interoperable with other software. Best-of-breed results in acquisition of separate software solutions for various operational and administrative functions.

Develop and Distribute the RFI or RFP

Once the requirements have been defined and documented, the organization should determine if they wish to initiate a **request for information (RFI)** or a **request for proposals (RFP)**. The RFI is used to ask vendors for information about their products and services. It is often used to obtain information from a large number of vendors to narrow the field of vendors to whom a RFP will be issued. The RFP is a more formal request to vendors to provide specific information about how they can meet the organization's specific requirements. In the RFP, the organization should describe the goals and priorities for the IT acquisition including technical and functional requirements.

A proposal committee of key stakeholders may be established at this point to assist in the RFP process. Similar to the project steering committee, the proposal committee should have broad representation of internal stakeholders, including all departments that will use or be affected by the EHR system. Representatives may include a **physician champion**, clinical departments (nursing, laboratory, radiology, and such), pharmacy, health information management, information technology, compliance, privacy and security, legal, finance, and purchasing. The physician champion is a physician tasked with the responsibility of representing the views of the physician users. AHIMA has published an RFI/RFP Template, which provides guidance for organizations. A sample from the template can be seen in table 6.2, while the entire RFI/RFP Practice Brief and Template are found in Appendices B and C of this book.

A vendor's response to an RFP will generally include a summary of all costs related to the project: hardware and software acquisition, technical support, consulting, staff training, and implementation services. The detail in the RFP allows for comparison across vendors on the proposed solutions. The RFP may also serve as the basis for the final contract, which is the legal agreement between the vendor and the organization.

Evaluate Vendor Options

Once the responses to the RFP are received, a side-by-side comparison or the proposals should be conducted. A matrix to compare the various vendor's proposals may be useful in facilitating the evaluation of the options. Table 6.3 provides an example of how an evaluation matrix might be used to compare different vendors across the required functionality. In evaluating options, it should be determined how the software will be delivered, whether in an **application service provider (ASP)** model whereby application services are accessed via the Internet or as an onsite application.

Hold Vendor Demonstrations

Based upon the results of the RFP comparison matrix, organizations will generally select three to five vendors to provide demonstrations of their technology. It is suggested the demonstrations should be on a live system with a number of internal stakeholders present to explore if and how the technology can meet the end-user's needs. Users should have the opportunity to ask for demonstrations of specific tasks and processes that will be used after the software is implemented. A selected, diverse sample of stakeholders should have a hands-on experience with the product during the demonstration.

Table 6.2 Sample of AHIMA RFI/RFP Template (partial for illustration only)

Functional User Requirements/Features	Available	Custom Developed	Future Development	Not Available
Authentication				
Does the system authenticate principals (i.e, users, entities, applications, devices, etc.) before accessing the system and prevent access to all nonauthenticated principals?				
Does the system require authentication mechanisms and can the system securely store authentication data/information?				
If user names and passwords are used, does the system require password strength rules that allow for a minimum number of characters and inclusion of alphanumeric complexity, while preventing the reuse of previous passwords, without being transported or viewable in plain text?				
Does the system have the ability to terminate or lock a session after a period of inactivity or after a series of invalid log-in attempts?				
Access Control				
Does the system inactivate a user and remove the user's privileges without deleting the user's history?				
Does the system prevent users with read and/or write privileges from printing or copying/writing to other media?				

Source: AHIMA 2010.

Table 6.3 RFP response comparison matrix

Functional User Requirements/Features (Available = 1; Custom Developed = 2; Future Development = 3; Not Available = 4)	Vendor A	Vendor B	Vendor C	Vendor D
Authentication				
Does the system authenticate principals (i.e., users, entities, applications, devices, etc.) before accessing the system and prevent access to all nonauthenticated principals?	1	1	1	1
Does the system require authentication mechanisms and can the system securely store authentication data/information?	1	1	1	1
If user names and passwords are used, does the system require password strength rules that allow for a minimum number of characters and inclusion of alphanumeric complexity, while preventing the reuse of previous passwords, without being transported or viewable in plain text?	1	1	2	3
Does the system have the ability to terminate or lock a session after a period of inactivity or after a series of invalid log-in attempts?	1	1	1	2
Access Control				
Does the system inactivate a user and remove the user's privileges without deleting the user's history?	1	1	3	1
Does the system prevent users with read and/or write privileges from printing or copying/writing to other media?	2	1	3	1

Source: AHIMA 2010.

Make Site Visits and Check References

Many organizations will elect to send members of their project steering committee or proposal committee to visit one or more potential vendor sites where the technology is in operation so they can obtain detailed information from end-users who have had the technology in place to support their business processes. Extensive reference checks with organizations that have used the vendor's products are recommended. Due to the evolving nature of the technology, it is recommended that both long-term and short-term users of the vendor's technology be contacted.

Vendors should also be asked to provide data regarding their customer satisfaction ratings and their customer service records. For example, KLAS reports provide a source of information about the potential vendors. KLAS is a company that evaluates vendor performance based upon input from providers about the technology and provides the results of their evaluations for a fee.

Evaluate Vendors

Given that EHRs are very expensive, it is important for organizations to evaluate any potential vendor thoroughly. This is a part of good governance and is often referred to as "due diligence." Persons in an organizational position with decision-making power must exercise that power carefully. One model for selecting an ambulatory EHR vendor suggests evaluating the goals of the clinic or practice as it relates to following four aspects of the EHR:

- **Functionality** addresses the features of the EHR product, including patient encounter documentation, automating and facilitating office workflow, decision support during patient encounters, and reporting that supports care management and template customization.

- **Usability** addresses the speed and ease of use, including goals about tasks that must be done fast, computer literacy of the practice staff, and the methods by which data will be entered.

- **Practicality** addresses costs including goals about price, internal resources to maintain the EHR, whether the EHR is integrated or interfaced with the practice management systems, and interfaces with labs.

- The **reputation** of the vendor should also be evaluated, including how established the vendor is, references from other clients, and confirmation that their software is certified (Anon 2009).

Rank Vendors and Costs

Once the vendors have been evaluated a ranking system should be used to evaluate the vendors on the functionality of the system and estimated cost. It is highly unlikely that one vendor will have all of the desired functionality at the lowest price. Organizations may have many requirements above and beyond the required criteria. The additional requirements should be prioritized so that a ranking system can be developed and utilized to assist in decision making. The top vendor should be selected and contract negotiations initiated based upon the overall ranking.

Conduct Contract Negotiations

Generally a contract from a software company will be written from the perspective of and to protect the software company. The Centers for Medicare and Medicaid Services (CMS) developed the Doctor's Office Quality–Information Technology (DOQ-IT) program to assist physician practices with EHR implementation activities. The DOQ-IT materials suggest that organizations request language changes to make the contracts more "equal." DOQ-IT contracting guidelines advise that purchasers look at a number of specific issues, including hardware and software, support, interfaces, training, implementation, and disaster recovery and planning. The language should be clear and understandable with specific terms defined. One important way an organization can protect itself is to include the vendor response to the RFP in the contract. This is where the vendor stipulated, usually with great specificity, what they could provide.

One of the challenges encountered in HIT and EHR contracting has been the insertion of "hold harmless" clauses in contracts. These clauses were designed to indemnify software vendors for malpractice or injury claims when the software may have been at fault or even to prevent healthcare providers from disclosing errors, bugs, design flaws, and other HIT-software-related hazards (Goodman et al. 2011). The 2011 American Medical Informatics Association Board Position Paper maintains that these clauses are unethical since they protect corporations at all times, sometimes to the detriment of patient safety and quality of care (Goodman et al. 2011). This is becoming a widespread and recognized concern as evidenced by the 2012 Food and Drug Administration Safety and Innovation Act, which charges the Food and Drug Administration, the ONC, and the Federal Communications Commission with developing "a report that contains a proposed strategy and recommendations on an appropriate, risk-based regulatory framework pertaining to health information technology, including mobile medical applications, that promotes innovation, protects patient safety, and avoids regulatory duplication" (US Government 2012).

Implementation

Implementing a new system or technology represents a significant change to any size or type of healthcare organization. Establishing a comprehensive project plan and schedule is required. This is often accomplished by an implementation team. This implementation team will generally include members of the project steering committee and the proposal committee, but will also include additional user representatives and individuals with the expertise to deploy the new system. The implementation team must forecast and senior management must dedicate the resources needed for the implementation.

It is also recommended that the implementation team include at least one champion, someone who is known and respected in the organization, who sees the new system as necessary to the achievement of the organization's goals, and who is passionate about implementing it. In many healthcare organizations, the EHR champion will be a highly regarded physician who assumes a leadership role with the medical staff and with other system users. The champion must also have strong verbal communication skills. The champion will often have to find ways to motivate many different people to utilize the new technology. Effective communication is critical to successful implementation.

Project Implementation Plan

It is important to have a project implementation plan for an EHR implementation project, just due to the size and scope. The project implementation plan should include the following elements:

1. Major tasks identified
2. Major milestones set
3. Estimated duration of each task
4. Dependencies among activities (for example, if one task must be completed before another can be started)
5. Resources and budget (including staff who will be devoted to the project)
6. Responsible individual or group for each task and milestone
7. Target dates for each milestone
8. Measures for evaluating completion and success (Wager et al. 2009)

A longer list might be utilized for an EHR or HIT implementation plan. It is important to remember that the plan often has to be modified as the project progresses. This should not be considered failure. It may be beneficial to think of the implementation as an opportunity to learn for the next implementation or upgrade.

Workflow and Process Analysis

The workflow process and analysis completed in the assessment phase of the system life cycle development documented the "as-is" of the healthcare practice. It is now very important to plan how technology either can or, of necessity, will evolve into the new workflows and processes. For example, in a hospital doctors or nurses may be required to enter orders that were once entered by unit clerks. This is because the new system will generate alerts for possible contraindications or provide other knowledge the clinician may need to deliver appropriate care. If this new and additional work is not acknowledged and accounted for the clinicians may become frustrated. Conversely, the new system may include tools that change the communication methods, that is, inboxes or alerts for abnormal lab results or other needed notifications that used to require phone calls. Everyone involved in the communication, unit clerk, diagnostic technician, and receiving clinician, including the physician, need to be involved in the planning for these new flows.

Install System Components

Before a project can go-live the hardware and software must be installed. This will include ensuring that there is adequate network infrastructure to support the new system and that required interfaces are built. Depending upon the penetration and use of information technology that already exist in the organization, this can be a minor upgrade or it can be a major part of the project, such as installing **computers-on-wheels (COWs)**, self-contained rolling carts containing a computer for access to the EHR on each unit. It is recommended that a test of the system's effectiveness be piloted in a small unit before the entire system is installed. This will allow for an evaluation of the system and the opportunity to address any issues or concerns.

Train Staff

Training is essential to the successful implementation of any new system. The vendor's role in training should have been defined in the contracting process. The implementation team must define who needs to be trained, who should do the training, how much training is required, and how the training will be accomplished.

The AHRQ Health Information Technology research portfolio recommends demonstration systems (Dixon and Zafar 2009). These are systems entirely separate from the planned production system. They allow clinicians and other users to practice prior to system implementation. In many cases, vendors will supply training as a part of the implementation. Most EHR training is online or in-person; however, users find the training to "be boring, too long or simply not helpful" (Behravesh 2010). Whether the vendors provide the training, the organization builds a demonstration system, or other methods are used, training is important and cannot be ignored.

Convert Data and Test the System

One of the decisions that should already have been made is the extent to which the organization will convert or incorporate **legacy data**, as well as the methods for doing so. Legacy data are existing data, some of which are on paper and some of which may already be digital. Whatever the current format, they must be converted to a format that is compatible with the new product or system. It is recommended that the process or product be tested to ensure that it will allow the data to be converted using a limited amount of data at first. All data should be backed up and cleaned prior to the conversion. There are processes outside the scope of this chapter that describe data cleaning in detail.

The amount of data to be converted would have been defined in the planning process but it is recommended that only as much data as must be accessed in the new system be converted. Very often this decision must be made with both clinical and administrative staff having input. Data conversion can be time consuming, expensive, as well as impact system response time, so it is recommended that the pros and cons of conversion be considered carefully. At a minimum, conversion should be scheduled outside of peak periods. Following the conversion, steps must be taken to validate that the data were successfully converted. Chapter 5 of this book includes steps and processes for data quality checking.

Communicate Progress

Throughout the system implementation, stakeholders should be kept apprised of the project status. This is important to ensure the various users begin to understand the project and do not get the feeling that it is happening in a vacuum. Communication can be accomplished through formal and informal methods including reports to major committees, e-mail blasts, updates in a newsletter, or posts on the company's website. The methods of communication will vary with the size and complexity of the organization and the project, but as many channels of communication as possible should be used to ensure that all stakeholders have timely and accurate information about the project. It is literally impossible to overcommunicate with a project of this impact and scope.

Plan for Go-Live Date

The go-live date is the date that the organization transitions from the old system to the new or initiates the transition from a paper to an electronic system. The targeted go-live date was identified when the project implementation plan was initiated.

The go-live date should be selected for a time period when workload is lower. In the inpatient setting, the date should be one for which there is a historically low census. In academic medical centers, the go-live would need to occur when interns, residents, and fellows are not in the first month of their training. Organizations could also decide to defer elective admissions and surgeries during the go-live time frame to ensure optimal deployment of staff and minimal interruption to patient care. In the ambulatory setting, organizations may elect to reduce the patient workload for a period immediately prior to, during, and following the conversion to allow time for training, learning the new system, and becoming proficient in using the system. Reducing the census or ambulatory workload has an economic effect that should be planned for as part of the implementation process.

Support and Evaluation

Changes will have to be made as any new system is implemented. The implementation team must respond quickly to identified problems or concerns to ensure that users remain confident in the system and feel supported by the organization. A specific individual or group should be assigned to address issues and the end-users should be advised to contact that person or group to report any problems or concerns. The implementation committee should establish a formal process to collect data regarding all reported problems to identify patterns and trends and opportunities to improve the system. AHRQ has published a *Health Information Technology Evaluation Toolkit* (Cusack et al. 2009). This toolkit is very helpful when developing monitors. It includes the consideration of feasibility of collecting the measure, as well as the science behind a measure. Figure 6.2 is a sample measure found in the toolkit. A team of researchers focused on evaluating CPOE and recommend 18 measures, including percentage of system downtime, mean response time, percentage of orders entered by physicians, percentage of orders entered as miscellaneous, and others (Sittig et al. 2007). As can be seen from this limited CPOE example, there are many measures that can be monitored for an EHR implementation. The entire team should participate in setting the measures, the most current research from resources such as the ONC and AHRQ websites should be utilized and, most importantly, the measures must be pertinent to the practice and the setting.

Figure 6.2   Sample HIT evaluation measure

Measure	Quality Domain(s)	Data Source(s)	Notes	Potential Risks
Preventable adverse drug events (ADEs)	Patient Safety Quality of Care	Chart review Prescription review Direct observations May also consider patient phone interviews Instrumenting the study database EMR	Need to distinguish between ADEs and MEs MEs can be divided by stage of medication Process: • Ordering • Transcribing • Dispensing • Administering • Monitoring Can be assessed in both inpatient and outpatient settings. ADEs are: • Idiosyncratic reactions • Drug-diagnosis interactions	Preventable ADEs are relatively common, especially if there is no clinical decision support (CDS) at the time of drug ordering. Many drug-drug and drug-diagnosis interactions can be avoided if CDS tools are available at the time or ordering of medications. Keep track of alerts that fire in a system with CDS, understanding that in a system without CDS those alerts will not be available; we can get an upper bound for preventable ADEs. It is hard to define what is meant by a "preventable ADE." Some idiosyncratic reactions are not preventable and it is impossible to predict who will get what reaction.

Source: AHRQ 2012.

The implementation committee should be careful to establish a mechanism to identify any unintended adverse consequences. This is now made easier with the recent publication of the *Unintended Consequences Guide (UCG)* published by RAND under contract with AHRQ (Jones et al. 2011). The guide is web-based and includes introductory information regarding the overall evaluation of health information technology. The main reason for this site, though, is to assist in the identification of unintended adverse consequences. It does this by educating users why these consequences can and do occur, as well as providing a template to assist with the identification and tracking of unintended consequences. Figure 6.3 is a screenshot of the Issues Log workbook, found in the section Identify Unintended Consequences. Early adopters have learned that it is important to monitor unintended consequences to protect patient safety and ensure user satisfaction.

⊙ Transition to a Completely EHR

The implementation of an EHR does not mean that paper patient records will cease to exist or that the use of paper in healthcare organizations will be a thing of the past. The continued need or requirement to utilize paper in conjunction with an EHR has a name. Patient records that are maintained in both paper and electronic formats are known as **hybrid** records. These records are the most difficult to manage because what is in paper and what is electronic may be constantly changing, while the organization will have to comply with the regulations for both paper records and EHRs. A study of 14 sites from across the United States found that continued use of paper was due to one of the following reasons:

- ⊙ Old uses are still valued.
- ⊙ New uses of paper have been identified.
- ⊙ Sometimes paper may be best (Dykstra et al. 2009).

The old uses of paper that are still valued run from the psychological including the familiarity of paper, which confers a level of comfort, to the social where clinical activities are organized around paper documents, such as intensive care unit flow sheets, and then to a natural resistance to or failure to change, meaning that paper is printed because "that is the way it has always been done."

The new uses of paper include the ability of paper to "fill the gaps" left by incompletely developed or implemented EHR software or functions that have yet to be standardized. One example is the advance directives of patients. Very often the EHR will include an advance directive indicator of Yes, No, or Unknown, but the advance directives will often be maintained in hard copy or, at most, scanned and retained as a PDF document. It is also standard for the downtime system to be paper based (Dykstra et al. 2009).

So, how can a paper patient record be better than an EHR? Well, paper is very versatile. In addition to the forms approved for the record, sticky notes can facilitate much clinical communication. Paper checklists and reminder lists are standard tools for healthcare. Although most of the regulatory hurdles to paper have been

Figure 6.3   Unintended Consequences Issues Log workbook

	**INTRODUCTION TO THE ISSUES LOG**: The issue log is a central repository of information about EHR-related unintended consequences. This Excel sheet is an example of what an Issue Log might look like, your organization may wish more or less functionality (for example, the ability to query, or allow users to submit issues via the web). This template should be adapted and modified to meet the needs of your organization.
	DESCRIPTION					**DISCOVERY**		
ID	Detailed Description	Date Time	EHR Module	Where was user?	What was user doing Trying?	Stage of Discovery	Discovered by	Notification method
1	CPOE calculated incorrect heparin dose. Dosing error was not identified and patient received an overdose of heparin	1/7/2011 13:45	CPOE	ED	Order entry	Production Use	End-User	internal report
2	Unable to place orders for transfer patients until they are admitted and registered. This delays care for critically ill transfer patients	1/18/2011 11:20	CPOE	Ped ICU	Order entry for transfer patients	Production Use	End-User	user complaint
3	Residents notes are excessively long and redundant. Notes from previous days have been copied and pasted	1/23/2011 14:05	Patient Notes	Med Surg	Review clinical notes	Upgrade	End-User	user complaint
	This set of items: Information about: who, what, why, where, when. This information will help you identify causes and remediate problems.					**This set of items**: Information about the stage at which the problem was discovered, and the manner of discovery		

IMPACT & CAUSATION					TRACKING & REMEDIATION				
Risks of care-process compromise	Care-process compromise that occurred	Probable cause	Risks of patient harm	Patient harm that occurred	Corrective Actions	Steps taken to date (time line)	Assigned To	Date Assigned	Progress
		Erroneous patient weight entered at triage	Clinicians may become over dependent on automatic dose calculator	Patient received wrong dose of heparin, and major bleeding occurred	Evaluate measures to reduce distractions while using the EHR. Removing Paper order forms from the ED within the month. Mandating MD CPOE use starting 6/12/2011. Providing 5 CPOE training sessions between the removal of the paper forms and the implementation of the CPOE mandate. Up staffing the ED for a month after the mandate and deskside support during peak ED hrs	3 of 5 CPOE training sessions conducted	CMIO	1/16/2011	On Track
Delayed care for transfer patients	Delayed care for transfer patients	Inability to place orders for un-registered patients	Delay in time sensitive treatment	None yet	Hospital executive, clinical, and IT leadership determining most appropriate policies for entering transfer patients into the EHR	Have set up a hotline in the nursing office. Realize this is temp. step.	Bob S and Sam Z	1/28/2011	Still working on problem. Report probable repair by 2/12
		Ease of cut and paste and insufficient training	Out of date & inaccurate or misleading notes can cause harm pts		Develop organizational policy on the use of copy and paste and strategies to audit copy and paste	Weekly meetings highlight good v. bad notes	Chief of Med and Chief of Surgery Dept.	2/15/2011	Have talked with head of medicine

This set of items: Information about the suspected causes of the problem, possible unintended consequences, as well as unintended consequences that have already occurred.

This set of items: Information about corrective actions planned to remediate the issue, status of steps taken, and individuals responsible addressed, some states may still require paper for specific purposes. States may require paper copies of documents for informed consent or resuscitation status (Dykstra et al. 2009).

Challenges when Handling Hybrid Records

The use of patient records that are part paper and part electronic is the most complicated since the requirements, regulations, and constraints of both types of records must be met. This especially becomes problematic when the patient record format may be constantly changing, as is the case with an organization involved in the active implementation of an EHR system. There must be a way for clinicians to know where the information is located, paper or electronic. If they are looking in the wrong place they may miss an abnormal lab result or act contrary to the provisions of an advance directive they could not find. Additionally, the facility will find it difficult to collect and aggregate data between two different systems, adding yet another layer of complexity to quality measure reporting.

A significant challenge exists with the definition of the legal EHR. This is the official record that the healthcare organization will release when it is requested by a third party such as an attorney or insurance company. Maintaining this definition can mean the creation of a "cheat sheet" to indicate which format is used for the different data and information types. This then results in increased time to compile the complete record. An additional challenge is the management of updates or addendums (Dimick 2008). One solution to these challenges is to scan the paper parts of the record so the entire record can be stored electronically.

Check Your Understanding 6.2

Instructions: Indicate whether the following statements are true or false (T or F).

1. The specific technology to be acquired is determined during the planning and analysis phase of the SDLC.

2. It is literally impossible to communicate too much information about the progress of an EHR project to internal and external stakeholders.

3. A request for information (RFI) is used to ask vendors for information about their products and services in order to narrow down the vendors to whom a request for proposals (RFP) will be issued.

4. Patient records that are maintained in both paper and electronic formats are known as hybrid records.

Instructions: Choose the best answer.

5. The role of a project manager is to
   a. Lead the steering committee
   b. Decide which technology should be acquired
   c. Keep the project on track
   d. All of the above
   e. a and c only

6. The legal health record has all but which of the following characteristics:
   a. Is the official record that the organization will release when requested by a third party
   b. May include both paper and electronic documents
   c. Is defined by the patient or their designated representative
   d. May result in increased time to compile a complete record

◉ Usability

The **International Organization for Standards (ISO)** is a worldwide nongovernmental organization that develops and publishes international standards. The ISO is a network of the national standards institutes of 162 countries that enables consensus to create solutions to meet business requirements and the broader needs of society (ISO 2012).

In standard 9241-11, the ISO defines the usability of a product as "the extent to which a product can be used by specified users to achieve specified goals with effectiveness, efficiency and satisfaction in a specified context of use" (ISO 2012). This means that usability cannot be measured as a property of the product itself, but only in relation to the context of its use: the physical and social conditions in which the product is being used (Svanaes et al. 2008). The usability measures proposed by ISO are

1. effectiveness or the extent to which the goals, whatever they may be, of the users are achieved (often this is measured as task completion);

2. efficiency or the resources needed to achieve the goal (for information technology this is usually measured as completion time); and

3. the user's subjective assessment of the product (Svanaes et al. 2008).

For medical informatics users, candidate tasks range from patient scheduling to clinical care to data reporting necessary for quality management and beyond. When using an EHR, efficiency might mean reducing common tasks to the fewest clicks or screens possible so that time and effort are not wasted. A user's subjective assessment may be more difficult to accomplish with a full-blown EHR, but this input can be well worth the trouble to ensure a high-quality product. Usability in healthcare IT must be considered in context because of the great diversity of users, their tasks, and the work environments (Svanaes et al. 2008). The healthcare delivery system is very heterogeneous; it is highly specialized, with many different professionals performing many different activities on varied patient groups.

EHR Vendors and Usability

While it is important for health informatics and information management professionals to have an appreciation for usability, the software developers, and EHR vendors are responsible for a large portion of the usability of the systems. A recent AHRQ-funded study interviewed various EHR vendors to determine their practices related to EHR usability (McDonnell et al. 2010).

As might be expected the EHR vendors expressed a commitment to developing usable EHR products for the market; however, formal usability testing, user-centered design processes, and development personnel with expertise in usability engineering are still rare (McDonnell et al. 2010). In 2009, the University of Texas Health Science Center School of Biomedical Informatics received a very large ONC grant to expand their cutting-edge work examining EHR software usability (NCCD 2013). This ongoing work will continue to be a growing area of focus for EHR implementation. Additionally, it was discovered that there are no standards for EHR vendors to collect and report usability issues that might impact patient safety (McDonnell et al. 2010). Usability is considered to be a competitive differentiator so little collaboration occurs between vendors.

Usability experts were allowed to review the interview findings and made the following recommendations regarding EHR usability:

1. Standards in Design and Development
   a. Increase the diversity of users surveyed for predeployment feedback. It was noted that most vendors use volunteers, hardly an unbiased sample. Most people who would volunteer enjoy testing technology and are not representative of the typical end-user.
   b. Support an independent body for vendor collaboration and standards development. As with much of healthcare, the health IT market does not meet the criteria for a full free market. All parties do not have equal access to information. Specifically, the buyer has a limited ability to determine whether the product meets their needs and, if they decide incorrectly, the cost of purchasing a different product is substantial.
   c. Develop standards and best practices in use of customization during EHR deployment. Some customization is necessary to support the needs of different healthcare organizations and different users within those organizations. However, more information is needed to understand which and how much customization is of benefit and which is not.

2. Usability Testing and Evaluation
   a. Encourage formal usability testing early in the design and development phase as a best practice. To quote Benjamin Franklin, "An ounce of prevention is worth a pound of cure." Correcting issues after the product has gone to market is much more expensive, especially for training and help desk support.
   b. Evaluate ease of learning, effectiveness, and satisfaction qualitatively and quantitatively. In essence, use the measures promulgated by the ISO. Be sure to include qualitative or contextual information.

3. Postdeployment Monitoring and Patient Safety
   a. Decrease dependence on postdeployment review supporting usability assessments. An EHR's usability is pervasive throughout the software. While smaller issues can often be corrected after deployment, major usability issues, which may be more of a threat to patient safety, will be much more difficult to fix.

    b. Increase research and development of best practices supporting designing for patient safety. Specifically, designing for patient safety needs to be incorporated from the beginning. Currently, vendors appear to monitor and design for patient safety in the late stages or during the release cycle.

4. Certification programs should be carefully designed and valid. Usability is complex and any certification would need to reflect that complexity. Assisting the EHR vendors to create usable products requires a process that identifies usable products, establishes and disseminates standards, and encourages innovation (McDonnell et al. 2010).

As with many other aspects of health information technology, the industry is learning that standards and collaboration are necessary in order to provide the support required to deliver safe, high-quality patient care.

EHR Usability Testing and Assessment

EHR usability and the evaluation of that usability is a part of implementing an effective, efficient EHR system. It is necessary to have a basis of understanding or a framework for examining the usability of systems.

ISO standard 25062 specifies the format for reporting usability testing. The format allows comparisons across technologies and includes the following elements:

- The description of the product
- The goals of the test
- The test participants
- The tasks the users were asked to perform
- The experimental design of the test
- The method or process by which the test was conducted
- The usability measures and data collection methods
- The numerical results (ISO 2012)

It would also be important to include a description of the use context of the test as described previously. This is because healthcare has multiple settings. By definition good usability for the ambulatory setting would be different than good usability for the acute care setting and so forth.

A framework for EHR usability, called TURF (Tasks, Users, Representations, and Functions) defines usability as how useful, usable, and satisfying a system is for the intended users to accomplish goals (Zhang and Walji 2011). TURF is based upon ISO 9241-11, but differs in some selected definitions ("effective" in the ISO and "useful" in TURF and "efficient" in ISO and "usable" in TURF). Under TURF, a system is usable if it is easy to learn, efficient to use, and error tolerant. Learnability is defined as the ease of learning and relearning, which can be measured by the amount of time and effort required to become skilled in performing the task (Zhang and Walji 2011). Other important components of the framework include efficiency, the amount of effort required to accomplish a task, and error tolerance, the ability of the system to prevent errors and recover from errors that do occur (Zhang and

Walji 2011). The TURF framework may be used to objectively measure usability and for evaluating and redesigning existing technologies to reduce the number of task steps and the time required to complete tasks. It will be very valuable as a method for organizing and discussing EHR usability. For example, the researchers applied the TURF framework in the analysis of a task to maintain an active medication allergy list, and reduced the task from 187 steps to 82.

With EHR implementation reaching significant levels across the United States and the world, the usability of these systems can no longer be ignored. The threat to patient safety and the waste of resources, especially clinician time, make a focus on EHR usability an imperative.

Check Your Understanding 6.3

Instructions: Indicate whether the following statements are true or false (T or F).

1. Usability cannot be measured as a property of a product itself, but only in relation to the context of its use.

2. The heterogeneous nature of the healthcare system requires that products be evaluated and tested for usability in the actual healthcare setting in which they will be deployed.

3. Learnability is not an important component of EHR usability.

4. Poor usability is generally not included as a threat to patient safety.

Instructions: Choose the best answer.

5. The ISO defines usability as
   a. Affordability—the ability of the organization to pay for the technology
   b. Effectiveness—the extent to which the goals of the users are achieved
   c. Efficiency—the resources needed to achieve the goal
   d. All of the above
   e. b and c only

⊙ Summary

Telephones, automobiles, and other technology have evolved from difficult-to-use novelties to widely accepted tools of the trade. Healthcare organizations need to use an EHR as a tool to achieve their strategic goals. However, healthcare is complex. The many internal and external stakeholders, the importance of the industry, where patient lives are at risk, and the regulated nature of the healthcare industry means implementation of an EHR requires careful planning at all levels of the organization. Using the SDLC process can be helpful. If the information technology is governed well, implementation of the EHR system will have its own cycle, which is incorporated into a larger, more extensive, health information technology system life cycle. Within the systems development cycle, implementation of the different components will be managed with a well-developed project plan.

Aside from these considerations, EHR implementations will need to incorporate careful planning for handling of a hybrid record, as well as usability assessment and testing, if the chosen system vendors do not provide usability results of their own. All in all, EHR implementation requires a multitude of personnel with different talents and skills all working towards the same goals.

REFERENCES

Agency for Healthcare Research and Quality. 2012. Health IT Evaluation Toolkit. http:// healthit.ahrq.gov/portal/server.pt/community/health_it_tools_and_resources/919/ health_it_evaluation_toolkit/27872.

AHIMA. 2010. RFI/RFP Template (Updated). http://library.ahima.org/xpedio/groups/ public/documents/ahima/bok1_047959.hcsp?dDocName=bok1_047959.

AHIMA. 2012. *Pocket Glossary for Health Information Management and Technology.* 3rd ed. Chicago, IL: AHIMA Press.

Anon. 2009. DOQ-IT University. *EHR Adoption and Implementation.* http://www.doqitu .org/EHR_Adoption/Implementation/L1P7.html.

Bass, A. 2003. Health-Care IT: A Big Rollout Bust. CIO.com. http://www.cio.com/ article/29736/Health_Care_IT_A_Big_Rollout_Bust.

Behravesh, B. 2010. Understanding the End User Perspective: A Multiple-Case Study of Successful Health Information Technology Implementation. ProQuest LLC.

Centers for Medicare and Medicaid Services. 2012. EHR Incentive Programs | Centers for Medicare & Medicaid Services. http://www.cms.gov/Regulations- and-Guidance/Legislation/EHRIncentivePrograms/index.html?redirect=/ EHRIncentivePrograms/

Corrao, N.J., A.G. Robinson, M.A. Swiernik, and A. Naeim. 2010. Importance of testing for usability when selecting and implementing an electronic health or medical record system. *Journal of Oncology Practice* 6(3):120–124. doi:10.1200/JOP.200017.

Cusack, C., C.M. Byrne, J.M. Hook, J. McGowan, E.G. Poon, and A. Zafar. 2009. Health Information Technology Evaluation Toolkit: 2009 Update (Prepared for the AHRQ National Resource Center for Health Information Technology Under Contract No. 290-04-0016). Agency for Healthcare Research and Quality. healthit.ahrq.gov/portal/ server.pt/gateway/.../09_0083_EF.pdf.

Dimick, C. 2008. Record limbo. Hybrid systems add burden and risk to data reporting. *Journal of AHIMA* 79(11):28–32.

Dimick, C. 2011. Meaningful use: Notes from the journey. *Journal of AHIMA* 82(10):24–30.

Dixon, B.E., and A. Zafar. 2009. *Inpatient Computerized Provider Order Entry (CPOE): Finding from the AHRQ Health IT Portfolio.* Rockville, MD: AHRQ National Resource Center for Health IT under Contract No. 290-04-0016.

Dykstra, R.H, J.S Ash, E. Campbell, D.F. Sittig, K. Guappone, J. Carpenter, J. Richardson, A. Wright, and C. McMullen. 2009. Persistent Paper: The Myth of "Going Paperless. *AMIA Annual Symposium Proceedings/AMIA Symposium,* pp.158–162.

Garrido, T., B. Raymond, L. Jamieson, L.L. Liang, and A.M. Wiesenthal. 2004. Making the business case for hospital information systems—A Kaiser Permanente investment decision. *Journal of Healthcare Finance* 31(2):16–25.

Goodman, K.W., E.S. Berner, M.A. Dente, B. Kaplan, R. Koppel, D. Rucker, D.Z. Sands, and P. Winkelstein. 2011. Challenges in ethics, safety, best practices, and oversight regarding HIT vendors, their customers, and patients: A report of an AMIA Special Task Force. *Journal of the American Medical Informatics Association* 18(1):77–81. doi:10.1136/jamia.2010.008946.

Griffith, J.R., and K.R. White. 2010. *Reaching Excellence in Healthcare Management.* Chicago: Health Administration Press.

Han, Y.Y., J.A. Carcillo, S.T. Venkataraman, R.S.B. Clark, R.S. Watson, T.C. Nguyen, H. Bayir, and R.A. Orr. 2005. Unexpected increased mortality after implementation of a commercially sold computerized physician order entry system. *Pediatrics* 116(6):1506–1512. doi:10.1542/peds.2005-1287.

International Organization for Standardization. 2012. About ISO. http://www.iso.org/iso/about.htm.

Jones, S.S., R. Koppel, M.S. Ridgely, T.E. Palen, S. Wu, and M.I. Harrison. 2011. *Guide to Reducing Unintended Consequences of Electronic Health Records Prepared by RAND Corporation Under Contract No. HHSA2902006000171, Task Order #5.* Rockville, MD: Agency for Healthcare Research and Quality. http://www.ucguide.org/index.html.

LaTour, K.M., S. Eichenwald Maki, and P. Oachs, eds. 2013. *Health Information Management: Concepts, Principles, and Practice.* Chicago, IL: AHIMA Press.

McDonnell, C., K. Werner, and L. Wendel. 2010. *Electronic Health Record Usability: Vendor Practices and Perspectives.* Rockville, MD: Agency for Healthcare Research and Quality.

National Center for Cognitive Informatics and Decision Making. 2013. The University of Texas Health Science Center School of Biomedical Informatics. http://www.uthouston.edu/nccd/projects/sharpc/index.htm.

Office of the National Coordinator, DHHS. 2011. Federal Health IT Strategic Plan (2011–2015) – Overview. http://healthit.hhs.gov/portal/server.pt?open=512&objID=1211&parentname=CommunityPage&parentid=2&mode=2.

Office of the National Coordinator, DHHS. 2012a. HealthIT.hhs.gov: ONC-Authorized Testing and Certification Bodies. http://healthit.hhs.gov/portal/server.pt/community/healthit_hhs_gov__onc-authorized_testing_and_certification_bodies/3120.

Office of the National Coordinator, DHHS. 2012b. HealthIT.hhs.gov: Certified EHR Solutions. http://www.healthit.gov/policy-researchers-implementers/certified-health-it-product-list-chpl.

Sittig, D.F., E. Campbell, K. Guappone, R. Dykstra, and J.S. Ash. 2007. Recommendations for Monitoring and Evaluation of In-patient Computer-based Provider Order Entry Systems: Results of a Delphi Survey. *AMIA … Annual Symposium Proceedings / AMIA Symposium. AMIA Symposium* 2007:671–675.

Svanaes, D., A. Das, and O.A. Alsos. 2008. The contextual nature of usability and its relevance to medical informatics. *Studies in Health Technology and Informatics* 136:541–546.

United States Congress. 2009. Health Information Technology for Economic and Clinical Health (HITECH) Act. *Code of Federal Regulations.* http://edocket.access.gpo. gov/2010/pdf/2010-17210.pdf.

United States Government. 2012. Food and Drug Administration Safety and Innovation Act. *United States Code..* http://www.gpo.gov/fdsys/pkg/BILLS-112s3187enr/pdf/ BILLS-112s3187enr.pdf.

Wager, K.A., F.W. Lee, and J.P. Glaser. 2009. *Health Care Information Systems: A Practical Approach on Health Care Management.* 2nd ed. San Francisco, CA: Jossey-Bass.

Yoon-Flannery, K., S.O. Zandieh, G.J. Kuperman, D.J. Langsam, D. Hyman, and R. Kaushal. 2008. "A qualitative analysis of an electronic health record (EHR) implementation in an academic ambulatory setting. *Informatics in Primary Care* 16(4):277–284.

Zhang, J. and M.F. Walji. 2011. TURF: Toward a framework of EHR usability. *Journal of Biomedical Informatics.* 44(6):1056–67.

Chapter 7

Healthcare Informatics and Decision Making

By Joanne Valerius

KEY TERMS

Alert fatigue
Clinical analytics
Clinical decision support system (CDSS)
Computer-assisted coding (CAC)
Computerized provider order entry (CPOE)

C-suite
Data analytics
Decision support system (DSS)
Electronic patient portals
Knowledge management (KM)
Natural language processing (NLP)
Unintended consequences

⊙ Introduction

Decisions are a part of daily living. Through repetition, rules, and regulations for safety and well-being, along with ongoing input from our environment, we may automatically respond to situations and make instant decisions, such as a fuel warning alert telling us to refuel. If we ignore the warning, we may be stranded. A red oil light might mean severe engine damage may occur if we do not pay attention immediately. Traffic lights flash warnings of when to walk and stop walking, and tell us when to go (green), slow down (yellow), and stop (red). There are laws and regulations that we are required to follow or we are penalized. In a complex changing environment, we are constantly adapting to the decisions we make and how they affect our future.

Healthcare also is a complex system that is constantly adapting to external and internal forces; making decisions may be instantaneous, such as cardiopulmonary resuscitation (CPR), which relies on automatic responses and trusted clinical protocols. Or, the decisions may involve long-term healthcare solutions with multiple factors that need human interaction as well as electronic interpretation of data. This chapter will examine the many ways that electronic **decision support systems (DSSs)**, both administrative and clinical, impact the healthcare environment and organization. A DSS is a computer-based system that gathers data from a variety of sources and assists in providing structure to the data by using various analytical models and visual tools in order to facilitate and improve the ultimate outcome in decision-making tasks associated with nonroutine and nonrepetitive problems (LaTour et al. 2013, 909). A DSS supports administrative decisions and may use many data sources such as reimbursement, utilization of services, and aggregate patient sociological data. **Clinical decision support systems (CDSSs)** can include alerts in the electronic health record such as an allergy to medications, reminders for preventive healthcare services, and links for providers to find references or order sets. CDSS is a special subcategory of clinical information systems that is designed to help healthcare providers make knowledge-based clinical decisions such as those previously mentioned (AHIMA 2012, 85).

Further, this chapter will explore the importance of knowledge management (KM) in a dynamic and ever-changing electronic system to enhance quality. KM is important to DSSs because through KM data are acquired and transformed into information, and then into understanding of the context (LaTour et al. 2013, 926).

In a dynamic and ever-changing healthcare system the focus is on the ability of organizations to enhance quality of patient care. Use of KM systems to support decisions at many levels in the healthcare organization is essential. Understanding how to extract the patient data from databases and data banks is key to provide feedback to improve patient care.

The use of electronic resources for assisting in making human decisions is evolving and naturally affects the current mindset to continue the development of new applications that will benefit patient safety and the quality of healthcare. In doing so, efficient and effective ways to utilize the financial resources that will affect the future of the management of healthcare finance and healthcare systems continue to be examined. The focus on CDSSs as EHRs are implemented has aided in improving the quality of patient care.

A CDSS should be designed to provide the

1. Right information
2. To the right person

3. In the right format

4. Through the right channel

5. At the right time (Osheroff et al. 2009)

The challenge to an organization is to analyze their systems to determine how these components can be provided. Each organization must be able to define the architectural components of their system, and determine the interoperability of software programs to talk with one another in order to provide the "rights" for a CDSS.

⊙ Knowledge Management

In this chapter, we will look at **knowledge management (KM)** systems as the tool to capture and disseminate electronic information for use in decisions at multiple levels of an organization. Figure 7.1 is one conceptual model of KM illustrating the complexity inherent in KM. This includes, however, the interdependencies of human relationships. One model of KM has determined that

a. "a knowledge artifact, that is, codified knowledge is in a format that is insufficient for fully effective knowledge use by practices (e.g., digital medical records);

b. a number of interdependent processes are necessary to manage knowledge;

c. there are social and technical dimensions to these processes as a result of knowledge being tacit (e.g., that knowledge conveyed in apprenticeships relationships) and being explicit (e.g. objects such as procedure manuals);

d. action emanates from the tacit dimension of knowledge and KM processes engaged in pursuit of organization's mission" (Orzano et al. 2008).

This model relies on the human resources to collaborate and build systems that provide the expectations of organizational performance. This model, applied to any

Figure 7.1 A conceptual knowledge management framework in healthcare

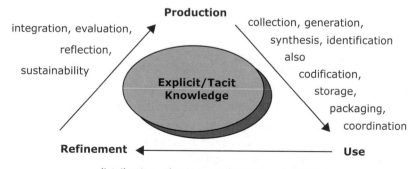

Social Context (structures, values, preferences)

Source: Lau 2004, 3.

healthcare environment, demonstrates an effective means to improve the quality of healthcare by accessing every employee and system in the organization. It reflects the importance of relationships, trust, and practice (social context) while having expectations for accessible technology and systems to process and generate needed information for decision making.

Check Your Understanding 7.1

Case: A large health maintenance organization (HMO) is finding that many former procedures and processes done onsite could be done remotely. This would lower the cost of overhead for the HMO. The chief operating officer has asked the director of health information management (HIM) to develop a plan to have more employees work remotely.

Currently, coders are working remotely. When coders were set up to work at home, issues around technology and access to needed software systems caused anxiety and slow down in revenue cycle processing. The HIM department manager was held accountable for the workflow slowdown caused by the technology breakdown.

Another area that could be considered for remote work is release of information. The department manager has identified that 80 percent of the release of information requests could be done remotely in secure settings. However, it is anticipated that the changeover to remote release of information will cause backlog for a month. Given the previous experience with remote coding, the department manager is pushing back against this idea.

Instructions: Answer the following questions on a separate piece of paper.

1. Using the model provided in figure 7.1, what needs to occur to make the process of remote release of information meet organizational performance standards?

2. Since technology was the cause for the workflow issues in remote coding, who would you plan to involve in the next remote project?

3. What steps could the department manager take to reduce the risk of backlog when implementing a new remote work area?

4. What other areas could be done remotely when using an EHR? If needed, search for journal articles that may recommend some options.

⊙ Administrative Uses of Decision Support Systems

Not all decisions in healthcare immediately affect the patient's safety or the quality of care delivered. However, eventually all decisions do affect the patient's encounter with the healthcare system, for example, the process of coding a diagnosis for reimbursement affects the patient. In the most advanced systems, a code could be generated from **natural language processing (NLP)** technology systems, which are sophisticated electronic systems reading the structured word-processed document. NLP is a technology that converts human language (structured or unstructured) into data that can be translated then manipulated by computer systems (AHIMA 2012, 283). This process, also known as **computer-assisted coding (CAC)**, will dramatically assist a medical coding specialist. In CAC the computer software extracts and translates transcribed or computer-generated free-text data into diagnosis and procedural codes for billing and coding purposes (LaTour 2013, 904). However, the critical analysis of a coding specialist is needed to review the medical record to validate a final decision for medical claims. Reminders and alerts about correct coding procedures also provide clues for decision making for the coder. Reminders to choose more specific codes, alerts that certain codes cannot be utilized for the principal diagnosis, and others have increased the reliability and accuracy of coded data.

The decision support tools like NLP, reminders, and alerts are a part of the many administrative DSSs that affect the workflow of information processing. These are essential to both the patient knowing their claim is processed, and the healthcare organization knowing the claim will be paid. No DSS replaces the coding specialist in making a final decision.

HIM relies on DSSs that can assist in daily operations. Through electronic portals, providers can be sent reminders for completion of health records. These reminders are built from the laws, rules, regulations, internal policy and procedures, and accreditation standards that healthcare organizations must follow. The tools for completing quantitative and qualitative analysis on an electronic record assist the health information specialist in completing these processes.

The **C-suite** (executive management, such as chief operating officer, chief information officer) as well as department managers, public health agencies, among others, rely on data collected and generated to make decisions about managing current programs, developing new programs, providing public information for the improvement of safety for patients, and increasing the quality of overall healthcare. DSSs provide financial as well as clinical information for administrative decision making. Reliance on DSS and other systems, data warehouses, and national repositories, have the potential to inform administrators of areas to improve efficiency and effectiveness in healthcare, which impacts the quality of healthcare for patients. Electronically generated reports and dashboards provide textual information as well as visual displays of specific data from the data warehouses. The more electronically readable, or structured, the data is, the greater the usability for decisions. Administrators will rely on the employees who can mine and statistically interpret the metadata, databases, and repositories that are rich informatics tools. This use of statistical analysis of data to make business decisions is called **data analytics** (LaTour et al. 2013, 525). Similarly, **clinical analytics** is mining discrete patient healthcare data such as laboratory results, medication, and genetics to make clinical decisions or to aid in translating data for research or further healthcare treatment.

Information available to the public provides consumers with the material necessary to make intelligent decisions about where to seek healthcare organizations or individual clinicians that will meet their standards for care, or will be covered by their healthcare insurers. Websites such as HealthGrades (http://www.healthgrades.com/), the Leapfrog Group (http://www.leapfroggroup.org/), and Hospital Compare (http://www.hospitalcompare.hhs.gov/) provide consumers with comparable information on hospitals and physicians. Sites such as Yelp and Angie's List also deliver feedback on providers; however, they may not be as authoritative as the previously mentioned sites. As with everything related to the Internet, these websites are continually evolving.

Electronic patient portals that provide access to personal health information are often available from a patient's healthcare organization. These portals provide patients with opportunities to view results of exams and treatment, and also provide alerts for preventive care. Figure 7.2 provides an example of these types of reminders from the Veterans Health Administration Blue Button portal. Patient education to access the portals is key to the ongoing success of engaging patients to

Figure 7.2 Preventive Care from Veterans Health Administration HealtheVet Blue Button Example

VA Wellness Reminders	
Source:	VA
Last Updated:	24 Sep 2012 @ 1134

Wellness Reminder	Due Date	Last Completed	Location
Body Mass >25 Alert	DUE NOW	UNKNOWN	DAYT29
Colon Cancer Screening	13 Aug 2015	13 Aug 2012	DAYT29
Influenza Vaccination	13 Aug 2013	13 Aug 2011	DAYT29
Elevated Cholesterol Alert	13 Aug 2013	13 Aug 2011	DAYT29
Eye Exam For Diabetes	13 Aug 2013	13 Aug 2011	DAYT29
Foot Exam For Diabetes	13 Aug 2013	13 Aug 2011	DAYT29
HbA1c for Diabetes	13 Aug 2014	13 Aug 2012	DAYT29
Elevated Blood Pressure Alert	DUE NOW	13 Aug 2009	DAYT29
Lipid Measurement (Cholesterol)	DUE NOW	13 Aug 2009	DAYT29
Pneumonia Vaccine	DUE NOW	UNKNOWN	DAYT29
Comments	Learn more about these Wellness Reminders by visiting My HealtheVet. Please contact your health care team with any questions about your VA Wellness Reminders.		

Source: Blue Button, Veterans Health Administration, 2013.

be aware of their responsibility in their own care. Finding out whether a patient has access to a computer, a mobile application, or other technology will be important to the use of an electronic system to alert patients. Of course, in all cases, patients' rights to privacy must comply with all federal (Health Insurance Portability and Accountability Act (HIPAA)) and state rules and laws integrated into any electronic communication system.

We will continue to look more closely at examples of systems that show the need for the interconnectedness of administrative and CDSSs. The importance of looking at organization-wide information systems to provide meaningful information as required by law and to enhance patient safety is imperative.

Check Your Understanding 7.2

Case 1: You are a new HIM director. The healthcare organization's chief executive officer (CEO) has asked you to pull data that a board subcommittee will use to plan for possible expansion of the emergency room. You have no experience in data analytics.

Instructions: Answer the following questions on a separate piece of paper.

1. What would be some of the first steps you would take on this project?
2. You decide to pull a team together to work on this project. Who will you ask to join the team?
3. What kind of data do you think you would need to pull?
4. Would you consider gathering any qualitative data such as interviews with the ED physicians and staff? Why or why not?
5. What are some ways to present the data to the board?

Case 2: You are the HIM supervisor of the release of information area in a small community hospital. Recently, an EHR has been implemented with a patient portal. You have been asked to lead a public service project on a campaign for patients to be more aware of the patient portal and the organization's healthcare website, which may improve their knowledge and provide alerts for preventative care. The population you are working with is rural, and the bandwidth of the Internet is slow and cumbersome for many of the patients. Some do not have access to the Internet unless they go to the public library or come to the hospital. The patient portal was developed to improve the quality of care and communication between the patient and the physician.

Instructions: Answer the following questions on a separate piece of paper.

6. Who will you involve in the project team?
7. How will you determine who has access to the patient portal?
8. What would you recommend to the team regarding access for those that have limited Internet access?
9. What types of decision support tools could help you with this project?
10. How will you provide education to the patients and the providers?

⊙ Clinical Decision Support Systems (CDSSs) to Improve Safety and Quality of Patient Healthcare

Electronic health record vendors and healthcare IT teams continue to build reminders and alerts that are intended to support the goals of patient safety and quality of healthcare. The health record is the primary communication tool for a healthcare team. Using CDSS tools to improve documentation in the health record is intended to improve patient safety and overall quality of healthcare. Alerting a clinician of a potential medication interaction or a nurse of a missed medication administration will contribute to the care of the patient. In addition, a CDSS can aid a healthcare provider in making decisions about treatment that can be used for an individual. In 2012, the federal government enacted legislation calling upon the Food and Drug Administration (FDA), the Federal Communications Commission (FCC), and the Office of the National Coordinator for Health Information Technology (ONC) to post on their websites, within 18 months, a strategy and recommendations for an "appropriate, risk based regulatory framework" for health IT, including mobile medical applications, that promotes innovation, protects patient safety, and avoids regulatory duplication (US Government 2012). KM systems, which generate up-to-date information on clinical protocols and disease management and can be incorporated into EHRs, are beginning to be viewed as applications that have a direct impact upon patient care and patient safety.

Disparity in Access to Information for CDSSs

One goal of a CDSS is to eliminate provider bias for care. For instance if a provider believes that a patient will not comply with medical management based on age, race, sexual preference, or other characteristics, information about options for treatment or medications may be withheld from them. A system-wide EHR could be used to objectively determine a patient's need for services. Alerts sent to patients and to providers simultaneously based on clinical protocols and using electronic data extraction could reduce bias. In addition, providing patients with information that relates specifically to their healthcare diagnosis contributes to improved care (Lopez et al. 2011).

Finding the best way to communicate with a patient will be essential to the use of CDSS that meets everyone's needs for information. Not all patients will have computers, apps on their mobile devices, or other technology to respond to alerts. Healthcare organizations that are sensitive to and seek ways to engage patients in their healthcare will need to develop strategies that reduce discrimination or disparities based on lack of electronic technology availability.

The Joint Commission (JC) encourages focused efforts in areas where significant health disparities occur (Haider et al. 2011). Disparities in healthcare continue to plague healthcare delivery systems and negatively impact patient safety and quality of care. Although equity in healthcare delivery has been emphasized in national reports such as Crossing the Quality Chasm, Unequal Treatment: Confronting the Racial and Ethnic Disparities in Healthcare, and the 2009 AHRQ National Healthcare Disparities Report it is evident that this ongoing divide needs to be lessened.

If we focus on the patient side of the issues, we can see that many HIT factors can influence ongoing patient care. The root causes emphasize the communication issues that interfere with patients accessing and complying with healthcare providers. In an area where consumers are encouraged to access their EHR, it is imperative that the tools for doing this will be available. If an alert system is in place, it is only as good as the access to the system. As we improve decision support tool access for one community, the potential for increased patient safety and quality of healthcare for others improves as well.

The CDSSs need strong leadership and executive management directives to develop strong, inclusive, patient-focused systems that also influence the efficiency and effectiveness of resources. Key to the advancement of a stellar CDSS is also the inclusion of clinician champions to lead the process. But clinicians are not the only practitioners who need to be included. Any department utilizing an electronic clinical system, such as pharmacy, radiology, nursing, and so on, needs to be a part of a dynamic team to lead the organization to a successful system. End-users of the system also need to be involved, such as HIM administrators, quality assurance administrators (and individuals within the department who manage quality assurance), and, perhaps most importantly, patients.

Research about Decision Support Systems

Research on the use of DSS is useful to study in order to understand how implementation and uses of EHRs can support or be a barrier to effective use of DDS. Informaticists who are involved in DSS will want to explore the plethora of articles that explore this area. Below are a few examples of the use of decision support tools (DSS or CDSS).

Long-Term Care

CDSS systems can be used in nonacute-care settings too. For example, one ongoing area of clinical concern in nursing homes is the issue of pressure ulcers. Pressure ulcers are often painful, hard to heal once developed, and can be a costly problem. A CDSS tool, On-Time QI for Pressure Ulcer Prevention (On-Time PrU) sought to design a program "...to leverage the knowledge of certified nursing assistant (CNA) staff and promote proactive care coordination and planning using IT" (Hudak 2011). The research shows that it takes 12 to 18 months to implement such a program across a nursing home. At-risk residents were reported on a Trigger Summary, which identified known risk criteria such as nutrition, incontinence, and others. The On-Time PrU focused on quality improvement processes. An important part of this CDSS tool was the integration of IT into the normal workflow of those caring for the patient. Further development of CDSS tools like the On-Time PrU benefit patient quality and safety and satisfaction of care, and reduce the cost of healthcare in this environment.

Genomics and Personalized Medicine

The need for CDSS in genomics and personalized medicine is being studied. Clearly, as more is known about the human genome and treatment of diseases, the impact of CDSS will grow. The use of CDSS is complicated when protocols change for treatment, and the knowledge is not uniformly communicated. The need for national and international data repositories of knowledge content is inevitable. The use of standard language such as Health Level 7 (HL7), the Systemized Nomenclature for Medicine (SNOMED), Logical Observations Identifiers Names and Codes (LOINC), Unified Medical Language system (UMLS), and others continues to be of importance in this area. Additionally, how information is collected so that it can be retrieved uniformly is of concern. The Nationwide Health Information Network (NwHIN) recognizes that CDSSs are important to the effective use of health information technology.

Current national and international informatics standards to support the national CDSS systems may conflict. However, many organizations continue to work collaboratively to reduce the conflicts in order to further the exchange of healthcare information and to support a national infrastructure. The government agencies include the Office of the National Coordinator, the Agency for Healthcare Research and Quality (AHRQ), the Veterans Health Administration, and the US Department of Health and Human Services along with many other governmental and nongovernmental agencies seeking to improve the secure exchange of health information to improve patient safety, and reduce the cost of healthcare. The need for standards continues to be a high priority for all stakeholder organizations. The evolution in this area is fast and students are encouraged to use journals and the Internet to determine the most current standards and regulations.

It is useful to visualize the use of CDSS in one disease to emphasize the importance of collaboration and accurate systems:

> ...an electronic health record (EHR) system could consider the gene expression profile of a patient's cancer biopsy and provide an individually-tailored prediction of how the patient is likely to respond to various therapeutic options... Over 90% of clinician-directed CDS interventions evaluated in randomized controlled trials have significantly improved patient care, provided that the CDS was delivered automatically as part of the clinician workflow, offered at the time and location of decision making, recommended a specific course of action, and used a computer to generate the recommendation (Kawamoto et al. 2009).

Specific skill sets are important to work with researchers to translate personalized and genomic information into meaningful information. Figure 7.3 presents skills that are identified as important. Continuing to develop skills in research will impact the advancement of the HIM professional in projects that relate specifically to decision support.

Figure 7.3   Skills for HIM Professionals in the Post-Genomic Era

Current Skills to Apply

- Policy and procedure development for managing patient health information to ensure its accuracy, integrity, privacy, and security (including investigating and resolving problems that may arise in the development of phenotype and genotype databases that involve breaches of patient information)
- Knowledge of EHR database systems design and their maintenance
- Knowledge of forms design, computer input screens, and clinical documentation tools and guidelines
- Knowledge of implementing industry standards for data sharing and interoperability
- Developing standardized healthcare data sets
- Knowledge of coding and classification systems
- Experience with organizational compliance to laws, rules, and regulations for licensure and accrediting agencies
- Knowledge of maintaining a master patient index and master client index
- Developing policies and procedures for release of medical information

Skills to Develop

- Statistics for data analysis, including calculus-based probability and statistics; statistical programming languages (SAS, S-Plus, R)
- Information science
- Computer science
- Knowledge of genetics

Source: Mendoza 2010.

Computer-Assisted Coding (CAC) in All Healthcare Settings

A report from the American Health Information Management Association (AHIMA) discussed the implications of ongoing changes in CAC (including the changing role of the coding specialist to that more of an editor, using critical thinking and decision-making skills). As mentioned earlier in this chapter, NLP has created advances in extracting key information that can be used to identify possible codes. Code numbers are used as secondary data for the revenue management cycle but also for data mining for registries, research studies, and administrative planning purposes. Accurate coding not only influences the capture of reimbursable claims, but also impacts the entire use of informatics for those secondary purposes.

CAC DSSs need to be designed so that the designated record set to be utilized for coding diagnoses and procedures is clearly utilized. This calls for a system that can track when appropriate documentation is entered into the electronic system. Additional tools such as this will assist in the coding process, lessening the need for physician queries. A CAC total package will include decision support tools of reminders and alerts that will contribute to meeting the government regulations related to the meaningful use of EHRs (Bronnert et al. 2010–2011). Overall, this report suggests that CAC can function to support the coding process in the following ways:

- Steamline the coding workflow
- Support clinical documentation improvement programs
- Facilitate data mining
- Create problem lists for physician review and validation
- Support ICD-10-CM education
- Provide Recovery Audit Contractor (RAC) audit trails (Bronnert et al. 2010–2011)

An important focus of CAC is the reduction in compliance risk because of the KM tools that are embedded in the system. Built-in fraudulent billing alerts, for instance, assures managers that misrepresentation for financial purposes is reduced or eliminated. Encoding systems will provide a magnitude of resources and references that provide up-to-date coding changes and appropriate application of the current and future payment and reimbursement models.

Community Mental Health

In an attempt to increase patient involvement in their care, a community mental health clinic compared the use of an electronic DSS to set goals with patients during care planning to promote shared decision making and greater awareness. The researchers found that case managers who used the system were more satisfied than those that did not. Client satisfaction in the process, however, did not improve with the DSS (Woltmann et al. 2011). The result of this study illustrates that although DSS can contribute to easing an operational function like goal setting in mental health settings, it does not necessarily have the same effect on patient satisfaction with their care. In this case, the management may need to determine if the DSS is appropriate for use or engage more patient input to improve the tool.

In another mental health study, EHR-based tools were used to screen for bipolar disorder for patients with depression. A screening instrument from the World Health Organization Composite International Diagnostic Interview (CIDI) was used as a clinical decision support tool embedded into the EHR to assist clinicians. When a patient with a diagnosis of depression was seen at an office visit, the screening tool automatically displayed for use. They found that "…widespread use of the CDS tool and a higher rate of diagnosis and medication prescription suggest that EHR-based CDS can be useful in improving the detection of bipolar disorder in patients with depression" (Gill et al. 2012, 289). Developing tools that are easily available to clinicians can improve the quality of care and patient safety.

Unintended Consequences of Clinical Decision Support Systems

When change occurs, such as reengineering a workflow or introducing a new technology, one cannot anticipate all of the repercussions that might occur from it. Human-computer interaction for many clinicians, informaticists, end-users, workflow managers, and others has been smooth after implementation of an EHR, while others have struggled with the change process.

Additionally, research in this area is finding that there are unanticipated and undesirable issues or problems, often described as **unintended consequences** of implementation. Electronic systems, and the human who interacts with them, are not error free, and new systems may inadvertently introduce new documentation errors, communication issues, and a dependence on the system that is unrealistic. One area that may not be considered is the shift in power, control, and autonomy affecting the provider-patient relationship.

In a preliminary study of **CPOE (computerized provider order entry)**, unintended consequences affecting clinicians during early implementation of the EHR were reported. CPOE consists of electronic prescribing systems that allow physicians to write prescriptions and transmit them electronically. This qualitative research provided a better understanding of the impact of the change in workflow and frustrations that impeded successful CPOE implementations (Ash et al. 2007). The AHRQ, tasked with research to improve the quality of patient care, published a publicly available Unintended Consequences Guide, which is available on the Internet (Jones 2011). The AHRQ guide uses the framework in Figure 7.4 to illustrate the variety of issues that must be considered related to unintended consequences, as well as the iterative nature of the process, which is never truly finished.

Figure 7.4   ITSA Framework

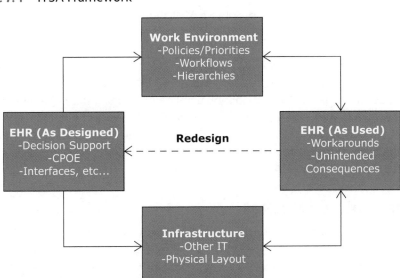

Source: Jones et al. 2013.

⊙ Quality

Unintended consequences of CPOE implementation have impacted quality of healthcare as found in some studies. Workflow and electronic system issues can seriously and negatively impact quality of care when implementing new electronic systems. The importance of analyzing workflow prior to, during, and after implementation cannot be emphasized enough. As project teams study the implementation of a system, it is essential to consider the precise timeliness of needed information. Reflecting on current practice (what works and what does not), human relationships (trust and effective communication), and the infrastructure of systems and human resources helps in completing a successful implementation that can impact patient safety and quality.

What continues to plague DSSs is the ability to have just-in-time information so decisions critical to patient care can be made in a timely manner. Determining who can turn alerts "off and on" and what happens when a clinician ignores an alert are other details that need to be determined. It is not only important to involve clinicians, information technology (IT), quality professionals, and others in the process of determining the policies and procedures for the facility. It is also imperative to involve legal counsel in this process. Some organizations have implemented CDSS committees in order to assist the set up of alerts, review their effectiveness, review issues, and ultimately ensure the most effective CDSS (Kuperman et al. 2005).

One of the areas that tends to be difficult to establish for some healthcare organizations is the definition of the legal health record and the implications of ignoring or working around alerts. If metadata is allowed in discovery, subpoenaed, and found admissible in a court of law, the decisions made to ignore alerts may find new legal ramifications. The court system will need to decide if and how the lack of alerts, content of DSS, and ignoring or working around alerts has affected the quality of care of a patient. As court decisions are made related to these issues, the power and autonomy concerns will be impacted. In a practice brief on defining the legal health record, AHIMA states, "At a minimum the EHR should include documentation of the clinician's actions in response to decision support. This documentation is evidence of the clinician's decision to follow or disregard decision support. The organization should define the extent of exception documentation required (e.g., what no documentation means)" (AHIMA 2011).

As health informatics and information management professionals, our knowledge about the legal system, the legal health record, and the access to metadata is needed as DSSs and CDSSs are developed and utilized. Our knowledge of laws, regulations, rules, and accreditation standards is essential to not only protect the safety of the patient, but also of the healthcare organization.

⊙ The State of the Art

In the article "Clinical Decision Support Systems: State of the Art," some of the ongoing issues related to time, speed, and ease of access and key issues are captured in table 7.1 (Berner 2009). The author points out that "while some of these issues have been addressed by research, there are no universally accepted guidelines regarding them, in part because clinicians often differ in their preferences....there are varying

Table 7.1   CDSS intent and key issues

CDSS Intent	Match to User's Intention	Key Issues
Reminder of actions user intends to do, but should not have to remember (automatic)	High	Timing
Provide information when user is unsure what to do (on demand)	High	Speed and ease of access
Correct user's errors or recommend user change plans (automatic or on demand)	Low	Automatic: timing, autonomy and user control over response On demand: speed, ease of access, autonomy, and user control over response

Source: Berner 2002.

clinical approaches that are justified" (Berner 2009). This points to the ongoing struggle for informaticists to construct a meaningful CDSS that will be effective across systems.

A remaining concern for informaticists, clinicians, IT professionals, and others is the intention of those using the DSS. For example, consider a hard stop alert intended to stop a clinician from ordering two medications that will interact; savvy clinicians may find ways to override the alert. This may be warranted by their intimate knowledge of the patient's current health situation. The art of medicine demands that the clinician has that independence to think critically about treatment. However, protecting the integrity of the legal health record by enforcing basic policies and procedures about tools such as alerts is essential. Clearly documenting who has the rights and responsibility to change alert tools further protects the facility. Conducting quality audits of alert overrides, for instance, can provide information that impacts patient safety.

The growth of the EHR and the use of CDSSs will continue to evolve. Some future perspectives for changes in CDSSs may be impacted by

- Payer initiatives to increase incentives for use of a CDSS
- Pay for performance and e-prescribing shift payment incentives to make use of a CDSS
    - Groups like Leapfrog and AHRQ encourage it
- Technological Developments
    - EMR vendors driving it
    - CCHIT developing standards across EHR systems
    - Internet knowledge systems becoming more available
    - Legislation demands it (Berner 2009)

DSSs, whether clinical or administrative, call for creative individuals to continue development and to manage the knowledge that is needed to keep current. This is time intensive and costly. Large academic hospitals, government facilities such as the Veterans Affairs Medical Centers, and large healthcare enterprises have traditionally taken the lead in development, research, and evaluation of systems. The benefits of the collective work provides smaller healthcare systems with hope for accessing DSSs that will also enhance their administrative and patient safety goals.

Check Your Understanding 7.3

Case: You sit on the health IT committee of your organization. A parallel committee on the legal health record meets separately and you also sit on that committee. You also sit on the quality management committee.

IT committee: The IT support personnel (does not include the chief information officer or the chief medical information officer) for physicians have been asked to "turn off" certain alerts in the CPOE because of ongoing complaints of **alert fatigue**. Alert fatigue is a commonly observed condition among physicians overwhelmed with large numbers of clinically insignificant alerts, thus causing them to "tune out" and potentially miss an important drug-drug or drug allergy alert (Jones 2011). IT decides to turn off the alerts requested by physicians. You discuss your knowledge about issues in malpractice litigation and voice concern about turning off the alerts without discussion with the legal health record and quality management committees. The IT staff do not consider this a problem and continue with the plan to turn off the alerts.

Instructions: Answer the following questions on a separate piece of paper.

1. Using the American Health Information Management Association Code of Ethics, available at http://www.ahima.org/about/ethicscode.aspx, discuss your ethical obligations in this situation.

2. Describe your responsibility to discuss the IT committee's action with the legal health record committee.

3. Describe your responsibility to discuss the IT committee's action with the quality management committee.

4. Should you contact the chief information officer directly?

5. Is it necessary to report this to your immediate supervisor or manager?

⊙ Summary

Throughout this chapter the ways that electronic DSSs impact the healthcare environment have been examined. A CDSS along with the rich administrative data in data repositories can benefit many decisions in a healthcare system. However, it is known that potential unintended consequences of implementing new systems affect individual autonomy, workflow, and clinical decisions. The impact of the DSS includes a partnership with patients. A benefit of a CDSS and DSS can be a reduction in risk in compliance and legal issues. But if alerts and reminders, for example, are ignored, an increase in risk may occur. The balance of individual critical thinking and KM tools through decision support continue to influence the role of the informatician in healthcare.

REFERENCES

AHIMA. 2011. Fundamentals of the legal health record and designated record set. *Journal of AHIMA* 82(2). Chicago: AHIMA Press. http://library.ahima.org/xpedio/groups/public/documents/ahima/bok1_048604.hcsp?dDocName=bok1_048604.

Ash, J., D. Sittig, E. Poon, K. Guappone, E. Campbell, and R. Dyskstra. 2007. The extent and importance of unintended consequences related to computerized provider order entry. *Journal of the American Medical Informatics Association* 14(4):415–423. doi:10.1197/jamia.M2373.

Berner, E. 2009. Clinical Decision Support Systems: State of the Art. Agency for Healthcare Research and Quality. Rockville, MD. Publication number: 09-0069-EF.

Berner, E.S. 2002. Ethical and legal issues in the use of clinical decision support systems. *Journal of Health Information Management* 16:4.

Blue Button. Veterans Health Administration. http://www.va.gov/bluebutton/.

Bronnert, J., B. Cassidy, S. Eichenwald-Maki, H. Eminger, J. Flanagan, M. Morsch, K. Peterson, K. Phibbs, P. Resnick, R. Schichilone, and G. Smith. 2011. CAC 2010-11 Industry Outlook and Resources Report. AHIMA.

Campbell, E., D. Sittig, K. Guappone, R. Dykstra, and J. Ash. 2007. Overdependence on technology: an unintended consequence of computerized provider order entry. *AMIA Annual Symposium Proceedings*, pp. 94–98.

Gill, J., Y.X. Chen, A. Grimes, and M. Klinkman. 2012. Using health record-based tools to screen for bipolar disorder in primary care patients with depression. *Journal of American Board of Family Medicine* 25:283–290. doi:10.3122/jabfm.2012.03.110217.

Haider, A. and P. Pronovost. 2011. Health information technology and the collection of race, ethnicity, and language data to reduce disparities in quality of care. *The Joint Commission Journal on Quality and Patient Safety* 37(10):435–436.

Hudak, S. and S. Sharkey. 2011. California Healthcare Foundation. Trendspotting: How IT Triggers Better Care in Nursing Homes. http://www.chcf.org/.

Jones, S.S., R. Koppel, M.S. Ridgely, T.E. Palen, S. Wu, and M.I. Harrison. 2011. *Guide to Reducing Unintended Consequences of Electronic Health Records Prepared by RAND Corporation Under Contract No. HHSA29020060001 71, Task Order #5*. Rockville, MD: Agency for Healthcare Research and Quality. http://www.ucguide.org/index.html.

Kawamoto, K. D. Lobach, H. Willard, and G. Ginsburg. 2009. A national clinical decision support infrastructure to enable the widespread and consistent practice of genomic and personalized medicine. *BMC Medical Informatics & Decision Making* 9:17. doi: 10:1186/1472-6947-9-17.

Kuperman, G.J., R. Diamente, V. Khatu, T. Chan-Kraushar, P. Stetson, A. Boyer, and M. Cooper. 2005. AMIA Annual Symp Proc. pp. 415–419 PMCID: PMC1560425.

LaTour, K.M., S. Eichenwald-Maki, and P. Oachs. 2013. *Health Information Management: Concepts, Principles, and Practice.* 4th ed. Chicago: AHIMA.

Lau, F. 2004. Toward a conceptual knowledge management framework in health. *Perspectives in Health Information Management* 1:8.

Lopez, L., A. Green, A. Tan-McGrory, R. King, and J. Betancourt. 2011. Bridging the digital divide in healthcare: The role of health information technology in addressing racial and ethnic disparities. *The Joint Commission Journal on Quality and Patient Safety* 37(10):437–445.3

Mendoza, M.C.B. 2010. HIM and the path to personalized medicine: Opportunities in the post-genomic era. *Journal of AHIMA* 81(11):38–42.

Orzano, J.A., C.R. McInerney, D. Scharf, A.F. Tallia, and B.F. Crabtree. 2008. A knowledge management model: Implications for enhancing quality in healthcare. *Journal of the American Society for Information Science & Technology* 59(3):489–505.

Osheroff, J.A, J.M. Teich, D. Levick, L. Saldana, F.T. Velasco, D.F. Sittig, K.M. Rogers, and R.A. Jenders. 2009. *Improving Outcomes with Clinical Decision Support: An Implementer's Guide.* 1st ed. Chicago: HIMSS.

United States Government. 2012. Food and Drug Administration Safety and Innovation Act. United States Code. http://www.gpo.gov/fdsys/pkg/BILLS-112s3187enr/pdf/BILLS-112s3187enr.pdf.

Woltmann, E., S. Wilkniss, A. Teachout, G. McHugo, R. Drake. 2011. Trial of an electronic decision support system to facilitate shared decision making in community mental health. *Psychiatric Services* 62(1). http://ps.psychiatryonline.org/article.aspx?articleID=102131.

RESOURCES

Agency for Healthcare Research and Quality. 2010. National Healthcare Disparities Report for 2009. Publication No. 10-0004. March. Washington, DC. Retrieved from http://www.ahrq.gov/research/findings/nhqrdr/nhdr09/nhdr09.pdf.

Ahmadian, L., M. van Engen-Verheul, F. Bakhshi-Raiez, N. Peek, R.Cornet, and N.F. de Keizer. 2011. The role of standardized data and terminological systems in computerized clinical decision support systems: Literature review and survey. *International Journal of Medical Informatics* 80(2):81–93. doi:10.1016/j.ijmedinf.2010.11.006.

Fossum, M., G. Alexander , M. Ehnfors, and A. Ehrenberg. 2011. Effects of a computerized decision support system on pressure ulcers and malnutrition in nursing homes for the elderly. *International Journal of Medical Informatics* 80:607–617. doi:10:1016/j.ijmedinf.2011.06.009.

Han, Y.Y., J.A. Carcillo, S.T. Venkataraman, R.S.B. Clark, S. Watson, T.C. Nguyen, H. Bayir, and R.A. Orr. 2005. Unexpected increased mortality after implementation of a commercially sold computerized physician order entry system. *Pediatrics* 116(6):1506–1512.

Kaplan, B. 2001. Evaluating informatics applications–Clinical decision support systems literature review. *International Journal of Medical Informatics* 64(1):15–37.

Kesselheim, A.S., K. Cresswell, S. Phansalkar, D.W. Bates, and A. Sheikh. 2011. ANALYSIS & COMMENTARY: Clinical decision support systems could be modified to reduce 'alert fatigue' while still minimizing the risk of litigation. *Health Affairs* 30:122310–2317.

Kohn, L.T., J.M. Corrigan, and M.S. Donaldson. 2001. Crossing the quality chasm: a new health system for the 21st century. Washington: Committee on Quality of Health Care in America, Institute of Medicine.

Learned Hand, J. *The T.J. Hooper*, 60 F.2d 737, 740 (2d Cir. 1932).

Osheroff, J.A., E.A. Pifer, D.F. Sittig, R.A. Jenders, and J.M. Teich. 2004. Clinical decision support implementers' workbook. Chicago: HIMSS. www.himss.org/cdsworkbook.

Smedley, B.D., A.Y. Stith, and A.R. Nelson. 2003. Institute of Medicine, Committee on Understanding and Eliminating Racial and Ethnic Disparities in Health Care. Unequal Treatment: Confronting Racial and Ethnic Disparities in Health Care. Washington: National Academies Press.

Data and Information Movement

By Susan H. Fenton

Learning Objectives

- Describe the history of health information exchange (HIE) in the United States
- List and define the different types of health information exchange organizational structures
- Explain the advantages and disadvantages of the different types of HIE consent models
- Analyze the issues and challenges encountered when securing provider and consumer acceptance of HIE
- Describe the difference between population and public health
- Discuss the use of HIE in relationship to Accountable Care Organizations

KEY TERMS

Accountable Care
   Organization (ACO)
Aggregated HIE
Data liquidity
Federated HIE
Health information exchange (HIE)
Interoperability

No-consent
Opt-out
Opt-out with exceptions
Opt-in
Opt-in with restrictions
Population health
Public health

⊙ Introduction

The increased adoption of electronic health records (EHRs) and other health information technology has resulted in ever-increasing amounts of health data and information. While this data and information is expected to be extremely useful and beneficial in the settings where created, the usefulness and benefits should increase if the data and information can be made available when and where they are needed.

The ubiquitous sharing of healthcare data and information was termed **data liquidity** by a group focusing on the need to think beyond EHRs (Penfield et al. 2009). They recommended two actions to improve the flow of healthcare information. First, the market needs to focus on **interoperability**, the ability of different systems to work together seamlessly. In health information, interoperability is expected to include transmitting the meaning of the data. The second action focused on the need for payment reform, so that participating providers are not penalized, but are rewarded for freely sharing health information (Penfield et al. 2009).

This chapter will explore the evolution of health information exchange (HIE) in the United States, its structural and organizational issues, efforts supporting national implementation in the United States, as well as provider and consumer perceptions. It will conclude with a discussion of the population health and public health benefits resulting from health information exchange.

The key to any "interoperability" or "health information exchange" is the existence of complete, publicly available standards. This chapter will not try to examine the many different technical standards that are evolving at a rapid pace. Readers are encouraged to refer to the latest ONC and CMS regulations and guidance, which can be accessed at the www.healthit.gov website.

⊙ Health Information Exchange

Health information exchange (HIE) is a term used both as a noun and verb. As a noun HIE refers to "an organization that supports, oversees, or governs the exchange of health-related information among organizations according to nationally recognized standards" (AHIMA 2012, 193). As a verb health information exchange refers to the actual "exchange of health information electronically between providers and others with the same level of interoperability, such as labs and pharmacies" (AHIMA 2012, 193). For the remainder of this chapter the word HIE will be used to refer to the organization while the words "health information exchange" will be used to refer to the action of exchanging the information.

Health information exchange is becoming commonplace in the United States since it was included in the provisions of the Health Information Technology for Economic and Clinical Health (HITECH) sections of the American Recovery and Reinvestment Act (ARRA) (US Government 2009). The legislation is being implemented via the Centers for Medicare and Medicaid Services EHR Incentive Program, which pays providers for their meaningful use (MU) of EHR technology. The plan for MU included the articulation of three stages so that providers could adopt EHRs and increase the functionality and interoperability over time. Stage 1 of

MU requires providers to have the ability to perform health information exchange (HHS 2010). Stage 2 of MU increases the requirements for health information exchange in multiple ways. Eligible providers (EPs) will need to participate in generating and transmitting prescriptions electronically; provide patients with the online ability to view, download, and transmit their health information; submit electronic data to immunization registries; and use secure electronic messaging to communicate with patients on relevant health information (CMS 2012). The Stage 3 requirements are in development. However, even beyond Stage 3, it is expected that the requirements and standards will continue to evolve. Health information professionals will need to monitor federal regulations related to EHR interoperability standards.

The Office of the National Coordinator for Health Information Technology (ONC) is providing assistance for establishing HIEs with the State Health Information Exchange Cooperative Agreement Program. Using this funding mechanism ONC is supporting "states' efforts to rapidly build capacity for exchanging health information across the health care system both within and across states" (ONC, DHHS, 2012). This section will discuss health information exchange; the history, challenges, and clinical and financial benefits; provider and consumer perceptions; as well as anticipated future efforts.

History of HIE

Health information exchange was not first conceived in the HITECH legislation. In fact, networks titled community health management information systems (CHMISs) were first established in 1990 through grants from the Hartford Foundation (Vest and Gamm 2010). CHMISs focused on the development of a centralized repository of clinical, demographic, and eligibility data. They experienced significant obstacles as they preceded the advent of widespread, reasonably priced, standards-based high-speed Internet access. Expensive hardware, software, and network connections were required for CHMISs, the lack of data standardization was an obstacle, and both patients and providers expressed privacy concerns (Vest and Gamm 2010).

A few years later saw the emergence of community health information networks (CHINs). These commercial initiatives focused on financial savings, with little emphasis on the public health benefits that might accrue. CHINs encountered problems when competitors limited the data sharing functionality to prevent any perceived loss of competitive advantage, the ability of vendors to charge fees, and differences in the fees charged different participants raised questions regarding any financial benefits (Vest and Gamm 2010). The main lesson from CHINs was that the benefits could not be assigned to one small group (in this instance, providers); they must be spread and shared across the healthcare industry.

The late 1990s and 2000s saw the rise of the regional health information organization (RHIO) in the healthcare industry. RHIOs are the immediate precursor to the HIE. An RHIO is a neutral, third-party organization that facilitates information exchange between providers within a geographical area. The obstacles to RHIO success were less about the technology. These organizations continued to experience problems identifying a sustainable business model, assuring privacy and security of the data, and overcoming the issue of competitor distrust. These same problems exist for HIEs today.

However, as previously stated, the HITECH legislation and MU regulations now mandate HIE functionality and its use. Researchers have proposed the following considerations for the continued development of US HIEs. They include

- ⊙ Adoption of an improved business model—perhaps with the increased use of quality incentives.
- ⊙ Acknowledgement of the public health benefits of health information exchange—this might include improved registries for chronic conditions and much better biosurveillance.
- ⊙ Monitoring of health information exchange activities so both providers and consumers trust that private health information is private and secure.
- ⊙ The setting of state borders as the standard geographical unit for HIEs (now operationalized by ONC). (Vest and Gamm 2010).

Structure and Adoption

Health information exchanges can have different technical and organizational structures. Given their history, no one clearly superior structure has emerged. It is reasonable to presume that HIE operations will become standardized in the future; however, the industry is still evolving related to HIEs.

Structure

There are two main technological approaches to HIEs. The first is an **aggregated HIE**. The aggregated HIE combines all of the data into a centralized repository with a master patient index (MPI) or record locator service. The different HIE participants query, or send a request to, the repository to obtain demographic, clinical, or other information (Hess 2011). It is easy to see how the aggregated HIE might be preferred by persons or local governments trying to maximize the public health benefits of HIEs; however, they present greater risks to the privacy and security of data. All of the data, some of it very detailed and potentially sensitive, must flow to the centralized repository.

The second type of HIE model is a **federated HIE**. Federated HIEs are designed as provider-to-provider networks using the Internet for connectivity, with no central repository of data (Hess 2011). A central entity maintains the MPI or record locator service, which is used to determine where patients have been treated previously and where their health information might exist. Providers send requests for data information directly to other providers. This type of arrangement may require an additional step; however, given the distributed maintenance of the data it is viewed as having stronger privacy and security protection.

The technical structure of the HIE is separate from the organizational structure of the HIE. HIEs tend to be one of three types: public, cooperative, or private. Public HIEs are entirely supported by state government agencies or are semi-independent, with governmental financial backing (Hess 2011). There is some consideration of HIEs as a public good, much as the road system (Vest and Gamm 2010). The case for the long-term governmental support of HIEs is, unfortunately, not an easy one to make. However, there are natural disasters, such as Hurricane Katrina, or epidemics, such as the outbreak of H1N1 (avian) flu, which support the public health benefit claims.

Cooperative HIEs arise when relationships are formed for the purpose of exchanging information between what are otherwise competing healthcare providers (Hess 2011). Sometimes these HIEs struggle with financial viability and sometimes they are quite successful. Often the difference rests on the community or geographical region's concerns. For example, hospitals in Austin, Texas came together to form the Integrated Care Collaborative (ICC). The original goal was to address mutual concerns related to "drug shopping" and the excessive use of area emergency rooms (ERs). Since all of the hospitals with ERs could easily see potential financial advantages, they agreed to contribute money to establish the HIE. The ICC has received governmental funding under the HITECH initiatives and is expanding its operations to other providers.

The third HIE model is the private HIE. This type involves a single, integrated delivery system (IDS) that connects all of its different providers with an "internal" HIE. One example is the Veterans Health Administration (VHA). For years VHA had aggregated their patient data; however, as the World War II veterans aged and began retiring or spending large parts of each year in different regions of the country, the need to transmit or exchange the data became a high priority. Over a decade or more VHA established the data and other standards that allowed them to be a pioneer in health information exchange. They are now undertaking efforts to include non-VHA data from non-VHA providers in their health information exchange efforts.

One additional, very important, aspect of structure and management for an HIE is the consent option chosen. Each HIE must determine how patients and consumers will consent or not consent to have their data and information transmitted by or included in HIE operations. A white paper prepared for the Texas Health Services Authority describes five generally accepted models for defining patient consent to participate in an HIE (Gray 2011). Each will be described here with the main points for each option described in table 8.1.

The **no-consent** model does not require any agreement on the part of the patient to participate in an HIE. HIEs that have adopted this model operate in states that explicitly allow this model via legislation. The major benefit of this option is that providers can be more certain that any data and information they are receiving is complete. This ensures they are not trying to make clinical decisions using incomplete data. However, this consent option does not mean patients have no rights. The HIEs using this option usually allow consumers to deny access to their data and information even if it is technically included in the HIE. This is the easiest consent option to administer as patients and consumers must take action to deny access. Providers must include the fact that they participate in an HIE in their Health Insurance Portability and Accountability Act (HIPAA) Notice of Privacy Practices that patients receive at their first visit (Gray 2011).

The **opt-out** model allows for a predetermined set of data to be automatically included in an HIE, but a patient may still deny access to information in the exchange. This model allows the consumer to prevent their data and information from inclusion in the HIE. Inclusion or exclusion is all or nothing for this option, that is, either all of the patient's information is included or it is all excluded. Issues to address in this model include the following:

⊙ Who will collect the necessary information for patients to opt out?

⊙ How will the opt-out information be communicated to the HIE and to other providers?

⊙ What processes can be implemented to handle cases where a patient changes his mind (Gray 2011)?

The **opt-out with exceptions** model makes the patient's information available in the exchange, but enables the patient to selectively exclude data from an HIE, limit information to specific providers, or limit exchange of information to exchange for specific purposes (Gray 2011). While this option is understandably attractive to patients, it is not yet clear how to implement this model from a technical standpoint, that is, it is very resource intensive. As well as raising questions about the completeness of the data, this option presents many of the challenges the opt-out model does (Gray 2011).

The **opt-in** model requires patients to specifically affirm their desire to have their data made available for exchange within an HIE. This option provides up-front control for patients since their data cannot be included unless they have agreed. Disadvantages of the opt-in model are primarily the administrative complexity of implementing such an approach. Issues the HIE must address include the following:

⊙ Who will obtain the consent?

⊙ Will one consent suffice for participation in the system as a whole or must each provider obtain consent for his or her own patients?

⊙ What process will be used to communicate the patient's consent?

⊙ What happens if a patient wants to withdraw his consent? Can his data be removed from the HIE or will the withdrawal of consent only be effective for data developed after the withdrawal of consent was given (Gray 2011)?

The **opt-in with restrictions** model allows patients to make all or some defined amount of their data available for electronic exchange. Patients may restrict how their data is used by allowing access only to specific providers, by allowing only specific data elements to be included, or by allowing data to be accessed only for specific purposes (Gray 2011).

As of this writing there is no single mandated consent option for HIE implementation. It is imperative that HIEs choose wisely as the ease of provider implementation, as well as consumer confidence in the HIE, may be impacted by the option chosen.

As will be explored, many HIEs in the United States have begun with governmental support and are trying to develop sustainable business models

Table 8.1   Health information exchange consent options

OPTION	PROS	CONS
No-consent model: does not require any agreement on the part of the patient Unknown: Notice requirements to patients; interface with an HIE requiring consent	Easier to administer; addresses provider concerns about incomplete information	Lack of patient control
Opt-out: a predetermined set of data are automatically included, unless the patient "opts-out" or denies access to the information.	Automatic inclusion of data for more complete data for providers, yet patients can restrict use	Procedures for documenting opt-out so providers know about it are unclear
Opt-out with exceptions: patient can choose level of participation. • Selective exclusion of personal health information (PHI) • Limited to certain providers • Limited to exchange for certain purposes	Much more patient control	Very, very difficult to implement
Opt-in: patients choose to include their data in an HIE. It is an all-in or all-out choice.	Patient has complete, up-front control; provides an opportunity to educate patients; may provide better record matching	Obtaining and communicating consent; questions as to how consent be revoked or withdrawn
Opt-in with restrictions: patient agrees up front, but can determine which data is shared, which providers can access it, or the purposes for which it can be accessed.	Patient control up front and very detailed	Very, very difficult to manage

using a combination of public and private support. The extent to which these efforts will be successful remains to be determined. As with all things in health information technology, HIEs are evolving quickly, sometimes in unexpected ways.

Adoption

The adoption of HIEs is now a part of the national initiatives to help healthcare adopt 21st century information technology. Specifically, as stated previously, the HITECH legislation provided funding for the State Health Information Exchange Cooperative Agreement Program (ONC, DHHS 2013). This section will explore levels of adoption of HIEs, how HIEs are used, as well as costs, benefits, and evaluation, concluding with the expected interaction between the states and the federal health information exchange.

Thanks in large part to federal funding, research over the years reveals ever-increasing levels of adoption, with the number of HIEs increasing from 35 to 44 over a 17-month period (Adler-Milstein et al. 2009, 2011). Given the difficulty of initiating these activities, this 25 percent increase is significant. However, these and other surveys of operational HIEs reveal a continued concern regarding sustainability and financial viability, with questions about clinical benefits remaining.

Overall, HIEs at the federal and state levels are focusing on a public-private collaborative structure. Although the National Health Information Network (NHIN) was established and supported by the Office of the National Coordinator, management of national health information exchange efforts was transferred to Healtheway, Inc. on October 10, 2012. Healtheway, Inc. states it is "is a community of public and private exchange partners who share information based upon a shared set of 'rules of the road' and a trust agreement, called the Data Use and Reciprocal Support Agreement (DURSA)" (Healtheway, Inc. 2012). State HIEs will become members of Healtheway, Inc., which will establish and support a portfolio of nationwide health information network standards, services, and policies (Healtheway, Inc. 2012). As technical standards, policies, and procedures are constantly changing, the reader is directed to the ONC website for the most up-to-date information.

The fact that HIE has been mandated as a significant part of MU and it is supported by funding does not provide one with any information regarding usage of the HIE, or financial or clinical benefits. Usage refers to the manner in which providers utilize HIEs. It is important to understand how HIEs are used within clinician workflow to continue to improve functionality and value. The most common type of HIE use is "encounter-based" (Vest et al. 2012). Studies have shown HIEs are often queried for information when patients are seen in clinics and report a history of other clinical care such as a physician visit or hospital stay (Frisse et al. 2012; Vest et al. 2012). Both studies reported unanticipated impacts upon workflow. For example, the Frisse research team found clinicians reporting additional work when sorting through their clinical data, the data from the HIE, and any paper forms (Frisse et al. 2012). Organizational factors rather than the HIE technology may impact use. For example, if the emergency department is not fully staffed the personnel may not take the time to query the HIE. Yet another study found that usage varied by user and workplace setting. Physicians and others under significant time pressures used the system less than nurses, public health, and other workers (Vest and Jasperson 2012). As with other new technologies, effective incorporation of HIE data and the processes for health information exchange into the delivery of high-quality healthcare will need to develop over time.

Evaluation of the use and utility of health information exchange is imperative as the country continues to implement them. One researcher who performed a meta-analysis summarized his findings with the statement "The extent of clinical HIE benefits to date is dependent upon the context of the HIE" (Joshi 2011). For example, though a community such as Austin, Texas might reap significant benefits by tracking patient usage of ERs via an HIE, the physicians in the ER actually see an increase in their work or, at the least, experience a potential delay in the timing of care delivery. Likewise, the benefit of the surveillance of epidemic or outbreaks is related to the size of the exchange system (Joshi 2011). HIEs can be used to improve patient care or it can have little impact upon patient care. Implementation and context makes a difference.

The relationship between cost savings and utilization of health information exchange is difficult to understand. One study did quantify an annual savings of $1.07 million in an emergency department utilizing health information exchange (Frisse et al. 2012). This is particularly noteworthy since other studies have been quick to point out that the perverse incentives in the US healthcare industry payment models have providers paying for HIT implementation and health information exchange efforts, while patients and payors reap the efficiency (financial) and quality benefits (Pevnick et al. 2012).

Development and evolution of HIEs is likely to continue for the foreseeable future. The final structures, technical and organizational, along with ultimate clinical and financial benefits, remain to be determined.

Stakeholder Perceptions

The ultimate success or failure of HIEs is dependent upon two important factors: (1) providers or users accessing the HIE and using the data and information; and (2) patients or consumers allowing their data and information to be transmitted across the HIE. This section will explore these factors.

Providers or Users

HIEs do not operate in a vacuum and must be supported by the healthcare organizations in a geographical region for success. Aside from the national mandate, health information exchange implementation will be more successful if the organizations believe it can bring value to themselves and their constituents. The value may be in the form of financial benefits, such as reduced duplicative laboratory testing, or enhancing the organizational reputation for technology use that contributes to the quality of patient care. Conversely, the organization may have concerns such as legal liability or loss of competitive advantage.

Of course, within each organization participating in an HIE are the users who must access the HIE in order for the benefits to be achieved. As described above, the HIE is either a central data repository of existing patient data or an index linked to historical patient data. Thus, any provider wishing to access data must request it from the HIE. It is important to understand how users, the physicians and nurses who use the HIE in their day-to-day work, feel about HIEs.

Similar to organizational stakeholders, clinicians perceive significant positive value from an HIE. In particular, clinicians noted benefits with HIE participation including better decision making, improved treatment planning, enhanced medication tracking, and an enriched physician-patient relationship (Hincapie et al. 2011). Given that HIEs are still evolving, many do not transmit or share complete EHR data. A consistent clinician request was for additional information to be included in the HIE (Gadd et al. 2011; Hincapie et al. 2011). One study focused on analyzing usage to evaluate HIE utility. As might be expected with most systems, usage ranged from minimal to intensive, sometimes dependent upon the setting, sometimes dependent upon the type of user (Vest and Jasperson 2012). The main take-away is that HIEs are similar to other HIT and will require human factors analysis and studies of usability to maximize utility.

The perceptions of organizational and provider participants in HIEs are important and will play an important role in their success or failure. The potential benefits in terms of patient health management are expected to accrue to society or geographical regions.

Consumer Perceptions

Consumers and patients must agree to participate and have their data included in HIEs in order for them to be successful. In some ways it seems odd that this might even be a concern. After all, many consumers use social media, such as Facebook, to share intimate personal information. Similarly, they use mobile banking and shop online, as well as using other advanced technologies that puts their data out on the Internet. However, health data and information is considered to be sensitive, especially if it is related to conditions such as substance abuse, addiction, or sexually transmitted diseases. That said, easing access to health information and even moving it across cities, regions, and countries could be of significant benefit to patients.

As stated previously, the Stage 2 MU standards have an increased emphasis on engaging consumers in their healthcare, with criteria calling for providers to offer patients ability to view, download, and transmit their health information online and to use secure electronic messaging to communicate with patients on relevant health information (CMS 2012). These requirements are consistent with findings that 51 percent of consumers trust their physicians' practice over a health plan, hospital, or the government to regulate the privacy and security of their electronic health information (Dhopeshwarkar et al. 2012). In a different study more than 75 percent indicated they might use personal health record (PHR) services to manage their electronic information with more than 80 percent supporting the electronic sharing of health information via an HIE (Patel et al. 2012). Between 78 and 80 percent of cancer patients, who often require sustained continuing care, perceived patient information access to their own records, as well as the sharing of information between providers, to be important functionality for EHRs (Beckjord et al. 2011). The consistent, most important concern for these various consumers was the privacy and security of their data and information (Dhopeshwarkar et al. 2012; Beckjord et al. 2011; Dimitropoulos et al. 2011; Patel et al. 2012). Chapter 13 of this book covers consumer informatics thoroughly; however, these findings demonstrate that consumers understand the benefits and are willing to be involved if the tools are available.

Check Your Understanding 8.1

Instructions: Match the HIE consent terms with the appropriate descriptions.

a. No Consent
b. Opt-in
c. Opt-in with exceptions
d. Opt-out
e. Opt-out with exceptions

1. _____ Data are automatically included though the patient can limit the data to specific types.

2. _____ Does not require any agreement on the part of the patient.

3. _____ Data are automatically included unless the patient chooses not to participate at all.

4. _____ Patient agrees up front, but can limit the data included.

5. _____ Patients choose to include their data in an HIE. It is an all-in or all-out choice.

Instructions: Answer the following question on a separate piece of paper.

6. Discuss the different issues and concerns providers and patients might have related to HIEs.

⊙ Aggregating Health Information

As described in the previous section, moving health information between providers for healthcare benefits patients as they seek and receive care in a variety of settings. However, the need also exists to move the detailed information from EHRs into central locations, or aggregate it, for other purposes. This section will discuss the aggregation of patient health data or information for **population health** and for **public health**.

Population Health

Population health can be defined as the level and distribution of disease, functional status, and well-being of a defined group of people with specified characteristics (Friedman and Parrish 2010). The specified characteristics might be treatment by a given physician organization or admission to a given hospital with a defined time frame (Friedman and Parrish 2010). This differs from public health because public health usually refers to all of the inhabitants of a given neighborhood, city, region, state, country or the world. Population health is not usually charged with responsibility for vital statistics, but focuses on overall well-being of the specified group of people.

Population health initiatives are currently being pursued by healthcare organizations to meet the goals of the Medicare Accountable Care Organization regulations (CMS 2011). **Accountable Care Organization (ACO)** contracts issued under these regulations attempt to provide financial incentives for reductions in unnecessary treatment, such as procedures and hospitalizations, while ensuring quality outcomes improve (Gourevitch et al. 2012). An ACO is an organization of healthcare providers accountable for the quality, cost, and overall care of Medicare beneficiaries who are assigned and enrolled in the traditional fee-for-service program (AHIMA 2012, 9). Research has revealed that 80 percent of all diseases result from a combination of individual behavioral factors (smoking, physical activity, and so on), the environment (pollution, access to health food, and so on), and social factors (housing, education, and so on) (Hardcastle et al. 2011). Thus, prevention strategies such as smoking cessation and the promotion of physical activity within a given population can measurably improve the health of a given population. The ACO regulations reward providers for helping their populations make healthy choices while reducing the use of healthcare services (Gourevitch et al. 2012).

These developments are important for the health information management profession since HIM is likely to be the one charged with ensuring ACOs are able to aggregate and use the organizational healthcare data as needed. This might mean activities such as establishing a centralized data warehouse or virtual data locator service; ensuring that all of the necessary data elements are standardized; protecting the privacy and security of the aggregated patient data; assuring the quality of the data; and, not least, manipulating and presenting the patient data to clinicians who provide the care and those who make the organizational decisions. In short, aggregated patient information is vital to population health and the success of the CMS ACOs.

Public Health

Public health exists at many different levels in healthcare. At its broadest, the World Health Organization (WHO) promulgates the International Classification of Diseases (ICD) to track the causes of mortality and morbidity across the entire planet. This is not as academic as it might seem since new strains of influenza emerge each year, HIV originated in the twentieth century, and traveling across the globe within hours makes it possible to spread disease in a very short time. Each country, in turn, performs its own public health surveillance, usually required by law. States and usually counties and large cities also have public health systems, which may have separate requirements. Generally, the requirements include a predefined list of notifiable diseases or treatments such as immunizations that healthcare providers must report to healthcare authorities. Figure 8.1 is the list of notifiable diseases, conditions, treatments, or laboratory results required to be reported to the US Centers for Disease and Control. This reporting is essential to

Figure 8.1   List of conditions, diseases, treatments, and laboratory results reported to the CDC

CSTE List of Nationally Notifiable Conditions
August 2012

This list indicates the nationally notifiable conditions for which health departments provide information to CDC. It specifies the manner and time frame in which the health department notifiies CDC. Local requirements for reporting to public health by healthcare providers, laboratorians and others generally include these conditions but may require reporting of additional diseases, syndromes or findings and may specify different time frames. For information on local reporting requirements, contact the city, county or state health department.

IMMEDIATE, EXTREMELY URGENT - Notification within 4 hours

Call CDC EOC at 770-488-7100 within 4 hours; follow-up with electronic transmission of report by the next business day

CONDITION	CASES REQUIRING NOTIFICATION
Anthrax	
Source of infection not recognized	Confirmed and probable cases
Recognized BT exposure/potential mass exposure	Confirmed and probable cases
Serious illness of naturally-occurring anthrax	Confirmed and probable cases
Botulism	
Foodborne (except endemic to Alaska)	All cases prior to classification
Intentional or suspected intentional release	All cases prior to classification
Infant botulism (clusters or outbreaks)	All cases prior to classification
Cases of unknown etiology/not meeting standard notification criteria	All cases prior to classification
Plague	
Suspected intentional release	All cases prior to classification
Paralytic poliomyelitis	Confirmed cases
SARS - associated coronavirus	All cases prior to classification
Smallpox	Confirmed and probable cases
Tularemia	
Suspected intentional release	All cases prior to classification
Viral Hemorrhagic Fevers*	
Suspected intentional	Confirmed and suspected cases

IMMEDIATE, URGENT - Notification within 24 hours

Call CDC EOC at 770-488-7100 within 24 hours; follow-up with report in next regularly scheduled electronic transmission

CONDITION	CASES REQUIRING NOTIFICATION
Anthrax	
Naturally-occurring or occupational, responding to treatment	Confirmed and probable cases
Brucellosis	
Multiple cases, temporally/spatially clustered	Confirmed and probable cases
Diphtheria	All cases prior to classification
Novel influenza A virus infection, initial detections of	Confirmed cases
Measles	Confirmed cases
Poliovirus infection, nonparalytic	Confirmed cases
Rabies in a human	Confirmed cases
Rabies in an animal	
Imported from outside continental US within past 60 days	Confirmed cases
Rubella	Confirmed cases
Viral hemorrhagic fevers*	
All cases other than suspected intentional	Confirmed and suspected cases
Yellow Fever	Confirmed and probable cases

STANDARD - Notification by electronic transmission

Submit within the next normal reporting cycle (i.e., within 7 days for NNDSS conditions)

CONDITION	CASES REQUIRING NOTIFICATION
Anaplasmosis	Confirmed and probable cases
Arboviral disease (Calif. serogroup, EEE, Powassan, SLE, WNV, WEE)	Confirmed and probable cases
Babesiosis	Confirmed and probable cases
Botulism	
Infant, sporadic cases	All cases prior to classification
Wound, sporadic cases	All cases prior to classification
Brucellosis	
Cases not temporally/spatially clustered	Confirmed and probable cases
Cancer	Confirmed cases[†]
Chancroid	Confirmed and probable cases
***Chlamydia trachomatis* infection**	Confirmed cases
Coccidioidomycosis	Confirmed cases
Cryptosporidiosis	Confirmed and probable cases
Cyclosporiasis	Confirmed and probable cases

(Continued)

Figure 8.1   List of conditions, diseases, treatments, and laboratory results reported to the CDC (*Continued*)

STANDARD - Notification by electronic transmission	
Submit within the next normal reporting cycle (i.e., within 7 days for NNDSS conditions)	
CONDITION	**CASES REQUIRING NOTIFICATION**
Dengue virus infections	Confirmed, probable and suspect cases
Ehrlichiosis	Confirmed and probable cases
Escherichia coli , Shiga toxin-producing (STEC)	Confirmed and probable cases
Foodborne disease outbreaks	Confirmed outbreaks[‡]
Giardiasis	Confirmed and probable cases
Gonorrhea	Confirmed and probable cases
Haemophilus influenzae, invasive disease	All cases prior to classification
Hansen's disease	Confirmed cases
Hantavirus pulmonary syndrome	Confirmed cases
Hemolytic uremic syndrome, post-diarrheal	Confirmed and probable cases
Hepatitis A, acute	Confirmed cases
Hepatitis B, acute	Confirmed cases
Hepatitis B, chronic	Confirmed and probable cases
Hepatitis B, perinatal infection	Confirmed cases
Hepatitis C, acute	Confirmed cases
Hepatitis C infection, past or present	Confirmed and probable cases
HIV Infection	Confirmed cases of HIV infection; perinatally exposed infants prior to classification
Influenza-associated mortality, pediatric	Confirmed cases
Lead, exposure screening test result	All test results[#]
Legionellosis	Confirmed and suspected cases
Leptospirosis	Confirmed and probable cases
Listeriosis	Confirmed cases
Lyme disease	Confirmed, probable and suspect cases
Malaria	Confirmed and suspected cases
Meningococcal disease (*Neisseria meningitidis*)	Confirmed and probable cases
Mumps	Confirmed and probable cases
Pertussis	All cases prior to classification
Pesticide-related illness, acute	Definite, probable, possible and suspicious cases
Plague	
All cases not suspected to be intentional	All cases prior to classification
Psittacosis	Confirmed and probable cases
Q Fever	Confirmed and probable cases
Rabies in an animal	
Animal not imported within past 60 days	Confirmed cases
Rickettsiosis, Spotted Fever	Confirmed and probable cases
Rubella, congenital syndrome	Confirmed cases
Salmonellosis	Confirmed and probable cases
Shigellosis	Confirmed and probable cases
Silicosis	Confirmed cases
Staphylococcus aureus infection	
Vancomycin-intermediate (VISA)	Confirmed cases
Vancomycin-resistant (VRSA)	Confirmed cases
Streptococcus pneumoniae , invasive disease (IPD)	Confirmed cases
Streptococcal toxic shock syndrome (STSS)	Confirmed and probable cases
Syphilis	Confirmed and probable cases
Tetanus	All cases prior to classification
Toxic shock syndrome (non-Strep)	Confirmed and probable cases
Trichinellosis (Trichinosis)	All cases prior to classification
Tuberculosis	Confirmed cases
Tularemia	
All cases other than suspected intentional release	Confirmed and probable cases
Typhoid Fever	Confirmed and probable cases
Varicella	Confirmed and probable cases
Vibrio cholerae infection (Cholera)	Confirmed cases
Vibriosis	Confirmed and probable cases
Waterborne disease outbreaks	All outbreaks[‡]

*Notifiable viral hemorrhagic fevers include those caused by Ebola or Marburg viruses, Lassa virus, Lujo virus, or new world Arenaviruses (Guanarito, Machupo, Junin, Sabia), and Crimean-Congo hemorrhagic fever

† Notification for all confirmed cases of cancer should be made at least annually

Notification for lead exposure screening results should be submitted quarterly for children and twice a year for adults

‡ Outbreaks are defined by state and local health departments, all situations deemed by a local or state health department to be an outbreak are notifiable

Source: CSTE 2012.

maintaining the public health whether through outbreaks of diseases such as H1N1 (avian) flu or fungal meningitis contracted by patients across the country after being treated with tainted medicine.

Historically, public health data reporting was done via entirely separate systems, such that hospitals reported with one format using one system, while physicians reported using entirely separate methods (Shapiro et al. 2011). Eleven potential use cases have been identified where health information exchange can be used to improve public health (Shapiro et al. 2011). Each type of use case is listed here, along with more explanation of the benefits of health information exchange.

1. **Mandated Reporting of Laboratory Diagnoses:** The cornerstone of public health surveillance, this reporting is resource-intensive when performed manually. Electronic reporting is difficult if local modifications require initial and ongoing custom interfaces. An HIE could assist with transmission and standardizing message formats.

2. **Nonmandated Reporting of Laboratory Data:** Not all diseases that might have public health significance are required to be reported, for example, influenza and gastrointestinal illnesses. HIEs could be set up to cooperate with the appropriate health authorities to support improved illness and prevention efficacy tracking.

3. **Mandated Reporting of Physician-Based Diagnoses:** As stated above, physician reporting is separate from laboratory and hospital reporting. Further, compliance ranges anywhere from 9 percent to 99 percent dependent upon the disease, provider training, and provider perception of the benefits. Effective use of HIE could ease the reporting burden on physicians while greatly increasing its reliability and validity.

4. **Nonmandatory Reporting of Clinical Data:** HIE could assist with syndromic surveillance monitoring of nonreportable, nondiagnostic data such as the chief complaints from emergency departments or sales of over-the-counter medicines. Combined with reportable data and analyzed using the latest software, public health authorities could detect and address outbreaks earlier and more effectively.

5. **Public Health Investigation:** Public health authorities often become aware of cases that require investigation. With the availability of HIE these authorities could use their legislated authority to perform these investigations.

6. **Clinical Care in Public Health Clinics:** In some jurisdictions public health authorities are required to provide healthcare. Having access to an HIE would enable these providers to access patient data needed for clinical care purposes.

7. **Population-Level Quality Monitoring:** A regional HIE that included all of the providers of a region (not an ACO) could measure the quality of care delivered to members of the community, as well as the relevant outcomes.

8. **Mass-Casualty Events:** If the HIE were designed to receive ongoing admission-discharge-transfer messages from registration systems, local disaster authorities could be empowered to allow designated centers to query the HIE in response to requests from families and loved ones of persons who are missing.

9. **Disaster Medical Response:** The VHA was one of a handful of large healthcare providers with internal health information exchange that was utilized to make their patients' data available soon after Hurricane Katrina destroyed

the New Orleans physical infrastructure. Obviously, exchanging the data and having it exist in multiple locations results in redundancies that can be very beneficial in an emergency.

10. Public Health Alerting: Patient Level: The use of health information exchange could make it easier for the public health authorities to track and ensure patients with designated conditions, such as tuberculosis or antibiotic resistant organism infections, were tracked and treated appropriately when presenting for healthcare by new providers.

11. Public Health Alerting: Population Level: HIEs could assist with provider alerts related to outbreak trends or necessary preventive services. If patients were also allowed access to an HIE portal they could receive the same alerts and information for their given areas. This might help control the outbreak, spread, or prevention of selected diseases and conditions (Shapiro et al. 2011).

While some project the public health benefits of health information exchange use, others are documenting real benefits and change. One set of researchers determined that bidirectional health information exchange between public health and clinical practice could improve decision making and public health for infants with pertussis (Fine et al. 2010). Researchers in Louisiana sought to address the incidence of HIV/AIDS, using a bidirectional public health information exchange to facilitate the identification of patients with HIV/AIDS who had been lost to follow-up. When the patients reported to any ambulatory or inpatient facility, the clinicians were alerted to attempt to reengage the patients in clinical care. It was successful for 82 percent of the patients (Herwehe et al. 2012).

The studies just reviewed demonstrate that the theory of HIE use in public health can become the reality. With regulations and careful controls to prevent abuses of patient-level information, the use of health information exchange holds the promise of improved health and higher quality care for all citizens.

Check Your Understanding 8.2

Instructions: Choose the best answer.

1. The public health benefits of HIE are the same as the population health benefits of HIE.
   a. True
   b. False

2. Which of the following is NOT a potential public health benefit of HIE.
   a. Financial payment reform
   b. Disaster medical response
   c. Public health alerting
   d. Nonmandated reporting of laboratory data

Instructions: Match the population or public health use of data to the correct example.

   a. The Accountable Care Organization monitors whether smokers are receiving counseling
   b. Ensuring patients receive their critical medications after a tornado hits the city
   c. Confirmed cases of HIV must be reported to the Department of Health
   d. The schools are being notified that there is an influenza outbreak in the state

   _____Mandatory laboratory result reporting

   _____Population health monitoring

   _____Disaster medical response

   _____Public health alerts

⊙ Summary

It is impossible to deliver the best healthcare unless the right person has the right information at the right time. As with all advances in healthcare, the implementation of health information exchange will not always be easy or without challenges; however, it can benefit the entire healthcare system and all patients. HIEs will require that technical, organizational, and policy infrastructure be implemented across the nation. Financial sustainability, as well as privacy and security particularly will be significant challenges to widespread adoption of HIEs. Health information exchange is not only a requirement for the meaningful use of EHRs, it is also a necessary part of ACO management of population health, and it can be effectively used to improve public health. Health information is an asset that can be important for the public. The ability to move health information within and between organizations is essential for our future.

REFERENCES

Adler-Milstein, J., D.W. Bates, and A.K. Jha. 2009. U.S. regional health information organizations: Progress and challenges. *Health Affairs* 28(2):483–492. doi:10.1377/hlthaff.28.2.483.

Adler-Milstein, J, D.W. Bates, and A.K. Jha. 2011. A survey of health information exchange organizations in the United States: Implications for meaningful use. *Annals of Internal Medicine* 154(10):666–671.

AHIMA. 2012. Pocket Glossary for Health Information Management and Technology. 3rd ed. Chicago: AHIMA Press.

Beckjord, E., R. Rechis, S. Nutt, L. Shulman, and B. Hesse. 2011. What do people affected by cancer think about electronic health information exchange? Results from the 2010

LIVESTRONG Electronic Health Information Exchange Survey and the 2008 Health Information National Trends Survey. *Journal of Oncology Practice* 7(4):237–241. doi:10.1200/JOP.2011.000324.

Centers for Medicare and Medicaid Services. 2012. Electronic Health Record Incentive Program—Stage 2; Health Information Technology: Standards, Implementation Specifications, and Certification Criteria for Electronic Health Record Technology, 2014 Edition; Revisions to the Permanent Certification Program for Health Information Technology; Final Rules. *Code of Federal Regulations.* http://www.gpo.gov/fdsys/pkg/FR-2012-09-04/pdf/2012-21050.pdf.

Council of State and Territorial Epidemiologists. 2012. List of Nationally Notifiable Conditions. www.cste.org/resource/resmgr/PDFs/CSTENotifiableConditionListA.pdf.

Department of Health and Human Services. 2010. Health Information Technology: Initial Set of Standards, Implementation Specificaton and Certifcation Criteria for Electronic Health Record Technology. *Code of Federal Regulations.* http://edocket.access.gpo.gov/2010/pdf/2010-17210.pdf.

Dhopeshwarkar, R.V., L.M. Kern, H.C. O'Donnell, A.M. Edwards, and R. Kaushal. 2012. Health care consumers' preferences around health information exchange. *Annals of Family Medicine* 10(5):428–434.

Dimitropoulos, L., V. Patel, S. Scheffler, and S. Posnack. 2011. Public attitudes toward health information exchange: Perceived benefits and concerns. *American Journal of Managed Care* 17:SP111–6.

Fine, A.M., B.Y. Reis, L.E. Nigrovic, D.A. Goldmann, T.N. LaPorte, K.L. Olson, and K.D. Mandl. 2010. Use of population health data to refine diagnostic decision-making for pertussis. *Journal of the American Medical Informatics Association* 17(1):85–90. doi:10.1197/jamia.M3061.

Friedman, D.J., and R.G. Parrish. 2010. The population health record: Concepts, definition, design, and implementation. *Journal of the American Medical Informatics Association* 17(4):359–366. doi:10.1136/jamia.2009.001578.

Frisse, M.E., K.B. Johnson, H. Nian, C.L. Davison, C.S. Gadd, K.M. Unertl, P.A. Turri, and Q. Chen. 2012. The financial impact of health information exchange on emergency department care. *Journal of the American Medical Informatics Association* 19(3):328–333. doi:10.1136/amiajnl-2011-000394.

Frisse, M.E. 2010. Health information exchange in Memphis: Impact on the physician-patient relationship. *Journal of Law, Medicine & Ethics* 38(1):50–57. doi:10.1111/j.1748-720X.2010.00465.x.

Gadd, C.S., Y.X. Ho, C.M. Cala, D. Blakemore, Q. Chen, M.E. Frisse, and K.B. Johnson. 2011. User perspectives on the usability of a regional health information exchange. *Journal of the American Medical Informatics Association* 18(5):711–716. doi:10.1136/amiajnl-2011-000281.

Gourevitch, M.N., T. Cannell, J.I. Boufford, and C. Summers. 2012. The challenge of attribution: Responsibility for population health in the context of accountable care. *American Journal of Public Health* 102(S3):S322–S324. doi:10.2105/AJPH.2011.300642.

Gray, P. 2011. Consent Options for HIE in Texas. Houston, Texas: Texas Health Services Authority. http://hietexas.org/resources/policy-guidance.

Hardcastle, L., K. Record, P. Jacobson, and L. Gostin. 2011. Improving the population's health: The Affordable Care Act and the importance of integration. *Journal of Law, Medicine & Ethics* 39(3):317–327. doi:10.1111/j.1748-720X.2011.00602.x.

Healtheway, Inc. 2012. Home. http://healthewayinc.org/.

Herwehe, J, W. Wilbright, A. Abrams, S. Bergson, J. Foxhood, M. Kaiser, L. Smith, K. Xiao, A. Zapata, and M. Magnus. 2012. Implementation of an innovative, integrated electronic medical record (EMR) and public health information exchange for HIV/AIDS. *Journal of the American Medical Informatics Association* 19(3):448–452.

Hess, J. 2011. The brave, new world of HIEs. *Hfm (Healthcare Financial Management)* 65(2):44–48.

Hincapie, A.L., T.L. Warholak, A.C. Murcko, M. Slack, and D.C. Malone. 2011. Physicians' opinions of a health information exchange. *Journal of the American Medical Informatics Association* 18(1):60–65. doi:10.1136/jamia.2010.006502.

Joshi, J. 2011. "Clinical value-add for health information exchange (HIE)." *Internet Journal of Medical Informatics* 6(1):1.

Office of the National Coordinator, DHHS. 2013. HealthIT.hhs.gov: State Health Information Exchange Program. http://healthit.hhs.gov/portal/server.pt/community/healthit_hhs_gov__state_health_information_exchange_program/1488.

Patel, V., R. Dhopeshwarkar, A. Edwards, Y. Barrón, J. Sparenborg, and R. Kaushal. 2012. Consumer support for health information exchange and personal health records: A regional health information organization survey. *Journal of Medical Systems* 36(3):1043–1052. doi:10.1007/s10916-010-9566-0.

Penfield, S.L., K.M. Anderson, M. Edmunds, and M. Belanger. 2009. Toward Health Information Liquidity: Realization of Better, More Efficient Care From the Free Flow of Health Information. Booz Allen Hamilton. http://www.boozallen.com/media/file/Toward_Health_Information_Liquidity.pdf.

Pevnick, J., M. Claver, A. Dobalian, S. Asch, H. Stutman, A. Tomines, and P. Fu. 2012. Provider stakeholders' perceived benefit from a nascent health information exchange: A qualitative analysis. *Journal of Medical Systems* 36(2):601–613. doi:10.1007/s10916-010-9524-x.

Shapiro, J., F. Mostashari, G. Hripcsak, N. Soulakis, and G. Kuperman. 2011. Using health information exchange to improve public health. *American Journal of Public Health* 101(4):616–623. doi:10.2105/AJPH.2008.158980.

United States Government. 2009. American Recovery and Reinvestment Act of 2009. http://frwebgate.access.gpo.gov/cgi-bin/getdoc.cgi?dbname=111_cong_bills&docid=f:h1enr.pdf.

US Department of Health and Human Services, Centers for Medicare and Medicaid Services, Medicare Program. 2011. Medicare Shared Savings Program: Accountable Care Organizations, Final Rule. http://www.gpo.gov/fdsys/pkg/FR-2011-11-02/pdf/2011-27461.pdf.

Vest, J., L. Gamm, R. Ohsfeldt, H. Zhao, and J. Jasperson. 2012. Factors associated with health information exchange system usage in a safety-net ambulatory care clinic setting. *Journal of Medical Systems* 36(4):2455–2461. doi:10.1007/s10916-011-9712-3.

Vest, J. and J. Jasperson. 2012. "How are health professionals using health information exchange systems? Measuring usage for evaluation and system improvement. *Journal of Medical Systems* 36(5):3195–3204. doi:10.1007/s10916-011-9810-2.

Vest, J.R., and L.D. Gamm. 2010. Health information exchange: Persistent challenges and new strategies. *Journal of the American Medical Informatics Association* 17(3):288–294. doi:10.1136/jamia.2010.003673.

Chapter 9

Using Healthcare Data and Information

By Christopher G. Chute and Susan H. Fenton

Learning Objectives

- Describe the different secondary uses of healthcare data and information
- Define unstructured data and structured data
- Delineate how natural language processing is used to support secondary uses of healthcare data and information
- Explain the opportunities and challenges encountered when using unstructured data for secondary uses
- List and briefly define the major datasets, classification systems, clinical terminologies, and other standards utilized for secondary data use

KEY TERMS

Classification system
Clinical phenotyping
Comparable and consistent
Healthcare Common Procedure Coding System (HCPCS)
Linearizations
Logical Observation Identifiers Names and Codes (LOINC)
Morbidity
Mortality

Natural language processing (NLP)
Ontology
Primary data use
RxNorm
Secondary data use
SNOMED-CT
Structured data
Terminology
Unstructured data
Vocabulary

⊙ Introduction

There are two main ways to utilize healthcare data. The most common is **primary data use** for direct patient care. The other is **secondary data use**. Secondary use of health data is the "non-direct care use of personal health information (PHI)" (Safran et al. 2007). Most persons involved in the healthcare industry are familiar with secondary data use for purposes such as public health reporting, reimbursement, and quality improvement. Less known are purposes such as provider certification or accreditation; disease management; determining best practices or clinical guidelines; detecting financial fraud; monitoring patient compliance; and identifying candidates for clinical trials or using electronic health record (EHR) data for clinical trials. In fact, one of the phrases often heard these days is "collect once, use many" to describe healthcare data that is collected for patient care purposes and then used to meet a myriad of additional requirements. Organizations describe "big data" to convey the message that the widespread implementation of health information technology (HIT) has resulted in extraordinarily large and detailed databases being made available for secondary data use.

Secondary data use is not possible without data collection. This chapter begins by discussing unstructured and structured data entry, including the data standards currently in use and under development. The final section is a discussion of the secondary data use.

⊙ Unstructured Data

Unstructured data is free text or string data. This does not mean that there is no organization to the data, just that it is not structured with specific data elements, allowable values, and so on. Unstructured data might be organized into data fields or text boxes such as the history of present illness portion of a History and Physical or the Progress Note for the physician's hospital visit or it might be a Procedure Note. However, this organization only conveys very general meaning and is usually only relevant regarding the type of documentation one can expect to find. Inferring meaning and effective interoperability from native, unstructured data is difficult. Unstructured data is more difficult to use for secondary data uses precisely because of this. However, unstructured data is often preferred since it enables providers to document details and nuance that are usually not available with structured data. Examples of when unstructured data are used in healthcare documentation include most provider notes during a course of care, the history of an illness, the description of a procedure, or any situation where the number of different permutations is almost infinite.

Given the difficulties associated with unstructured data two questions naturally come to mind:

1. Why would one choose to use unstructured data?
2. If one uses unstructured data, how can it be used most effectively?

The short answer to the first question is that unstructured data contains the detail, in fact, the nuance, which is the "art" of medicine. The answer to the second question is the effective implementation of natural language processing.

Natural Language Processing (or Understanding)

Natural language processing (NLP) (or natural language understanding (NLU)) "is a technology that converts human language (structured or unstructured) into data that can be translated then manipulated by computer systems (AHIMA 2012, 283). Within the field of computer or information science, an **ontology** is a common vocabulary organized by meaning that allows for an understanding of the structure of descriptive information that facilitates a specific topic or domain (Giannangelo 2010).

NLP is a branch of artificial intelligence that uses computer algorithms and statistical probabilities to convert human free text into computer-readable forms and formats. The NLP processor or software receives the language and, if necessary, parses or separates it to help with the understanding. NLP programs have codified language structure and can often use the context of the word or sentence to help with the understanding. NLP has been in existence for a long time, only recently being refined to the point where it can be widely incorporated into everyday use and applications. Anyone who has used a smart phone with voice recognition assistance is using NLP. The more technical details of NLP are beyond this text; however, informaticians should be aware of the current uses and utility of NLP in healthcare.

A major use of NLP in healthcare is to support high-quality patient care. NLP was used to identify methicillin-resistant *Staphylococcus aureus* in Veterans Affairs Medical Centers over a 20-year period (Jones et al. 2012). Algorithms were developed that were able to determine tumor status from MRI reports at levels comparable to humans (Cheng et al. 2010). The methods developed in these and other studies will assist clinicians and researchers where needed data are inaccessible due to documentation methods or the data come from multiple, nonstandard, sources.

A related clinical use of NLP is for the discovery of point-of-care data. Previous research has revealed that clinicians have many questions each day which require knowledge-based answers (Ely 2004). Indeed, the provision of evidence-based support is one of the major tasks of today's EHRs. The resource most clinicians turn to when seeking health-related knowledge is MEDLINE, the index of medical literature citations created and maintained by the National Library of Medicine. However, while MEDLINE might be an extremely authoritative source of medical information, it is not easily used when clinicians are in a hurry when providing patient care.

Researchers are also using NLP for biosurveillance purposes within hospitals as well as across geographic regions or countries. A NLP tool was used to examine electronic emergency department (ED) patient records in an effort to identify patients who might carry community-acquired infections, thus posing an infection risk to other patients in the hospital (Gerbier et al. 2011). Other researchers focused on the ability of NLP to improve public health biosurveillance by identifying potential flu cases from encounter notes as opposed to the traditional chief complaint structured data fields (Elkin et al. 2012). This type of use of NLP is important to continued improvement in the timeliness of tracking diseases and providing adequate care as patients present for care.

NLP can also provide support in the administrative realms of healthcare, specifically for assigning the International Classification of Disease (ICD) and Current Procedural Terminology (CPT) codes required for payment for services. Studied for decades with varying degrees of success (Stanfill et al. 2010), computer-assisted coding (CAC) is experiencing widespread adoption as the United States implements ICD-10-CM/PCS and other more detailed standards for the effective use of EHRs (Hartman et al. 2012).

Unstructured data may be more difficult to use. Healthcare is just beginning to develop methods and procedures to use it accurately and appropriately; however, it is important to continue to allow and even encourage the use of unstructured data in healthcare. Unstructured data provides detail. When providers are forced to use structured data over unstructured data they are forced to make their clinical documentation fit into preconceived categories. Once this occurs the detail around the clinical event is lost forever. It can never be regained. Healthcare must develop methods and processes to convert unstructured data to structured data for secondary use purposes.

Check Your Understanding 9.1

Instructions: Choose the best answer.

1. NLP is used for which of the following?
   a. Tracking diseases and biosurveillance purposes
   b. Developing algorithms in support of high-quality patient care
   c. Providing knowledge-based answers for clinicians
   d. All of the above are uses of NLP

2. Primary data use is required for which of the following?
   a. Direct patient care
   b. Public health reporting
   c. Provider certification or accreditation
   d. Monitoring patient compliance

Instructions: Match the terms with the appropriate descriptions.

   a. Use of PHI for other than direct care
   b. Turns speech or text into computable data
   c. Common vocabulary organized by meaning that allows for understanding

1. _____ Ontology
2. _____ NLP
3. _____ Secondary data use

⊙ Coded and Structured Data

Structured data, also called discrete data, is binary, machine-readable data in discrete fields, with limitations on what can be entered into the field (LaTour et al. 2013, 951). Whether these data are in the form of specific, allowable text entries or numerical representations, they are preferred for the majority of secondary data uses. In and of itself, the use of structured data does not translate to automatic usability. Structured data comes in many different flavors and formats, some of which rise to the level of standards; others do not. Because healthcare is a very complex business, there are many concepts and ideas that must be accessed, combined, manipulated, and shared. Healthcare information systems use vocabularies, terminologies, and classification systems. A **vocabulary** is a dictionary of terms; that is, words and phrases with their meanings. A **terminology** is a set of terms representing a system of concepts, usually around a specific domain such as healthcare. Finally, a **classification system** arranges or organizes like or related entities (Giannangelo 2010). This section will explore code sets, classification systems, clinical terminologies, as well as other data set standards important to health informatics and the interoperability of health information. The discussion of value sets can be found in Chapter 5.

Healthcare Code Sets

Healthcare code sets are defined as "any set of codes used for encoding data elements, such as tables of terms, medical concepts, medical diagnostic codes, or medical procedure codes" (US Congress 1996). This very broad definition encompasses a wide array of different data types from demographics such as race, ethnicity, state, and country to very detailed clinical data elements such as clinical findings, procedures, or laboratory results. It is important for the array of code sets to be standardized so that data can be easily shared between organizations.

The Office of the National Coordinator (ONC) in the Department of Health and Human Services (HHS) is advised on HIT standards (including code sets) development and adoption by a federal advisory committee (FACA) known as "the HIT Standards Committee." One subgroup of the HIT Standards Committee is the Vocabulary Task Force, with the specific charge to "identify gaps, issues and needs for clinical and administrative vocabulary solutions within the scope of the HIT Standards Committee; to develop recommendations to the HIT Standards Committee for methods, actions, and/or programs to mitigate, manage, or solve these vocabulary concerns" (ONC, HHS 2013). The recommendations made by the HIT Standards Committee and its subgroups, if adopted, are ultimately included in the meaningful use EHR certification criteria. The remainder of this chapter will describe many of the different HIPAA and other code sets that have been adopted or are under consideration for adoption by the HIT Standards Committee.

Classification Systems

Classification systems have a wide range of uses in healthcare, including the collection and reporting of public health data; the design and administration of healthcare reimbursement systems; and the development and use of quality measures and other performance measures. Within the United States, the most commonly used classification system is the ICD.

International Classification of Diseases

Since 1999 the United States has used the tenth edition of the ICD (ICD-10) as developed by the World Health Organization (WHO) for **mortality** reporting, that is, for reporting the cause of death on death certificates. These mortality data are used to present the characteristics of those dying in the United States, determine life expectancy, and compare mortality trends with other countries. These are key indicators of the public health of a geographical region or country. Additional information on US mortality data can be found at http://www.cdc.gov/nchs/deaths.htm.

ICD-9-CM

The United States uses a derivative of the WHO version of ICD for reporting **morbidity**, diseases or conditions for which patients seek treatment. The US National Center for Health Statistics creates a "Clinical Modification" to provide additional detail. The ninth edition, ICD-9-CM, will be utilized in the United States for coding the diagnoses and conditions for all healthcare services provided through September 30, 2014. ICD-9-CM contains approximately 12,000 codes for diagnoses and 4,000 codes for inpatient procedures. Volume 1 of the ICD-9-CM is the Tabular List of diagnosis codes with the codes presented in their hierarchical arrangement. Volume 2 is the Alphabetic Index for the diagnosis conditions and injuries. Volume 3 of ICD-9-CM is for inpatient procedures and includes both the Tabular List and the Alphabetic Index.

The diagnosis codes are formatted with three digits before the decimal point and a maximum of two digits following the decimal point, or XXX.XX. The majority of the codes are entirely numeric, though an E or a V code may be used in the first position for two supplementary classifications. The ICD-9-CM procedure codes are formatted with two digits before the decimal point and a maximum of two digits following the decimal point, XX.XX. No alpha characters are used with the procedure codes. As with the diagnosis codes, the procedure codes are organized in a hierarchy. If a procedure cannot be found within the specified chapter, it might be in 00 – Procedures and Interventions, Not Elsewhere Classified. This section was added as the number of procedures utilized in healthcare has exceeded the available space in other sections.

ICD-9-CM codes are not just assigned as the different providers decide. The ICD-9-CM Coordination and Maintenance Committee is a FACA charged with maintaining and updating ICD-9-CM, as well as developing instructions and guidelines for consistent and accurate assignment of ICD-9-CM codes (CDC 2013a). The public committee meetings are held twice a year at the Centers for Medicare and Medicaid Services (CMS) Headquarters in Baltimore, MD. The ICD is a publicly created and publicly maintained classification system. As such, there are no licensing fees associated with its use.

Transition to ICD-10-CM/PCS

On October 1, 2014, the United States will officially adopt the tenth edition, ICD-10-CM, for all disease and injury coding in inpatient and outpatient healthcare settings (HHS 2012). On the same date ICD-10-PCS, the Procedural Coding System, will also be adopted for all procedures performed on inpatients (HHS 2012). Many countries have already made the transition to a version of ICD-10 for diagnostic coding within their healthcare system. Therefore, adopting ICD-10-CM/PCS will enable greater comparability between the United States and other countries, as well as within the United States between mortality and morbidity codes.

In developing ICD-10-CM, the United States implemented many structural and organizational changes, as well as greatly expanding the detail included in the system. The structural changes in ICD-10-CM include a total of 21 chapters (see table 9.1); expansion from a maximum of five digits to a maximum of seven digits (see figure 9.1); the inclusion of alpha characters as the initial digit for all codes and as a seventh digit code extension when applicable; and the use of a dummy placeholder X when necessary. The organizational changes include the incorporation of factors influencing health status and external causes (both supplemental in ICD-9-CM) into the main classification; the sense organs and nervous system disorders have been separated; injuries are now grouped by body part not injury type; the excludes notes have been moved to the beginning of each chapter; and postoperative complications are in the procedure-specific body system chapters. Finally, ICD-10-CM contains approximately 69,000 codes with additional detail such as laterality (when appropriate); expanded injury, diabetes, and complication codes; as well as a seventh character extension used to indicate initial encounter, subsequent encounter or sequelae, as appropriate. As with ICD-9-CM, users of ICD-10-CM will have some idea of what the code is representing by virtue of the structure of ICD-10-CM.

Unlike morbidity and mortality diagnostic reporting, which is led by the World Health Organization (WHO), no such international standard exists for procedures. Thus, CMS contracted with 3M Health Information Systems to develop ICD-10-PCS, a procedural coding system for inpatient procedure reporting in the United States. ICD-10-PCS has a seven-character alphanumeric structure, with each character having many different possible values, as the letters and numbers are mixed throughout the code. The different sections of ICD-10-PCS can be found

Figure 9.1 Format of ICD-10-CM

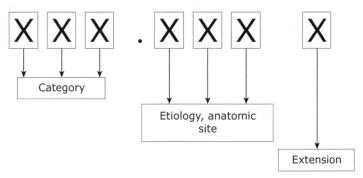

Table 9.1   ICD-10-CM chapter titles

CHAPTER	TITLE	CATEGORIES
1	Certain infectious and parasitic diseases	A00–B99
2	Neoplasms	C00–D49
3	Diseases of the blood and blood-forming organs and certain disorders involving the immune mechanism	D50–D89
4	Endocrine, nutritional and metabolic diseases	E00–E89
5	Mental and behavioral disorders	F01–F99
6	Diseases of the nervous system	G00–G99
7	Diseases of the eye and adnexa	H00–H59
8	Diseases of the ear and mastoid process	H60–H95
9	Diseases of the circulatory system	I00–I99
10	Diseases of the respiratory system	J00–J99
11	Diseases of the digestive system	K00–K94
12	Diseases of the skin and subcutaneous tissue	L00–L99
13	Diseases of the musculoskeletal system and connective tissue	M00–M99
14	Diseases of the genitourinary system	N00–N99
15	Pregnancy, childbirth and the puerperium	O00–O9A
16	Certain conditions originating in the perinatal period	P00–P96
17	Congenital malformations, deformations and chromosomal abnormalities	Q00–Q99
18	Symptoms, signs and abnormal clinical and laboratory findings, not elsewhere classified	R00–R99
19	Injury, poisoning and certain other consequences of external causes	S00–T88
20	External causes of morbidity	V01–Y99
21	Factors influencing health status and contact with health services	Z00–Z99

Source: CDC 2013b.

in table 9.2. As you can see, the first character can either be alpha or numeric. The digits 0–9 and the letters A–H, J–N, and P–Z are used. O and I are omitted to avoid confusion with 0 and 1. Figure 9.2 shows the meaning of each of the seven characters from section to body system to root (or main) operation to body part to approach to device to qualifier. Within each section the different characters have different valid entries resulting in a total of over 72,000 valid inpatient procedure codes.

The move to ICD-10-CM and ICD-10-PCS is a huge transition for the United States, estimated to cost many billions of dollars across the healthcare system. It is needed to ensure that the codes used to represent and evaluate the activity of the industry remain current, just as occurs with the use of new surgical tools and methods.

Table 9.2   Sections of ICD-10-PCS

Section	Title
0	Medical and Surgical
1	Obstetrics
2	Placement
3	Administration
4	Measurement and Monitoring
5	Extracorporeal Assistance and Performance
6	Extracorporeal Therapies
7	Osteopathic
8	Other Procedures
9	Chiropractic
B	Imaging
C	Nuclear Medicine
D	Radiation Oncology
F	Physical Rehabilitation and Diagnostic Audiology
G	Mental Health
H	Substance Abuse Treatment

Source: CMS 2009.

Figure 9.2   Meaning of characters for medical and surgical procedures

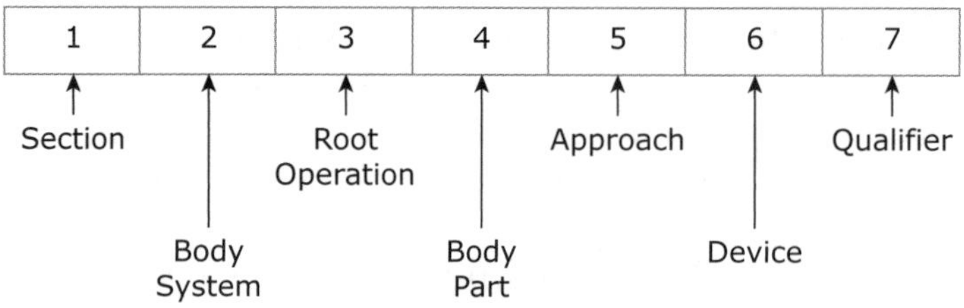

Moving to ICD-11

The present revision process of the ICD, its eleventh overall, is underway at the World Health Organization in Geneva. ICD-11 promises substantial improvements over historical rendering, embracing a tripartite structure of

1. An ontological core in partnership with the Systemized Nomenclature of Medicine (SNOMED).

2. A Foundation Layer of richly interlinked concepts with explicit preferred terms, fully specified terms, synonyms, definitions, and detailed attributes.

3. Several **linearizations** deriving from the Foundation Layer that will resemble the traditional mutually exclusive and exhaustive coding structure of historical ICD tabular versions. A linearization is "a subset of the ICD-11 foundation component, that is

   o fit for a particular purpose: reporting mortality, morbidity, or other uses
   o jointly exhaustive of the ICD universe (foundation component)
   o composed of entities that are mutually exclusive of each other
   o each entity is given a single parent" (WHO 2013)

The most important linearization will be the standard derivative used for morbidity coding in hospitals and clinical care. A proper and much smaller subset of this linearization will be used for mortality coding. Distinct from these will be specific linearizations for primary care, low-resource delivery environments in developing countries, and various specialty derivatives such as neurology, cancer, or psychiatry. Finally, the historical pattern of nations creating their own national modifications, such as the American ICD-10-*CM* (where the CM is the US Clinical Modification), can correspondingly be accommodated by nations invoking their own derivatives from the Foundation Layer of ICD-11, the advantage being that since all linearizations derive from the Foundation Layer, establishing linkages and mapping between and among virtually all linearizations—morbidity, mortality, specialty, primary care, or national derivations—can be achieved by mapping through the Foundation Layer in a hub and spoke model, rather than creating "point to point" mappings among the permutations.

An additional feature of ICD-11 will be its use of postcoordination for many attributes in order to avoid the excessive repetition evident in ICD-10-CM for many injury patterns. For example, each injury has a separate code for initial encounter, subsequent encounter, and sequela. Postcoordination means that the terms with modifiers are created as they are needed rather than the developers of the classification trying to conceive of all possible permutations for inclusion in the classification. Parameters such as severity, stage, detailed anatomy, acuity, or topography (for example, laterality, anterior, distal, and so on), could be rendered using postcoordination rather than creating hundreds of precoordinated terms for each of the combinations on such dimensions. Nevertheless, to maintain longitudinal continuity with historical versions of ICDs, the ICD-11 mortality linearization will retain the approximate level of precoordination evident in ICD-10.

The developers of ICD-11 recognize that postcoordination opens the possibility for multiple ways to code the same concept, for example postcoordinating a disease and severity when a precoordinated version of disease by severity might exist. To avoid violating the requirement that a statistical classification must have mutually exclusive categories (to avoid counting the same things twice or separately in different categories), ICD-11 introduces a body of "sanctioning rules" that are intended by be computationally executed, not manually practiced, since there will likely be many thousands of such rules. An example of such a sanctioning rule might be mapping a postcoordinated expression of renal failure and a severity code to its corresponding precoordinated version.

An interesting speculation as one proposal to obviate a proliferation of national modifications is to consider that some modes of precoordination would be required or prohibited as a set of restrictions, for example the United States might require the postcoordination of laterality where appropriate. Building on the notion that national modifications of ICD may become simply various linearizations derived from the Foundation Layer of ICD-11, a country's transition to ICD-11 can be facilitated by rendering their current system—such as ICD-10-CM in the United States—as a linearization of the ICD-11 Foundation Layer (this is technically straightforward), and simply evolving that linearization to become incrementally closer to the standard ICD-11 Morbidity Linearization over time. This provides a nondisruptive pathway for graceful adoption of the new revision without the abrupt transformation we witness around ICD-10-CM adoption in the United States today.

Clinical Terminologies

It is implausible that a single terminology or classification can or should function as the only or even as the major reference set for all the complexities of clinical information. Clearly, laboratory or genomic data are not well suited to representation in any version of the ICD, even the ever-versatile ICD-11. Thus, many purpose-specific terminologies are widely used today. Ideally, these would form nonoverlapping, complementary, and comprehensive enumerations of major clinical concepts; we have yet to reach quite that state but progress does continue. Here we comment on the more common terminologies.

Healthcare Common Procedure Coding System

The **Healthcare Common Procedure Coding System (HCPCS)** consists of two levels or systems. Level I is the CPT, a large, well-curated catalog of clinical and surgical procedures maintained by the American Medical Association as a proprietary and copyrighted resource. Its primary purpose is to enable the classification of resource categories or reimbursement, though it has levels of detail and granularity that support its reuse for secondary analyses such as quality improvement or comparative effectiveness research. While comprehensive, it is lacking for coherent overall structure, hierarchy, or conceptual organization, rendering its facile adoption for secondary use sometimes challenging.

Level II of the HCPCS is maintained by CMS. CMS creates and administers the Level II HCPCS codes as alphanumeric identifiers for products, supplies, and services not included in CPT. The codes consist of a leading alpha character followed by four numbers. They are used primarily for claims processing.

SNOMED-CT

The SNOMED developed over 40 years ago by the College of American Pathologists merged with the Clinical Terms (CT) vocabulary from the United Kingdom to create the modern SNOMED-CT we have today. **SNOMED-CT** is a logically organized and massive terminology, mostly ordered by a formal description logic, which permits SNOMED-CT to benefit from the classifying reasons developed by computer science and the fields of formal ontology and logic. Each entry in SNOMED-CT contains a concept identifier, a description that helps define the concept and relationships or attributes for the entry (IHTSDO 2013). It has highly detailed and granular characterization of diseases, findings, symptoms, anatomies, manifestations, and many related axes. Figure 9.3 is an illustration of the multiple granularities available in SNOMED-CT. It is properly regarded as the largest, most complex, and comprehensive terminology about clinical medicine ever. Architecturally, it is intended for postcoordinated application, though many precoordinated terms occur and are disambiguated by description-logic driven equivalences. SNOMED-CT today contains more than 310,000 separate, active, concepts, which when combined in postcoordinated expressions can render a nearly unbounded number of clinical descriptions. Finally, SNOMED-CT use in the United States is expected to grow because SNOMED-CT is specified as an acceptable standard for several Stage 2 meaningful use requirements (ONC 2013).

LOINC

Logical Object Identifiers Names and Codes (LOINC) comprise a dictionary of laboratory codes and clinical test descriptors, originated by Regenstreif Institute and funded by federal support grants as a public resource for the common good. It is publicly usable without any fees or licenses. Laboratory codes are synthesized from a six-part naming model: analyte (for example, sodium), property (for example, concentration), timing (for example, a moment or integrated over a defined period), sample type (for example, blood serum), scale (for example, quantitative), and optionally method. The largest part of LOINC is laboratory codes, with nearly 30,000 in the database as of publication. Variations on this six-part model are also used for clinical measurements (for example, blood pressure) and clinical scales or survey instruments (for example, the Glasgow Coma Scale). Selected examples

Figure 9.3   Multiple levels of granularity in SNOMED-CT

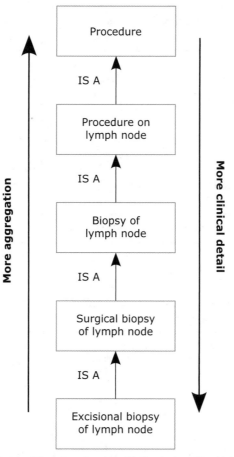

Figure reprinted by kind permission of the International Health Terminology Standards Development Organisation (*www.ihtsdo.org*).

from the LOINC tables are found in figure 9.4. LOINC was originally adopted as the payload for a Health Level 7 (HL7) clinical message, but is now endorsed as the preferred coding for laboratory data specified by emergent meaningful use regulations for the US HHS (ONC 2013).

RxNORM

As LOINC is for laboratory codes, **RxNorm** is for drug names. Created and curated by the National Library of Medicine, and updated weekly, RxNorm is the corresponding meaningful use specification for pharmaceutical names and codes in the United States. RxNorm is actually a relatively sophisticated database that enumerates "orderable drugs" such as Chewable Amoxicillin Tablet, 250 mg, as well as linking these to their component medicines (Amoxicillin), trade name variations, and active ingredients. It is the first publicly usable enumeration of drugs and ingredients without copyright or usage restrictions.

Figure 9.4 Selected Examples from LOINC Tables

LOINC #	Long Common Name	CLASS	Class Override
6019-4	Almond IgE Ab [Units/volume] in Serum	Allergy	Allergy
6020-2	Alternaria alternata IgE Ab [Units/volume] in Serum	Allergy	Allergy
19000-9	Vancomycin [Susceptibility]	ABXBACT	Antibacterial susceptibility
7059-9	Vancomycin [Susceptibility] by Gradient strip (E-test)	ABXBACT	Antibacterial susceptibility
38483-4	Creatinine [Mass/volume] in Blood	Chem	Chem
2160-0	Creatinine [Mass/volume] in Serum or Plasma	Chem	Chem
35591-7	Creatinine renal clearance predicted by Cockcroft-Gault formula	Chem	Chem

This material contains content from LOINC® (http://loinc.org). The LOINC table, LOINC codes, and LOINC panels and forms file are copyright © 1995–2012, Regenstrief Institute, Inc. and the Logical Observation Identifiers Names and Codes (LOINC) Committee and available at no cost under the license at http://loinc.org/terms-of-use.

Other Data Set Standards

This section has emphasized terminology, vocabularies, and classifications, though illustrated only a few. Additionally, there are information model and messaging standards that provide syntax to complement the raw semantics of controlled terms, or put another way, the context for the words. A detailed discussion of these standards is beyond the scope of this chapter, but includes simple structures such as HL7 Version 2 bar-delimited ASCII strings as well as the more elegant Consolidated Clinical Data Architecture specification more recently emergent from HL7 and destined for meaningful use health information exchange (HIE). Perhaps the most promising initiative presently underway is the Clinical Information Modeling Initiative (CIMI), which is unifying the midlevel modeling of structures for clinical observations such as a blood pressure measurement among previously competing groups. As the healthcare industry continues to develop its ability to effectively exchange data the standards will likewise evolve.

Metadata

In order to use data and information appropriately, it is important to understand metadata. Metadata are "descriptive data that characterize other data to create a clearer understanding of their meaning and to achieve greater reliability and quality of information. Metadata consist of both indexing terms and attributes. Data about data: for example, creation date, date sent, date received, last access date, last modification date" (AHIMA 2012, 269). Metadata are essential for a full understanding of the underlying data. For example, without metadata such as the creation or modification date, it may be impossible to determine which version of ICD-9-CM was used for coding a record. This is essential to ensure the code is interpreted correctly. Other metadata such as the access date are important for legal reasons such as ensuring no breach of confidentiality has occurred. Finally, metadata can simply help explain the data or information by defining the data element or specifying the length of the field or providing the values that are allowed to be entered in the field. Metadata about the data can even change over time. For example, a healthcare organization may have specified metadata related to its EHR data; however, if the EHR data is transmitted a new metadata field could be added to indicate the healthcare organization as the source of the data. Metadata is one of those hidden, necessary tools for effective use of data and information.

Check Your Understanding 9.2

Instructions: Choose the best answer.

1. Which of the following is utilized in the United States for reporting the cause of death on death certificates?
   a. ICD-10
   b. SNOMED-CT
   c. LOINC
   d. RxNORM

2. Which of the following have a wide range of uses in healthcare, including the development and use of quality and performance measures?
   a. Code sets
   b. Classification systems
   c. Clinical terminologies
   d. Data set standards

Instructions: Indicate whether the following statements are true or false (T or F).

3. ICD-11 is currently in development and includes plans for graceful evolution from ICD-10.

4. Data without metadata are just as easy to understand as data with metadata.

5. SNOMED-CT is a detailed clinical terminology with over 310,000 unique concepts.

◉ Secondary Data Uses of the Future

Historically, the primary and virtually only use of clinical data was for care providers to document the progress and details of a specific patient for their own records and to share with partnering healthcare providers. However, in this era of increasingly coordinated, cooperative, and preventive care, the use of clinical findings and outcomes across large numbers of patients may emerge to be the more important use of information from a societal perspective. Broadly labeled "secondary use," these practices involve data quality metrics, population-based guideline application, best evidence discovery, adverse event detection, comparative effectiveness analyses, and clinical and outcomes research of many varieties including clinical trials and observational epidemiology. Perhaps the single most important modality of secondary use is the identification of patients for whom a particular rule or guideline should "fire," commonly called clinical decision support. Thus aggregated patient information analyses and monitoring can improve the quality of care for an individual patient, by predicting and avoiding drug-drug or drug-disease interactions, inappropriate tests or treatments, or overlooked results and implications.

Big Data

One of the concepts that is evolving in the present and for the foreseeable future is "big data." Big data is defined as "high-volume, high-velocity and high-variety information assets that demand cost-effective, innovative forms of information processing for enhanced insight and decision making" (Gartner 2013). The first differentiator for big data is the sheer size the databases. Large hospital systems are accumulating terabytes of data every year, with Accountable Care Organizations and others wanting to combine the databases to be able to utilize the richness of all of the data. The CMS databases from 1965 to present would qualify as big data. The second issue is the speed with which the data needs to and does move around the system. This will continue to accelerate as HIE organizations become more prevalent and are more widely used. The third characteristic of big data is the variety of the data. The industry is beginning to seek ways to combine individually identifiable patient record information with genomic data, staffing data, or other types of data, which adds to the complexity of the data. In particular, it may be difficult to find tools that can handle such a wide variety of data. Big data is and will continue to be a focus for health informatics professionals.

Central to any secondary use is the principle of transforming heterogeneous clinical data into **comparable and consistent** representations. Comparable and consistent data has been normalized or transformed so that they conform to the designated standards. Absent such transformation, clinical data is not comparable, and cannot contribute to the myriad benefits of secondary uses. An example of data normalization is the use of NLP coupled with controlled terminologies to transform unstructured information into structured and semantically consistent forms that can sustain inferencing. More sophisticated forms include the practice of high-throughput **clinical phenotyping** from electronic medical records using validated phenotyping algorithms to identify patients for a particular study. Clinical phenotyping involves determining which observable characteristics are applicable for a given subset of patients (SHARP-C 2013). For example, researchers need to be able to identify patients and their relevant characteristics for inclusion or exclusion for numerators or denominators of quality metrics, inclusion criteria for clinical trials, appropriateness for a clinical decision support rule, or selection for a research cohort to further understand best practices and outcomes. Meaningful use is bringing the

United States closer to achieving comparable and consistent clinical data among practitioners, though most would agree that we have some distance yet to go.

⊙ Summary

Secondary data, whether collected in an unstructured format using NLP and then processed, or entered in a very proscribed, structured format, is a primary driver for the implementation and use of health information technology. Data standards such as classification systems and clinical terminologies, among others, assist in using the data efficiently and effectively. These data standards combined with developing analytical processes and tools will help to manage the very large, or big, databases being created with the widespread implementation of EHRs. Turning the masses of data that are being collected into information will occupy many health informatics and information management professionals for the next decade or more.

REFERENCES

AHIMA. 2012. *Pocket Glossary for Health Information Management and Technology.* 3rd ed. Chicago: AHIMA Press.

Centers for Disease Control and Prevention. 2013a. ICD—ICD-9-CM—Coordination and Maintenance Committee. http://www.cdc.gov/nchs/icd/icd9cm_maintenance.htm.

Centers for Disease Control and Prevention. 2013b. International Classification of Diseases, Tenth Revision, Clinical Modification (ICD-10-CM). http://www.cdc.gov/nchs/icd/icd10cm.htm.

Centers for Medical and Medicaid Services. 2009. ICD-10-PCS. http://www.cms.hhs.gov/ICD10.

Cheng, L.T., E.J. Zheng, G.K. Savova, and B.J. Erickson. 2010. Discerning tumor status from unstructured MRI reports—Completeness of information in existing reports and utility of automated natural language processing. *Journal of Digital Imaging: The Official Journal of the Society for Computer Applications in Radiology* 23(2):119–132.

Department of Health and Human Services. 2012. Administrative Simplification: Adoption of a Standard for a Unique Health Plan Identifier; Addition to the National Provider Identifier Requirements; and a Change to the Compliance Date for the International Classification of Diseases, 10th ed. (ICD-10-CM and ICD-10-PCS) Medical Data Code Sets (CMS-0040-F). *Federal Register.* https://s3.amazonaws.com/public-inspection.federalregister.gov/2012-21238.pdf.

Elkin, P.L., D.A. Froehling, D.L. Wahner-Roedler, S.H. Brown, and K.R. Bailey. 2012. Comparison of natural language processing biosurveillance methods for identifying influenza from encounter notes. *Annals of Internal Medicine* 156(1 Pt 1):11–18.

Ely, J.W. 2004. Answering physicians' clinical questions: Obstacles and potential solutions. *Journal of the American Medical Informatics Association* 12(2):217–224. doi:10.1197/jamia.M1608.

Gartner, Inc. 2013. Big Data Definition | Gartner. *IT Glossary.* http://www.gartner.com/it-glossary/big-data/.

Gerbier, S., O. Yarovaya, Q. Gicquel, A.L. Millet, V. Smaldore, V. Pagliaroli, S. Darmoni, and M.-H. Metzger. 2011. Evaluation of natural language processing from emergency department computerized medical records for intra-hospital syndromic surveillance. *BMC Medical Informatics and Decision Making* 11:50.

Giannangelo, K., ed. 2010. *Healthcare Code Sets, Clinical Terminologies, and Classification Systems.* 2nd ed. Chicago: AHIMA.

Hartman, K., S.C. Phillips, and L. Sornberger. 2012. Computer-assisted coding at the Cleveland Clinic: A strategic solution. Addressing clinical documentation improvement, ICD-10-CM/PCS implementation, and more. *Journal of AHIMA.* 83(7):24–28.

Health Story Project. 2013. http://www.healthstory.com/.

International Health Terminology Standards Development Organization. 2013. SNOMED-CT User Guide. http://ihtsdo.org/fileadmin/user_upload/doc/.

Jones, M., S.L. Duvall, J. Spuhl, M.H. Samore, C. Nielson, and M. Rubin. 2012. Identification of methicillin-resistant *Staphylococcus aureus* within the nation's Veterans Affairs Medical Centers using natural language processing. *BMC Medical Informatics and Decision Making* 12:34.

LaTour, K., S. Eichenwald Maki, and P. Oachs (eds.). 2013. *Health Information Management: Concepts, Principles, and Practice,* 4th ed. Chicago: AHIMA.

Logical Observation Identifiers Names and Codes (LOINC®). 2013. http://loinc.org/.

Office of the National Coordinator, HHS. 2013. Vocabulary Task Force | Policy Researchers & Implementers | HealthIT.gov. http://www.healthit.gov/policy-researchers-implementers/vocabulary-task-force.

Safran, C., M. Bloomrosen, W.E. Hammond, S. Labkoff, S. Markel-Fox, P.C. Tang, and D.E. Detmer. 2007. Toward a national framework for the secondary use of health data: An American Medical Informatics Association white paper. *Journal of the American Medical Informatics Association* 14(1):1–9. doi:10.1197/jamia.M2273.

SHARP-C Project. 2013. Division of Informatics. http://informatics.mayo.edu/sharp/index.php/HTP_Research.

Stanfill, M.H., M. Williams, S.H. Fenton, R.A. Jenders, and W.R. Hersh. 2010. A systematic literature review of automated clinical coding and classification systems. *Journal of the American Medical Informatics Association* 17(6):646–651. doi:10.1136/jamia.2009.001024.

United States Congress. 1996. *Health Insurance Portability and Accountability Act of 1996.* http://aspe.hhs.gov/admnsimp/pl104191.htm#1171.

World Health Organization. 2013. The International Classification of Diseases, 11th Revision. www.who.int/classifications/icd11/.

RESOURCES

American Medical Association. 2013. Current Procedural Terminology. http://www.ama-assn.org/ama/pub/physician-resources/solutions-managing-your-practice/coding-billing-insurance/cpt.page.

Health Level Seven International. 2013. http://www.hl7.org/.

International Health Terminology Standards Development Organization. 2013. SNOMED CT. http://www.ihtsdo.org/snomed-ct/.

Mayo Clinic Informatics: CIMI. 2013. http://informatics.mayo.edu/CIMI/index.php/Main_Page.

U.S. National Library of Medicine, National Institutes of HealthRxNorm. 2013. RxNorm. https://www.nlm.nih.gov/research/umls/rxnorm/.

World Health Organization. 2013. International Classification of Diseases. http://www.who.int/classifications/icd/revision/icd11betawhattoexpect.pdf.

Chapter 10

Privacy for Healthcare Informatics

*By Desla Mancilla,
Jacqueline Moczygemba,
and Susan H. Fenton*

Learning Objectives

- Explain the purpose of the HIPAA Privacy Rule
- Describe the focus of the Administrative Simplification provisions within the HIPAA Privacy Law
- Discuss how the HITECH Act modifies HIPAA
- Identify persons or entities that are governed by HIPAA and the HITECH Act
- Explain the meaning of a healthcare transaction and cite examples
- Explain the meaning of deidentified health information and list the data elements that must be removed to ensure a patient's health record is deidentified
- Discuss the type of information that is protected under HIPAA
- Articulate the meaning of ePHI and electronic media
- Discuss an individual's right regarding access to PHI
- Describe uses and disclosures permitted by HIPAA law
- Cite examples of incidental use and disclosure of PHI
- Articulate the core elements of a valid authorization
- Explain the minimum use requirement and note the exceptions to the requirement
- Articulate the importance of the Notice of Privacy Practices document and the required contents
- Examine the HITECH extensions that modified HIPAA's accounting of disclosures requirement
- Describe the relationship between the HIPAA Privacy Rule and the Genetic Information Nondiscrimination Act

KEY TERMS

Access
Accounting of disclosures
Administrative Simplification
American Recovery and Reinvestment
  Act (ARRA)
Authorization
Business associate (BA)
Business associate agreement (BAA)
Covered entity
Deidentified information
Designated record set
Electronic media
Electronic protected health
  information (ePHI)
Health Information Technology for
  Economic and Clinical Health
  (HITECH) Act

Health Insurance Portability
  and Accountability Act of 1996
  (HIPAA)
Health plan
Healthcare clearinghouse
Healthcare provider
Limited data set
Minimum necessary
Notice of Privacy
  Practices (NPP)
Office for Civil Rights
Operations
Payment
Protected health information (PHI)
Transaction
Treatment
Workforce

⊙ Introduction

Throughout history, consumers of healthcare have been concerned about the privacy of their health information. In general, most American citizens understand that the communications between a patient and his or her physician are confidential. However beyond this, most citizens would probably agree they have little understanding about their rights to access their health information and furthermore, who else has a legal right to the information. State laws have provided some privacy protections, but nuances exist that challenge both patients and the healthcare professionals who provide treatment. Coupled with the need for federal privacy standards and greater efficiencies in the US healthcare system, industry leaders have worked on solutions to these salient challenges for decades.

In an effort to improve the efficiency and effectiveness of the nation's healthcare system, the **Health Insurance Portability and Accountability Act of 1996 (HIPAA)** was enacted by the United States Congress and signed into law by President Bill Clinton (HIPAA 1996). HIPAA is a complex federal law; for the purposes of this textbook chapter, the content and discussion focus on the **Administrative Simplification** section of Title II, and even more specifically, the privacy and security of health information. In addition to the HIPAA Privacy, Security, and Enforcement Rules, Title II or the HIPAA Administrative Simplification Rule also includes rules and standards for transactions and code sets, and identifier standards for employers and providers. HIPAA was updated in 2009 with the passage of American Recovery and Reinvestment Act (ARRA), which included the Health Information Technology for Clinical and Economic

Health (HITECH) legislation, and much more recently with the issuance of the 2013 HIPAA Omnibus Rule. All will be addressed in this chapter.

⊙ HIPAA Privacy Rule

The **Office for Civil Rights** of the Department of Health and Human Services has been given responsibility for the oversight and enforcement of the HIPAA regulations. As stated in the Office for Civil Rights (OCR) Privacy Rule Summary:

> A major goal of the HIPAA Privacy Rule is to assure that individuals' health information is properly protected while allowing the flow of health information needed to provide and promote high quality health care and to protect the public's health and well-being. The Rule strikes a balance that permits important uses of information, while protecting the privacy of people who seek care and healing. Given that the health care marketplace is diverse, the Rule is designed to be flexible and comprehensive to cover the variety of uses and disclosures that need to be addressed (OCR 2003).

Since the Privacy Rule was originally issued there have been many changes in the healthcare industry as well as technology so that the HIPAA Privacy Rule now includes regulations to update the HIPAA Breach Notification Rule; to modify the HIPAA Privacy Rule to include the provisions of section 105 of Title I of the Genetic Information Nondiscrimination Act (GINA) of 2008; and to try to increase the workability of the HIPAA regulations for covered entities and business associates (BAs) (OCR 2013).

⊙ Focus of HIPAA Privacy Regulations

The Administrative Simplification provisions within HIPAA focus on the adoption of standards for the electronic transmission of financial and administrative transactions, national identifiers, privacy, and security. With the expectation of reducing costs and administrative burdens, Congress also recognized that advances in electronic technology could erode the privacy of a person's health information. Taking this into consideration, Congress incorporated into HIPAA legislation that mandated the adoption of federal privacy protections for individually identifiable health information. The HIPAA Privacy Regulations address the use and disclosure of protected health information (PHI). The United States Department of Health and Human Services (HHS) published the final HIPAA Privacy Rule in December 2000, which was later modified in August 2002 (OCR 2003). Health plans, healthcare clearinghouses, and healthcare providers had to comply with the HIPAA Privacy Rule by April 14, 2003, with the exception of small health plans, which were given an additional year.

In the years that followed enactment of HIPAA, some privacy advocates criticized the federal legislation as a "paper tiger" (Belfort 2009). Examples of some criticisms were that privacy and security rules do not apply to many organizations that routinely handle large amounts of health information and the potential sanctions are not sufficiently severe except in rare cases of criminal conduct (Belfort 2009). Congress responded to these issues with the passage of the **Health Information Technology for Economic and Clinical Health (HITECH) Act**, which was enacted as part of the **American Recovery and Reinvestment Act (ARRA)** of 2009. The HITECH Act strengthens enforcement of the rules promulgated under HIPAA. This chapter covers federal legislation on privacy of health information originally enacted under HIPAA and subsequently expanded and strengthened with the passage of the HITECH Act and most recently, with the issuance of what is known as the HIPAA Omnibus Rule in January 2013 (OCR 2013).

⊙ Basics of the HIPAA Privacy Regulations

While the HIPAA privacy regulations are only one part of the original law, they are very complex, especially after the various expansions and clarifications. In order to fully understand them, it is important to understand the definitions and other foundations upon which the regulations are built.

Covered Entities and Workforce

All of the various HIPAA privacy regulations apply to covered entities and all BAs of covered entities. A **covered entity** is a healthcare provider, health plan, or healthcare clearinghouse that transmits health information in electronic form in connection with healthcare transactions (OCR 2003). Under HIPAA, a **healthcare provider** is any person or organization who furnishes, bills, or is paid for healthcare in the normal course of business (OCR 2003). Healthcare providers include persons such as doctors, dentists, nurses, and therapists as well as entities such as hospitals, clinics, urgent care centers, pharmacies, and institutions (OCR 2003). A **health plan** is an individual or group plan that provides, or pays the cost of, medical care (OCR 2003). Examples of a health plan include group health plans, health insurance issuers, health maintenance organizations (HMO), Medicare Part A or Part B, and the Medicaid program. A **healthcare clearinghouse** is defined by HIPAA as a public or private entity, including a billing service, repricing company, community health management information system, or community health information system, and "value-added" networks and switches, that do either of the following functions:

1. Processes or facilitates the processing of health information received from another entity in a nonstandard format or containing nonstandard data content into standard data elements or a standard transaction.

2. Receives a standard transaction from another entity and processes or facilitates the processing of health information into nonstandard format or nonstandard data content for the receiving entity (OCR 2003).

When applying HIPAA, covered entities must also consider members of their workforce who may not be limited only to employees. The Privacy Rule defines **workforce** as "employees, volunteers, trainees, and other persons whose conduct, in the performance of work for a covered entity (CE) or BA, is under the direct control of such covered entity or business associate, whether or not they are paid by the covered entity or business associate" (OCR 2013). An example of nonpaid workforce would be a health information technology (HIT) or health information management (HIM) student who is completing a professional practice experience in the hospital setting.

Healthcare Transactions

The HIPAA law also delineates the meaning of healthcare transactions. **Transaction** means the transmission of information between two parties to carry out financial or administrative activities related to healthcare (OCR 2003). This definition applies to transmissions of electronic health information. Examples of healthcare transactions include healthcare claims or equivalent encounter information, health claim status, eligibility for a health plan, or health plan enrollment/disenrollment. Figure 10.1 provides a list of healthcare transactions affected by HIPAA.

Business Associates

The term "business associate" has a very specific meaning for covered entities when complying with HIPAA. **Business associates (BAs)** essentially are all entities that are not members of the workforce, but are providing a service or performing a task on behalf of a CE with the expectation or possibility that they will have access to PHI. The full definition can be found in figure 10.2. Examples of typical BAs of the health information department are an outsourced medical transcription company and coding or reimbursement consultants. The individuals performing these functions are

Figure 10.1   Healthcare transactions

1	Healthcare claims or equivalent encounter information
2	Healthcare payment and remittance advice
3	Coordination of benefits
4	Healthcare claim status
5	Enrollment and disenrollment in a health plan
6	Eligibility for a health plan
7	Health plan premium payments
8	Referral certification and authorization
9	First report of injury
10	Health claims attachments
11	Other transactions the Secretary may prescribe by regulation

Source: OCR 2003.

not members of the facility's workforce but they use or disclose health information to perform their respective duties on behalf of the CE. The newly expanded definition explicitly includes health information organizations that will be involved in exchanging information electronically. The new definition also carries the BA obligation out to BA subcontractors so that everyone or anyone handling PHI on behalf of a CE should consider themselves a BA.

Once a person or organization is identified as a business associate, the CE must initiate a **business associate agreement (BAA)** that meets all of the HIPAA

Figure 10.2 Definition of HIPAA business associate

Business associate:

1. Except as provided in paragraph (4) of this definition, business associate means, with respect to a covered entity, a person who:

    i. On behalf of such covered entity or of an organized health care arrangement (as defined in this section) in which the covered entity participates, but other than in the capacity of a member of the workforce of such covered entity or arrangement, creates, receives, maintains, or transmits protected health information for a function or activity regulated by this subchapter, including claims processing or administration, data analysis, processing or administration, utilization review, quality assurance, patient safety activities listed at 42 CFR 3.20, billing, benefit management, practice management, and repricing; or

    ii. Provides, other than in the capacity of a member of the workforce of such covered entity, legal, actuarial, accounting, consulting, data aggregation (as defined in § 164.501 of this subchapter), management, administrative, accreditation, or financial services to or for such covered entity, or to or for an organized health care arrangement in which the covered entity participates, where the provision of the service involves the disclosure of protected health information from such covered entity or arrangement, or from another business associate of such covered entity or arrangement, to the person.

2. A covered entity may be a business associate of another covered entity.

3. *Business associate* includes:

    i. A Health Information Organization, E-prescribing Gateway, or other person that provides data transmission services with respect to protected health information to a covered entity and that requires access on a routine basis to such protected health information.

Source: OCR 2013.

requirements, including the most recent. Covered entities should utilize the help of legal counsel to ensure that the BAA clearly documents the requirements of the BA "to implement administrative, physical, and technical safeguards that reasonably and appropriately protect the confidentiality, integrity, and availability of the PHI that it creates, receives, maintains, or transmits on behalf of the covered entity" (45 CFR § 164.308(b)(1) and 164.314). Other areas to be addressed in the agreement include the role of agents or subcontractors who are provided PHI; safeguards to protect the PHI; procedures for the reporting of security incidents of which it becomes aware; and authority of the covered entity to terminate the contract if the BA violates a material term of the contract. With an acceptable BAA in place, covered entities may lawfully disclose PHI to BAs who perform services for the covered entity.

Before HITECH came into force, BAs who failed to properly protect patient information were liable to the covered entities via their BAA, but they did not face governmental penalties. The HITECH Act expands HIPAA data privacy and security requirements to include the BAs of covered entities. Under the HITECH Act, a person or organization identified as a BA is now directly subject to the following HIPAA privacy requirements:

- Impermissible uses and disclosures
- Failure to provide breach notification to the CE
- Failure to provide access to a copy of electronic PHI either to the CE or individual
- Failure to disclose PHI to the Secretary as required to investigate or determine the BAs compliance
- Failure to provide an accounting of disclosures (OCR 2013)

Check Your Understanding 10.1

Instructions: Indicate whether the following statements are true or false (T or F).

1. The Privacy Rule is the name given to the 1996 HIPAA law, its regulations, the HITECH Act, and other related regulations.
2. If a business associate contracts with another party for services and they have access to PHI, they are not subject to HIPAA.
3. The only covered entities, as defined by HIPAA, are healthcare providers, health plans, and healthcare clearinghouses.
4. Only persons who are paid by the covered entity are considered to be members of the workforce.
5. Business associates must comply with all provisions for the Privacy Rule.

⊙ What Information Is Protected under HIPAA?

To better understand the HIPAA Privacy Rule and the goal of ensuring individuals' protection of health information, it is important to examine the meaning of **protected health information (PHI)** because this fundamental term is used throughout much of the legislation. PHI is defined in the rule as "individually identifiable health information that is transmitted by electronic media, maintained in electronic media, or transmitted or maintained in any other form or medium" (45 CFR § 160.103). A three-part test to determine whether or not information meets the definition of PHI is as follows:

1. The information must either identify the person or provide a reasonable basis to believe the person could be identified from the information given.

2. The information must relate to one's past, present, or future physical or mental health condition; the provision of healthcare; or payment for the provision of healthcare.

3. The information must be held or transmitted by a CE or its BA (Brodnik et al. 2012, 220–221).

Furthermore, the Privacy Rule provides guidance on what is not PHI and specifically addresses personnel and educational records. Health information noted in education records covered by the Family Educational Rights and Privacy Act (FERPA), 20 USC § 1232g, and employment records held by a CE in its role as employer are exempt from the rule (OCR 2013). As an example, employee physical examination reports contained within personnel files would not be subject to the Privacy Rule (Brodnik et al. 2012).

Another point to consider when interpreting the Privacy Rule is that the information must be "created or received" by a CE. Therefore, information that a patient communicates to his or her doctor is covered, but information that is created or received by another party other than a CE is not protected under HIPAA. An example of this would be a patient disclosing health information to a family member or friends. In this instance, HIPAA does not prevent the family or friends from disclosing the health information to others (Sullivan 2004).

Deidentification of Protected Health Information (PHI)

The Privacy Rule does not restrict the use or disclosure of **deidentified health information**. In the Privacy Rule summary, HHS explains that

> deidentified health information neither identifies nor provides a reasonable basis to identify an individual. There are two ways to de-identify information; either: (1) a formal determination by a qualified statistician; or (2) the removal of specified identifiers of the individual and of the individual's relatives, household members, and employers is required, and is adequate only if the covered entity has no actual knowledge that the remaining information could be used to identify the individual (OCR 2003).

45 CFR § 164.514(b) provides a distinct list of data elements that a CE can remove to ensure that a patient's information is deidentified. The 18 data elements

are listed in figure 10.3. Some examples of where deidentified health information is useful are research, decision support, and education in health professions.

Figure 10.3   Requirements for deidentification of PHI

To meet the intent of HIPAA 45 CFR 164.514 (b)2, the following identifiers of the individual or of relatives, employers, or household members of the individual, are removed:

1   Names

2   All geographic subdivisions smaller than a State, including street address, city, county, precinct, zip code, and their equivalent geocodes, except for the initial three digits of a zip code if, according to the current publicly available data from the Bureau of the Census:
(1) The geographic unit formed by combining all zip codes with the same three initial digits contains more than 20,000 people; and
(2) The initial three digits of a zip code for all such geographic units containing 20,000 or fewer people is changed to 000

3   All elements of dates (except year) for dates directly related to an individual, including birth date, admission date, discharge date, date of death; and all ages over 89 and all elements of dates (including year) indicative of such age, except that such ages and elements may be aggregated into a single category of age 90 or older

4   Telephone numbers

5   Fax numbers

6   Electronic mail addresses

7   Social security numbers

8   Medical record numbers

9   Health plan beneficiary numbers

10   Account numbers

11   Certificate/license numbers

12   Vehicle identifiers and serial numbers, including license plate numbers

13   Device identifiers and serial numbers

14   Web Universal Resource Locators (URLs)

15   Internet Protocol (IP) address Numbers

16   Biometric identifiers, including finger and voice prints

17   Full face photographic images and any comparable images; and

18   Any other unique identifying number, characteristic, or code except a code used for Reidentification purposes

Source: OCR 2003.

In November 2012 the HHS OCR released guidance to ensure the deidentification of PHI meets the intent of the HIPAA Privacy Rule. Figure 10.4 is a graphic depicting the two acceptable methods. The first method requires an expert to use statistical or scientific methods to ensure there is a very small probability of any identification of the individuals. The second method requires that the 18 data elements listed in figure 10.3 be removed. However, the second method also requires that there be no actual knowledge that the residual data can identify an individual (OCR 2012). For example, if the data were deidentified by the second method, yet retained a rare diagnosis code for a very small population of people, it is possible the person might be able to be recognized so the data would not be "deidentified" according to HIPAA.

Reidentification

A covered entity is allowed to have a policy and procedure in place for reidentifying information that had been previously deidentified. A code or other means of record identification can be used provided that the code is not derived from information about the individual and cannot be translated in some manner to identify the individual. Furthermore, the CE cannot use or disclose the code for any other purpose and must not divulge the mechanism for Reidentification (45 CFR § 164.514).

Electronic Protected Health Information (ePHI)

In looking at the privacy and security of patient health information, we must also consider **electronic protected health information (ePHI)**. ePHI is "individually identifiable health information that is transmitted by electronic media or maintained

Figure 10.4   Two HIPAA privacy rule deidentification methods

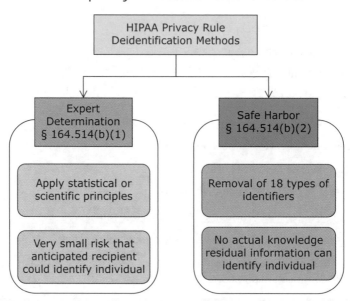

Source: OCR 2012.

in electronic media" (45 CFR § 160.103). The HIPAA Security Rule, discussed in detail in chapter 11, is a key law written to protect ePHI and to provide guidance for how electronic health information can be accessed appropriately (Brodnik et al. 2012).

HIPAA sets forth clear definitions of **electronic media**, which is helpful for interpreting the intent of the legislation. Electronic media is defined as

1. Electronic storage material on which data is or may be recorded electronically, including, for example, devices in computers (hard drives) and any removable/transportable digital memory medium, such as magnetic tape or disk, optical disk, or digital memory card;

2. Transmission media used to exchange information already in electronic storage media. Transmission media include, for example, the Internet, extranet or intranet, leased lines, dial-up lines, private networks, and the physical movement of removable/transportable electronic storage media. Certain transmissions, including of paper, via facsimile, and of voice, via telephone, are not considered to be transmissions via electronic media if the information being exchanged did not exist in electronic form immediately before the transmission (OCR 2013).

⊙ Uses and Disclosures of PHI

It is important to distinguish between the concepts of use and disclosure as emphasized in the HIPAA Privacy Rule. "Use means, with respect to individually identifiable health information, the sharing, employment, application, utilization, examination, or analysis of such information within an entity that maintains such information" (45 CFR § 160.103). "Disclosure means the release, transfer, provision of access to, or divulging in any other manner of information outside the entity holding the information" (OCR 2013). This section will examine uses and disclosures required by HIPAA as well as those that are permitted by the legislation.

Individual Rights Regarding Access to PHI

45 CFR § 164.524 addresses an individual's right of **access** to "inspect and obtain a copy of protected health information about the individual in a designated record set, for as long as the protected health information is maintained in the designated record set." Furthermore, 45 CFR § 164.501 defines the **designated record set** as

A group of records maintained by or for a CE that is:

i. The medical records and billing records about individuals maintained by or for a covered healthcare provider;

ii. The enrollment, payment, claims adjudication, and case or medical management record systems maintained by or for a health plan; or

iii. Used, in whole or in part, by or for the CE to make decisions about individuals.

While an individual has a right to access PHI, there are exceptions in this section of the law. Exceptions include

1. Psychotherapy notes

2. Information compiled in reasonable anticipation of a civil, criminal, or administrative action or proceeding

3. PHI subject to the Clinical Laboratory Improvements Amendments of 1988, 42 USC § 263a, to the extent the provision of access to the individual would be prohibited by law

4. PHI that is exempt from the Clinical Laboratory Improvements Amendments of 1988, pursuant to 42 CFR § 493.3(a)(2) (45 CFR § 164.524).

Upon receipt of an individual's request to access PHI, the CE must respond in a timely manner. The law allows 30 days from the receipt of the request to fulfill an individual's request. Additionally, covered entities are allowed a 30 day extension but must provide a written statement to the individual that includes the reason for the delay and a date in which the CE will complete the request. This applies to all requests, whether the information is maintained electronically, on paper or offsite (OCR 2013).

Grounds for Denying an Individual's Access to PHI

45 CFR § 164.524 includes language about denying an individual access to PHI. There are two forms listed in the law: (1) unreviewable grounds for denial and (2) reviewable grounds for denial. Examples of unreviewable grounds for denial include psychotherapy notes, correctional institutions or providers acting under the direction of a correctional institution, in some research studies, PHI obtained from someone other than a provider under promise of confidentiality, or PHI contained in records subject to the Federal Privacy Act. In these situations, a CE may deny an individual access without providing the individual an opportunity to review or appeal the denial. Health professionals are urged to read and examine the law carefully, as well as consult with their legal counsel, before denying access.

Uses and Disclosures Permitted by HIPAA

According to the 2013 HIPAA Omnibus Rule, a CE is permitted, but not required, to use and disclose PHI, without an individual's authorization, for the following purposes or situations:

i. To the individual;

ii. For treatment, payment, or healthcare operations, as permitted by and in compliance with § 164.506;

iii. Incident to a use or disclosure otherwise permitted or required by this subpart, provided that the covered entity has complied with the applicable requirements of §§ 164.502(b), 164.514(d), and 164.530(c) with respect to such otherwise permitted or required use or disclosure;

iv. Except for uses and disclosures prohibited under § 164.502(a)(5)(i), pursuant to and in compliance with a valid authorization under § 164.508;

v. Pursuant to an agreement under, or as otherwise permitted by, § 164.510; and

vi. As permitted by and in compliance with this section, § 164.512, § 164.514(e), (f), or (g) (OCR 2013).

In examining these six items further it is reasonable to infer that purpose (i) simply means that a CE may disclose PHI to the individual (or the individual's representative) who is the subject of treatment. It is the next five purposes that bear further discussion.

Treatment, Payment, and Healthcare Operations (TPO)

For one to understand permitted uses and disclosures involving TPO, it is important to understand the meaning of each term.

Treatment is the provision, coordination, or management of health care and related services for an individual by one or more health care providers, including consultation between providers regarding a patient and referral of a patient by one provider to another (OCR 2003).

Payment encompasses activities of a health plan to obtain premiums or to determine or fulfill its responsibility for coverage and provision of benefits under the health plan, and furnish or obtain reimbursement for health care delivered to an individual and activities of a health care provider to obtain payment or be reimbursed for the provision of health care to an individual (OCR 2013).

Health care **operations** are any of the following activities: (a) quality assessment and improvement activities, including outcomes evaluation, patient safety activities, population-based activities, protocol development, and case management and care coordination; (b) competency assurance activities, including provider or health plan performance evaluation, credentialing, and accreditation; (c) conducting or arranging for medical reviews, audits, or legal services, including fraud and abuse detection and compliance programs; (d) specified insurance functions, such as underwriting, enrollment, premium rating, related to the creation, renewal, or replacement of health insurance or benefits, along with risk rating and reinsuring risk relating to healthcare claims; (e) business planning, development, management, and administration; and (f) business management and general administrative activities of the entity, including but not limited to: deidentifying protected health information, creating a limited data set, and certain fundraising for the benefit of the covered entity (OCR 2003, 2013).

An example of treatment would be the freedom of healthcare providers from two separate organizations involved in an individual's care to discuss an individual's diagnosis, treatment, and prognosis. Another example is that of a relative who arrives at a pharmacy to pick up a prescription for an individual. By asking for a specific prescription, the relative verifies that he or she is involved in the individual's care (Sullivan 2004).

Examples of payment activities include billing, claims management and collection, utilization review, and reviewing healthcare services for medical necessity, coverage, or justification of charges. The 2013 HIPAA Omnibus Rule finalized regulations giving patients the right to request that their PHI not be disclosed to a health plan if they pay out of pocket in full for the services or items (OCR 2013). A provider who accepts the payment and provides the service is compelled to abide by this request.

As noted above there is a broad list of activities that fall under HIPAA's definition of healthcare operations. In addition, organizations should clearly distinguish activities considered to be operations and include examples of such in the Notice of Privacy Practices (NPP) discussed later in the chapter.

Some providers may obtain consents to use or disclose PHI for TPO purposes. The HIPAA Privacy Rule does not require a provider to obtain consent for TPO; however, it is important to note that consents cannot be used in situations where a patient authorization is required under the HIPAA Privacy Rule. Authorizations and their validity are discussed later in the chapter.

Uses and Disclosures with Opportunity to Agree or Object

Under the HIPAA Privacy Rule, an individual has the opportunity to informally agree to his or her information being included in a facility directory. The patient is usually asked if they wish to have their information included; if there is no objection by the individual, the directory information may include the individual's name, location in the facility, condition stated in general terms, and religious affiliation.

A separate "opportunity to object" arises when family and friends are with the patient who is being treated. An individual may also informally agree to a CE disclosing to the individual's family, other relative, or close friend PHI directly relevant to that person's involvement in the individual's care or payment for care (45 CFR § 164.510).

The 2013 HIPAA Omnibus Rule expanded this section to now include the release of PHI for assistance in disaster relief. PHI can also be released regarding a deceased person when the person requesting the information was involved in the healthcare of the patient before he or she died (OCR 2013).

Incidental Use and Disclosure

Based on established practice in healthcare communications and various environments, there is the potential risk for an individual's health information to be disclosed incidentally. An example of this might occur in the emergency department when a patient overhears a discussion or exchange between providers regarding the patient in the next treatment room. A use or disclosure of this nature is permitted as long as the CE has adopted reasonable safeguards required by the HIPAA Privacy Rule. Examples of reasonable safeguards for protecting an individual's health information include speaking quietly when discussing a patient's condition with family members in a public area such as a waiting room and avoiding the use of patient names in public places. In addition, proactive measures such as posting signs to remind employees to protect patient confidentiality are also reasonable safeguards (OCR 2003).

Public Interest and Benefit Activities

Another important consideration of use and disclosure of health information relates to national priority issues whereby there are important uses of health information outside the context of direct patient care and treatment. Twelve public interest purposes are identified in the Privacy Law and each is explained fully in section 42 CFR § 164.512 as special conditions or limitations may apply.

Limited Data Set

A **limited data set** is "protected health information from which certain specified direct identifiers of individuals and their relatives, household members, and employers have been removed" (OCR 2003). Limited data sets may be used for research, public health, or healthcare operations provided that the recipient of the data set enters into a data use agreement. The use agreement requires the recipient to safeguard the health information.

Authorized Uses and Disclosures

As a general rule, an individual's written **authorization** must be obtained by the CE for the disclosure of PHI unless the PHI meets an exception stated in the Privacy Rule where an authorization is not required. As previously discussed, an example of where an authorization would not be required is one of the 12 public interest purposes such as reporting an adverse event or product defect to comply with FDA regulations. One purpose of the authorization is to ensure that the CE and the individual fully understand the confidential relationship boundaries and what information is to be disclosed. The "minimum necessary" requirement is discussed later in the chapter.

Furthermore, the authorization must be written in plain language and must contain certain core elements, one of which is a statement that specifies that treatment, payment, enrollment, or eligibility for benefits cannot be denied because an individual declines to sign an authorization (45 CFR § 164.508). There are other core elements that must be included in a valid authorization. Figure 10.5 provides a list of the core elements for a valid authorization.

Invalid or Defective Authorizations

Health information professionals have always been diligent in reviewing a patient authorization to determine its validity. The HIPAA Privacy Rule distinctly explains that an authorization is not valid if the expiration date has passed or the expiration event is known to have occurred, the authorization is incomplete and lacks one or

Figure 10.5   Core elements for a valid authorization

Description of Information
This description must identify the information to be used or disclosed in a specific and meaningful fashion. For example, the request should specify what is wanted, such as "the discharge summary and the operative report," rather than asking for "any and all information." Providing the time frame for the information that is to be released (for example, hospitalization from 6/1/13 to 6/5/13) also provides a more specific description of the desired information.

Name of Person or Entity Authorized to Use or Disclose
The authorization must include the name or other specific identification of the person(s) or class of persons authorized to use or disclose the information. For example, the name of a hospital that is disclosing a patient's health information must be included.

Recipient of Information
The Privacy Rule requires that the authorization include the specific person(s) or class of persons (by name or other specific identification) to whom the covered entity may make the disclosure, such as an insurance company. This information should be verified by checking the patient demographic information that is collected on admission. If the insurance company information does not match, the patient should be contacted for clarification.

Purpose of Disclosure
Although the Privacy Rule requires that this element be present on authorizations, the patient is not required to provide a statement of purpose, and "at the request of the individual" is sufficient per the Privacy Rule.

Expiration
The Privacy Rule requires that an expiration date or expiration event (for example, "at the end of the research study" or "none") that relates to the individual or the purpose of the use or disclosure be included on the authorization.

Signature and Date
The patient must sign and date the authorization. It is essential that the signature be compared with one already existing in the medical record for validation purposes. A patient's personal representative may sign the authorization in lieu of the patient provided that a statement is included that describes that person's authority to act for the patient.
Although it is best practice for an authorization to be completed and dated after the date of the service (so that information is not created after the authorization was signed), the Privacy Rule does not prohibit predated

authorizations as long as the authorization encompasses the category of information that is later created and the authorization has not expired or been revoked. In summation, "the covered entity may use or disclose PHI that has been identified in the authorization regardless of when the information was created" (HHS 2007).

Statement of Right to Revoke
An authorization must contain a statement of the individual's right to revoke the authorization in writing and the exceptions to the right to revoke, together with a description of how the individual may revoke it.

Statement of Redisclosure
An authorization must include a statement that information used or disclosed pursuant to the authorization may be subject to redisclosure by the recipient and, subsequently, would no longer be protected by the Privacy Rule.

Statement of Eligibility
A statement in the authorization must specify that treatment, payment, enrollment, or eligibility for benefits cannot be denied because an individual declines to sign the authorization.

Copy Provided
A copy of the signed authorization is provided to the individual when authorization for use or disclosure is sought by the covered entity.

Source: Adapted from 45 CFR 164.508(c)(1–4).

more core elements, or the authorization is known by the CE to have been revoked (45 CFR §164.508(b)(2)).

Who Can Authorize Access to PHI?
One might question who can authorize access to PHI? First and foremost, the person who consented to the treatment can also authorize access to the PHI. Often, this is an adult patient who is mentally and physically competent can authorize the disclosure. Other parties who can authorize access include

- A parent, guardian, or custodian of a minor patient under 18 years of age
- A parent, guardian, or custodian of an incompetent patient
- Legal healthcare representative
- Power of attorney for healthcare
- Personal representative or executor or administrator of a deceased patient's estate

Health informatics professionals will need to be aware of any state laws governing consent to treatment and access to PHI.

Authorization for Psychotherapy Notes

In general an authorization is required for psychotherapy notes with the exception of carrying out the following treatment, payment, or healthcare operations listed in 45 CFR §164.508(a)(2):

i. To carry out the following treatment, payment, or health care operations:
   A. Use by the originator of the psychotherapy notes for treatment;
   B. Use or disclosure by the covered entity for its own training programs in which students, trainees, or practitioners in mental health learn under supervision to practice or improve their skills in group, joint, family, or individual counseling; or
   C. Use or disclosure by the covered entity to defend itself in a legal action or other proceeding brought by the individual; and

ii. A use or disclosure that is required by Sec. 164.502(a)(2)(ii) or permitted by Sec.164.512(a); Sec. 164.512(d) with respect to the oversight of the originator of the psychotherapy notes; Sec. 164.512(g)(1); or Sec.164.512(j)(1)(i).

Psychotherapy and other types of records, including those related to substance abuse, mental health, and other sensitive conditions, may be subject to either federal or state regulations above and beyond the HIPAA regulations.

Minimum Use Requirement

Many organizations in years prior to HIPAA implementation had best practices and guidelines in place to limit the unnecessary sharing of medical information. With the passage of HIPAA, more guidance was given. Covered entities must have policies and procedures in place that limit the protected information disclosed to the amount reasonably necessary to achieve the purpose of the disclosure. Policies and procedures should be designed to balance an individual's privacy against the legitimate need for information to accomplish the intended purpose of the use, disclosure, or request. One of the greatest challenges with implementing the **minimum necessary** standard is defining what is "reasonably necessary" and determining how minimum necessary uses, disclosures, and requests will be managed in the future with less paper. The minimum necessary standard requires covered entities to evaluate their practices and enhance safeguards as needed to limit unnecessary or inappropriate access to and disclosure of PHI (45 CFR §164.502(b)). Covered entities should also have policies and procedures in place for handling disclosures made on a routine or recurring basis. These documents guide the organization in achieving compliance with the Privacy Rule and ultimately, balance an individual's privacy against the legitimate need for information requested by the outside entity.

HIPAA carves out some exceptions to the minimum necessary requirement. The requirement does not apply to:

⊙ Disclosures to or requests by a healthcare provider for treatment

⊙ Uses or disclosures made to the individual

- Uses or disclosures made pursuant to an authorization
- Disclosures made to the Secretary of HHS
- Uses or disclosures that are required by law
- Uses or disclosures that are required for compliance with other applicable requirements of HIPAA (45 CFR §164.502)

Check Your Understanding 10.2

Instructions: Indicate whether the following statements are true or false (T or F).

1. In order to be compliant with HIPAA, all releases of PHI require a signed authorization to be legal.
2. Patients have an unconditional right to access their health information.
3. Appropriately deidentified health information is not subject to the HIPAA regulations.
4. If a patient revokes their authorization for releasing information the covered entity or business associate can no longer rely on that authorization for releasing PHI.
5. The minimum necessary standard presumes that all information in a record needs to be included when any information is requested.

⊙ Preemption of State Law

At times, health information professionals may find it impossible to comply with both state and federal laws regarding privacy standards. When that happens, one of the laws must necessarily preempt or take precedence over the other law. HIPAA addresses this in 45 CFR § 160.202. The Privacy Rule does not preempt or supersede stricter or more stringent state statutes if the statutes provide individuals with greater privacy protections or give individuals greater rights with respect to their PHI. State law will also prevail if it meets one or more of the following purposes pursuant to 45 CFR §160.203:

A. A determination is made by the Secretary of HHS that the provision of state law is necessary to prevent fraud and abuse related to payments for healthcare, ensure appropriate state regulation of insurance and health plans to the extent authorized by law, state reporting on healthcare delivery or costs, or to serve a compelling need related to public health, safety, or welfare and the intrusion into privacy is warranted when balanced against the need.

B. The purpose of state law is to regulate the manufacture, registration, distribution, dispensing of any controlled substances.

C. Where state law provides for the reporting of disease, injury, child abuse, birth, or death or for the conduct of public health surveillance, investigation, or intervention.

D. Where state law requires a health plan to report or provide access to information for management audits, financial audits, program monitoring and evaluation, or the licensure or certification of facilities or individuals.

In short, as with most things related to the HIPAA Privacy Rule, whether the state or federal law has precedence is complex and must be considered on a case-by-case basis with a different decision applicable in each state.

⊙ Administrative Requirements for Covered Entities

There are several administrative requirements that must be met to be in compliance with HIPAA and the HITECH Act. These requirements include policies and procedures to comply with the HIPAA Privacy Rule, an NPP, data safeguards, mitigation protocol, designation of a privacy officer, workforce training, and accounting of disclosures.

Notice of Privacy Practices

The **Notice of Privacy Practices (NPP)** is an essential document regarding an individual's "right to receive adequate notice of how a covered entity may use and disclose his or her protected health information. The notice also must describe the individual's rights and the covered entity's legal duties with respect to that information" (AHIMA 2011b). The NPP is an important tool to help patients understand their rights. The recent update to the HIPAA regulations included requirements for organizations to notify consumers that their data may be used for fundraising and that consumers must be notified if a breach of unsecured health information occurs (OCR 2013).

Safeguards

Another requirement of covered entities is to ensure appropriate administrative, technical, and physical safeguards to protect the privacy of PHI (45 CFR §164.530(c)). Examples of reasonable safeguards for paper records include isolating and locking file cabinets or record storage rooms. For computers that maintain personal health information safeguards may include passwords and firewalls. Other safeguards might include the use of cubicles, dividers, shields, curtains, or similar type barriers to provide privacy for patient-staff communications in a large clinic intake area (Sullivan 2004). Lastly, covered entities must be cognizant of any other types of reasonable safeguards that can limit incidental uses and disclosures.

Training

All members of the workforce need training in HIPAA policies and procedures regarding PHI to carry out their job functions. Furthermore, the CE must document the training it provides. Training may be provided through various formats that might include live instruction, video presentations, or interactive software programs (Sullivan 2004). Workforce members will need subsequent training when policies and procedures are revised to reflect changes in the law.

Privacy Official

According to 45 CFR § 164.530(a)(1), a CE must designate a person to be responsible for developing and implementing privacy policies and procedures. Health information professionals are well suited for this role given their knowledge and expertise in managing health information. There must also be a contact person or office responsible for receiving complaints. The contact person is responsible for responding to complaints and providing information about privacy practices covered in the NPP.

Accounting of Disclosures: HIPAA and HITECH

One of the purposes of the original HIPAA law was to provide individuals with a right to an **accounting of disclosures** regarding PHI. Disclosure is defined as "the release, transfer, provision of access to, or divulging in any other manner of information outside the entity holding the information" (45 CFR § 164.501). Thus, an accounting of disclosures is a listing of all of the disclosures made outside of the entity holding the information. This section will examine reporting requirements found in the original HIPAA law and recent modifications found in the HITECH Act. Since April 2003, HIPAA-covered entities have had to account for disclosures of PHI. The original HIPAA law gives an individual the right to receive an accounting of disclosures made anytime within six years prior to the individual's request. Exceptions to the accounting of disclosures rule are

1. For treatment, payment, or healthcare operations
2. Individual is given his or her own PHI
3. Incidental or otherwise permitted or required
4. Pursuant to an authorization
5. For use in a facility directory
6. To meet national security or intelligence purposes
7. To correctional institutions or law enforcement officials
8. Disclosure made as part of a limited data set
9. Disclosure that occurred before the HIPAA privacy compliance date (45 CFR 164.528(a)(1))

Information that must be included in the accounting report is the date of disclosure, name and address of the entity or person who received the information, and a brief statement of the purpose of the disclosure or, in lieu of such statement, a copy of a written request for disclosure (45 CFR §164.528(b)). The time to respond to a request for accounting is 60 days and may be extended once by no more than 30 days. A CE cannot charge a fee for the first accounting request by an individual. For each subsequent request, a reasonable, cost-based fee may be charged. Documentation regarding accounting of disclosures must be kept for six years (45 CFR §164.528(d)).

The HITECH Act of 2009 gave individuals new rights regarding the accounting of disclosures. Requirements regarding accounting of disclosures from the HITECH legislation included

- The requirement that disclosure to carry out treatment, payment, and healthcare operations is no longer exempt from a report of disclosures if disclosure is made through an electronic health record (EHR).

- Shortening the accounting of disclosure requirement to disclosures made during the three years prior to the request.

- Requiring, in situations where a BA makes a disclosure via an EHR for purposes of treatment, payment, and healthcare operations on behalf of the CE, to either be included in the report on disclosure by the CE, or for the CE to provide requestor with a list of all BAs in the requested time period (this is later changed in the requirements).

- The requirement that HHS promulgate regulations governing what information is to be collected about the disclosures taking into account the interests of the individual versus the administrative burden on the provider of the accounting.

- The specific requirements for an accounting of disclosures will be issued in an accounting of disclosures regulation and included in EHR certification criteria.

- The compliance date requirements for the rule specifying that "HIPAA CEs that have acquired an EHR after January 1, 2009 is January 1, 2011, or the date that it acquires an EHR, whichever is later. For CEs that acquired EHRs prior to January 1, 2009, the effective date is January 1, 2014. The statue authorized the Secretary to extend both of these compliance deadlines to no later than 2013 and 2016, respectively" (AHIMA 2011a).

In May 2011, the OCR published a Notice of Proposed Rulemaking regarding accounting of disclosures that includes a proposal for a new "access" report. The access report

> would be easier for covered entities to maintain and more likely to provide individuals with the information they want. The report would not distinguish between use and disclosure; instead it would identify anyone inside or outside the facility who accessed an individual's information. The report would be restricted to protected health information contained within the individual's designated record set and existing in electronic format (Heubusch 2011).

Since this is a proposed rule, the next step would be for OCR to proceed to an interim final rule that would be subject to modification or issue a final rule. Health professionals will need to monitor the federal register for further changes regarding accounting of disclosures.

Individual Rights Regarding Health Information

Since its creation, AHIMA has been committed to protecting the privacy of a patient's health information. Based on state and federal laws, consumers have many rights. AHIMA is committed to the advocacy and protection of consumers with regard to their health information. In September 2011, AHIMA published the *Consumer Health Information Bill of Rights*, a model for protecting health information principles. These principles, described fully in figure 10.6, include the right to view and obtain a copy, request limitations on the uses and releases, be informed about breaches, know who receives the health information and how it used, as well as expect the information to be private and secure. They also include the right to request changes to health information, have that information be accurate and complete, and file a complaint or report a violation related to health information (AHIMA 2011b).

Figure 10.6   AHIMA Bill of Rights

1. **The right to view and/or obtain a copy of your health information**

   You have the right to read and review the information used by healthcare professionals to make decisions about your care. Access can be requested at any time, including while you are receiving care. You have the right to obtain a copy of your health information in a timely manner in accordance with state and/or federal laws.

2. **The right to accurate and complete health information**

   You have the right to expect the information used to make decisions about your healthcare is accurate and complete. The delivery of quality healthcare depends upon accurate and complete health information. Inaccurate or incomplete health information can prevent you from clearly understanding your overall health and can prevent you from receiving the care you need.

3. **The right to request changes to your health information**

   You have the right to identify and request changes or additions to your health information when you believe information is incorrect or incomplete. It is up to your provider whether or not the requested change or addition will be made to the health record. However, your written request for changes or additions will remain with your health record.

4. **The right to know who receives your health information and how it is used**

   You have the right to a notice that explains how your health information is used. Your healthcare provider must give you a Notice of Privacy Practices that describes the possible uses and disclosures of your health

   (Continued)

Figure 10.6   AHIMA bill of rights (*Continued*)

information. You have a right to an accounting of disclosures (as required by law), which is a summary listing of who has received your information.

5. **The right to request limitations on the uses and releases of your health information**

   You have a right to request a limit on the medical information released to others involved in your care or the payment of your care. Your provider has the right to deny the request, but must provide you with a reason if it cannot be met. However, a request to keep information from your healthcare insurer must be granted if you pay for the service in full at time of delivery.

6. **The right to expect your health information is private and secure**

   You have the right to expect that protections are in place to keep your health information confidential and secure from unauthorized persons. You have the right to expect that your health information is exchanged securely across organizations. You also have the right to request that your provider contact you in the manner you prefer.

7. **The right to be informed about privacy and security breaches of your health information**

   You have the right to expect that organizations will hold staff responsible for any improper access, use, or release of your health information. You have the right to expect that a breach of your health information will be investigated as required by law and that you will be notified of harmful breaches and assisted accordingly.

8. **The right to file a complaint or report a violation regarding your health information**

   You have the right to file a complaint about the way your health information is handled including, but not limited to, privacy and security concerns. You have a right to expect a timely response and resolution. A complaint or violation can be reported to the organization and/or other state or federal agency.

Source: AHIMA 2009.

Genetic Information

Genetic testing has become almost commonplace in healthcare. However, genetic information is not always understood, even by healthcare professionals. Because of the complexities of the information, as well as the potential consequences, GINA was passed in 2008. GINA prohibits discrimination based on genetic information by health insurers related to eligibility, coverage, underwriting, or premium-setting decisions (Brodnik et al. 2012). Employers, employment agencies, labor organizations, and others are also prohibited from using genetic information for making employment decisions (Brodnik et al. 2012, 344–345). This law has now been included in the 2013 HIPAA Omnibus regulation to reconcile any differences. It is essential for allowing continued development of genetic and genetic testing technologies, while protecting healthcare consumers.

Check Your Understanding 10.3

Instructions: Indicate whether the following statements are true or false (T or F).

1. The designated privacy official is required to work full-time on health information privacy.

2. A state law can preempt HIPAA if it is stricter or gives the patients more rights.

3. GINA does not prevent employers from using employee genetic information when making hiring and firing decisions.

4. The requirement for maintaining an accounting of disclosures includes any and all verbal communications in a healthcare facility.

5. As an organization AHIMA is committed to protecting patients' rights related to their health information.

⊙ Summary

The privacy of health information is essential to all parties involved in healthcare. Privacy must be assured for the patients to trust that their data will not be misused by providers or others. The concepts, regulations, and guidance are continually evolving and, unfortunately, there are very few hard and fast rules. In line with that, the new HIPAA regulations have updated the time frame for compliance with new privacy regulations to 180 days (OCR 2013). CEs and BAs will need to remain informed so they can remain in compliance. Ensuring the data is released to only authorized parties requires an in-depth knowledge of federal and state laws and regulations, as well as the ability to analyze and apply the regulations thoughtfully. It is most important that the data be available when and where they are needed.

REFERENCES

42 CFR 493.3(a)(2): Laboratory requirements. 2013.

45 CFR 160.103: Definitions. 2013.

45 CFR 160.202: Definitions. 2013.

45 CFR 160.203: General rule and exceptions. 2013.

45 CFR 164.308(b)(1): Administrative safeguards. 2013.

45 CFR 164.501: Definitions. 2013.

45 CFR 164.502: Uses and disclosures of protected health information: General rules. 2013.

45 CFR 164.502(b): Uses and disclosures of protected health information: General rules. 2013.

45 CFR 164.508: Uses and disclosures for which an authorization is required. 2013.

45 CFR 164.508(a)(2): Uses and disclosures for which an authorization is required. 2013.

45 CFR 164.508(b)(2): Uses and disclosures for which an authorization is required. 2013.

45 CFR 164.510: Uses and disclosures requiring an opportunity for the individual to agree or to object. 2013.

45 CFR 164.514: Other requirements relating to uses and disclosures of protected health information. 2013.

45 CFR 164.514(b)(2): Other requirements relating to uses and disclosures of protected health information. 2013.

45 CFR 164.524: Access of individuals to protected health information. 2013.

45 CFR 164.528(a)(1): Accounting of disclosures of protected health information. 2013.

45 CFR 164.528(b): Accounting of disclosures of protected health information. 2013.

45 CFR 164.528(d): Accounting of disclosures of protected health information. 2013.

45 CFR 164.530(a)(1): Administrative requirements. 2013.

45 CFR 164.530(c): Administrative requirements. 2013.

AHIMA. 2009. Consumer Health Information Bill of Rights. http://library.ahima.org/xpedio/groups/public/documents/ahima/bok1_049282.pdf.

AHIMA. 2011a. Analysis of the NPRM HITECH Accounting of Disclosures. http://www.ahima.org/downloads/pdfs/advocacy/Analysis_of_the_NPRM_HITECH_AoD%28fin%29.pdf.

AHIMA. 2011b. "Notice of Privacy Practices (Updated)." (Updated February 2011). http://library.ahima.org/xpedio/groups/public/documents/ahima/bok1_048808.hcsp?dDocName=bok1_048808.

Belfort, R. 2009. HITECH Raises the Stakes on HIPAA Compliance. http://www.manatt.com/news.aspx?id=8912

Brodnik, M., L. Rinehart-Thompson, and R. Reynolds. 2012. *Fundamentals of Law for Health Informatics and Information Management*, 2nd ed. Chicago: AHIMA.

Centers for Medicare and Medicaid Services (CMS), Office of E-Health Standards and Services (OESS). 2008. HIPAA Compliance Review Analysis and Summary of Results. http://www.hhs.gov/ocr/privacy/hipaa/enforcement/cmscompliancerev08.pdf.

Department of Health and Human Services, Office for Civil Rights. 2003. Protected Health Information. http://www.hhs.gov/ocr/privacy/hipaa/understanding/training/udmn.pdf.

Guidance on Risk Analysis Requirements under the HIPAA Security Rule. 2010. http://www.hhs.gov/ocr/privacy/hipaa/administrative/securityrule/rafinalguidancepdf.pdf

Health Insurance Portability and Accountability Act of 1996. Public Law 104-191.

Heubusch, K. 2011. Access report: OCR tries subtraction through addition in accounting of disclosure rule. *Journal of AHIMA* 82(7):38–39.

HIPAA Administrative Simplification Statute and Rules. http://www.hhs.gov/ocr/privacy/hipaa/administrative/index.html.

HIPAA Compliance Review Analysis and Summary of Results. 2008. http://www.hhs.gov/ocr/privacy/hipaa/enforcement/cmscompliancerev08.pdf.

HIPAA Privacy Rule, Part 160, 2007. http://www.access.gpo.gov/nara/cfr/waisidx_07/45cfr160_07.html.

LaTour, K., S. Eichenwald-Maki, and P. Oachs. 2013. *Health Information: Management Concepts, Principles, and Practice*, 4th ed. Chicago: AHIMA.

Office for Civil Rights, Department of Health and Human Services. 2012. Guidance Regarding Methods for De-identification of Protected Health Information in Accordance with the Health Insurance Portability and Accountability Act (HIPAA) Privacy Rule. http://www.hhs.gov/ocr/privacy/hipaa/understanding/coveredentities/De-identification/hhs_deid_guidance.pdf.

Office for Civil Rights, Department of Health and Human Services. 2013. Modifications to the HIPAA Privacy, Security, Enforcement, and Breach Notification Rules under the Health Information Technology for Economic and Clinical Health Act and the Genetic Information Nondiscrimination Act; Other Modifications to the HIPAA Rules. *Federal Register* 78(17) 5566–5702.

Office for Civil Rights, Department of Health and Human Services. 2003. Summary of the HIPAA Privacy Rule. http://www.hhs.gov/ocr/privacy/hipaa/understanding/summary/privacysummary.pdf.

Recent Changes to HIPAA—the HITECH Act. 2009. http://www.lifespanrecycling.com/site/content/articles/RecentChangestoHIPAA-theHITECHAct.pdf.

Sullivan, J. 2004. HIPAA: A practical guide to the privacy and security of health data. Hartford: American Bar Association.

RESOURCES

Breach Notification Rule 2009. http://www.hhs.gov/ocr/privacy/hipaa/administrative/breachnotificationrule/index.html.

Brocato, L., S. Emery, and J. McDavid. 2011. Keeping compliant: Managing rising risk in physician practices. *Journal of AHIMA* 82(11):32–35.

Department of Health and Human Services. 2011. HIPAA Privacy Rule Accounting of Disclosures under the Health Information Technology for Economic and Clinical Health Act. *Federal Register* 76(104):31426–31449.

Security for Health Information

By Desla Mancilla,
Jacqueline Moczygemba,
Susan H. Fenton, and
Sue Biedermann

Learning Objectives

- Differentiate between addressable and required implementation specifications
- Describe what a security risk analysis entails
- Differentiate between the concepts of vulnerabilities, risks, and threats
- Provide examples of administrative, physical, and technical safeguards
- Appreciate the foundational importance of confidentiality, integrity, and availability in regard to the HIPAA Security Rule
- Articulate the HIPAA Security Rule complaint and enforcement process
- Identify the agencies responsible for HIPAA Security Rule enforcement
- Describe civil and criminal penalties and the tiered penalty approach
- Explain how HITECH modifies the HIPAA Security Rule
- Define medical identity theft
- Discuss the potential impacts of medical identity theft on patients and other stakeholders
- Describe the steps required for conducting a business impact analysis
- Delineate the concerns, challenges, and potential solutions involved in preparing a full-fledged information and organizational disaster preparedness plan

KEY TERMS

Administrative safeguards
Addressable implementation
   specifications
Availability
Breach
Break the glass
Business continuity plan (BCP)
Business impact analysis
Civil penalties
Cold site
Confidentiality
Criminal penalties
Disaster recovery plan (DRP)
Encryption
Health Information Technology for
   Economic and Clinical Health
   (HITECH) Act
HIPAA Enforcement Rule

Hot site
Integrity
Medical identify theft
Office for Civil Rights (OCR)
Physical safeguards
Recovery point objective (RPO)
Recovery time objective (RTO)
Red flags
Required implementation specifications
Risk
Sanctions policy
Security incident
Security Risk Analysis
Technical safeguards
Threat
Vulnerability
Warm site

⊙ Introduction

While there are many similarities between the Privacy and Security Rules, there are also notable differentiators. Where the HIPAA Privacy Rule protects all "individually identifiable health information," in any form or media, whether electronic, paper, or oral, the Security Rule is singularly concerned with electronic protected health information (ePHI). The Security Rule covers all ePHI created, received, maintained, or transmitted by an organization (Guidance on Risk Analysis 2010). This chapter will introduce specific guidelines to assure compliance with the security of the electronic health information. The enforcement of the guidelines will be covered as well as guidelines for handling breaches if they occur. HIPAA requires that we not only protect the patient identifiable health information but also requires that the information be available as needed in the delivery of care. Protection against medical identify theft and disasters are two considerations for a facility to ensure that they will be able to have the correct information available in a timely manner to support patient care.

Security Rule

The Security Rule is grounded in the same "reasonable" language as its Privacy Rule counterpart. The required standards include required and addressable implementation specifications that are intended to provide covered entities (CEs) and business associates (BAs) with flexible, scalable, technology-neutral solutions and alternatives for complying with the standards. **"Required" implementation specifications** are not optional, but must be implemented in conformance with the regulation. The term "addressable" implementation specification does not imply that the specification is "optional." **Addressable implementation specifications** should be implemented unless an organization determines that the specification is not reasonable and appropriate. If this is the case, then the organization must document why it is not reasonable and appropriate and adopt an equivalent measure if it is reasonable and appropriate to do so (45 CFR § 164.306(d)(3)).

In addition to the extensive language in the Rule intended to secure ePHI, a **security incident** is defined as the attempted or successful unauthorized access, use, disclosure, modification, or destruction of information or interference with system operations in an information system (45 CFR § 164.304). This definition is important as it serves as the method by which to evaluate reported Security Rule violations.

The foundational basis of a CE's and BA's information security program rests on its identification and management of potential risks to ePHI. The Security Rule outlines a broad set of regulations that include administrative, technical, and physical safeguards intended to ensure confidentiality, integrity, and availability of ePHI. Even in the best of situations, risk can turn into reality. For this reason, the Security Enforcement Rule outlines penalties and enforcement for violations of the Rule. Building on HIPAA, the **Health Information Technology for Clinical and Economic Health (HITECH) Act** outlines breach notification requirements and starts to lay the groundwork for additional protections as healthcare moves toward an integrated health information exchange environment.

⊙ Security Risk Analysis

The HIPAA Security Rule requires full evaluation of the methods, operational practices, and policies used by the CE to secure ePHI (45 CFR §§ 164.302–318). CEs and BA obligations in regard to risk analysis are outlined in 45 CFR § 164.308(a)(1)(ii)(A). The **Security Risk Analysis** process provides CEs and BAs with the structural framework upon which to build their HIPAA Security Plan. CEs and BAs are required to conduct a Security Risk Analysis "to evaluate risks and vulnerabilities in their environment and to implement reasonable and appropriate measures to protect against reasonably anticipated threats or hazards to the security or integrity of the e-PHI" (Guidance on Risk Analysis 2010).

The value of a risk analysis stems from its uniqueness to the specific organization in which it is conducted. Every organization is different and every risk analysis should reflect the unique and complex interrelationships between a multitude of systems, processes, and policies that in combination result in that specific organization's HIPAA Security Plan. For this very reason, the Security Rule is not prescriptive in requiring any specific method or approach for conducting the risk assessment. The Risk Analysis Final Guidance Document spells out some essential questions organizations should consider during the risk analysis process (Guidance on Risk Analysis 2010). These questions arise from the National Institute of Standards and Technology (NIST) Special Publication (SP) 800-66 and include the following:

⊙ Have you identified the ePHI within your organization? This includes ePHI that you create, receive, maintain, or transmit.

⊙ What are the external sources of ePHI? For example, do vendors or consultants create, receive, maintain, or transmit ePHI?

⊙ What are the human, natural, and environmental threats to information systems that contain ePHI? (NIST SP 800-66 2008).

Vulnerabilities

The ultimate goal of the risk analysis process is to guide organizations in the decisions made and actions taken to comply with the Security Rule's standards and addressable or required implementation specifications. Although necessary to put the risk analysis discussion in context, the concepts of **vulnerability**, threats, and risks are not expressly defined in the Security Rule. The Risk Analysis Guidance Document again refers to the NIST SP 800-66 document to frame the risk analysis discussion. Vulnerability is defined as an inherent weakness or absence of a safeguard that could be exploited by a threat (AHIMA 2012, 431). Vulnerabilities are grouped into either technical or nontechnical categories with technical vulnerabilities reflecting inappropriate information systems protective methods. Nontechnical vulnerabilities are demonstrated by such things as policy and procedure weaknesses.

Threats

A **threat** is the potential for exploitation of a vulnerability or potential danger to a computer, network, or data (AHIMA 2012, 410). Threats are grouped into three categories: natural, human, and environmental. Examples of natural threats are often weather related and include tornados, floods, and the like. Human threats are broad in nature and can be intentional or unintentional. Access to information by unauthorized individuals is a good example of a human threat since this can occur through intentional actions of the user, or can result from an accidental key entry error that exposes information to an unauthorized user. Environmental threats center on power failure, chemical, or other environmental agents with the potential to damage electronic data.

Risks

Risk is the probability of incurring injury or loss, the probable amount of loss foreseen by an insurer in issuing a contract, or a formal insurance term denoting liability to compensate individuals for injuries sustained in a healthcare facility (AHIMA 2012, 370).

Securing ePHI can be very costly and time consuming. It may not be possible to eliminate some threats and in those cases organizations must determine the extent of effort needed to reduce and mitigate the remaining risk. Figure 11.1 represents a typical project management tool used to assist in the evaluation of the likelihood and impact of risks. As one can see from this illustration, when there is a low probability of the occurrence of a risk and the impact of the potential risk is low, the risk would then be considered to be a low-level risk. Conversely, if the probability of the risk is high along with a high impact due to the risk, the risk would then be considered critical.

Risk Analysis Methods

The Security Rule intentionally leaves the methods for conducting the required risk analysis to the discretion of the entity. Regardless of the methods selected for conducting and documenting the risk analysis, the Security Rule does mandate several elements that must be included in the analysis:

- ⊙ Define the Scope of the Risk Analysis
- ⊙ Collect Data Collection
- ⊙ Identify and Document Potential Threats and Vulnerabilities
- ⊙ Assess Current Security Measures
- ⊙ Determine the Likelihood of Threat Occurrence
- ⊙ Determine the Potential Impact of Threat Occurrence
- ⊙ Determine the Level of Risk
- ⊙ Finalize Documentation
- ⊙ Perform Periodic Review and Updates to the Risk Assessment (45 CFR § 164.308(a)(1))

Figure 11.1 The risk impact/probability chart

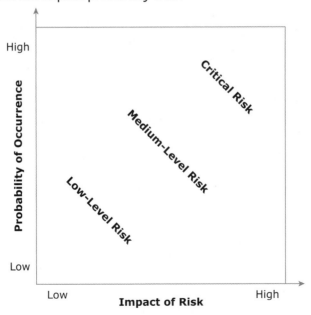

Reproduced with permission from MindTools.com.

Even though these elements must be included, they are to be considered a guide and a communication of the expectations. A healthcare facility should first consider its own characteristics and environment before proceeding with their risk analysis. Once this has been completed they can then determine the best way to conduct a risk analysis specific to their facility and situation while maintaining compliance with the mandated elements.

⊙ HIPAA Security Rule Safeguards

The Security Rule outlines a variety of safeguards necessary to ensure appropriate management and protection of ePHI. Working in concert, administrative, physical, and technical safeguards can produce the intended outcome of preserving the confidentiality, integrity, and availability of ePHI. While the intent and approach of each of these forms of safeguards vary greatly from one another, each form is necessary.

⊙ Administrative Safeguard Standards

Administrative safeguards are administrative actions such as policies and procedures and documentation retention to manage the selection, development, implementation, and maintenance of security measures to protect ePHI and manage the conduct of the CE's or BA's workforce in relation to the protection of that information (AHIMA 2012, 15; HIPAA Security Series 2007a).

Security Management Process Standard

The administrative safeguards comprise over half of all the safeguards included in the Security Rule. Many believe the administrative safeguards are the most difficult to address as they rely heavily on human involvement to ensure compliance with the safeguards. The first standard in the administrative safeguards section of the Security Rule is the security management process, which is found at 45 CFR §164.308(a)(1). This broad standard has four required implementation specifications that include the previously discussed risk analysis, a required risk management element, a required sanctions policy, and a required information systems activity review element. The risk management implementation specification picks up where risk analysis left off and outlines how the identified risks will be managed. Two critical factors in the risk management process include communication of security processes and leadership involvement with risk mitigation.

The **sanctions policy** must outline how cases of noncompliance will be addressed within the organization knowing that even with a strong risk management plan, the potential for noncompliance (either intentional or nonintentional) still exists. Some of the components a sanctions policy should include are a discussion of the significance of noncompliance, examples of noncompliance, and a sliding scale of discipline based on the severity of the act of noncompliance.

The implementation specification requires CEs to "Implement procedures to regularly review records of information system activity, such as audit logs, access reports, and security incident tracking reports" (HIPAA Security Series 2007a). Today's information systems have the ability to track and record a multitude of user activities, but unless specific measures are enacted by the organization to review these tracking progeny, security violations could go unnoticed. This implementation specification advises CEs to consider not only the technical abilities of their systems to create audit logs and reports, but also to address the nontechnical use of these tools through policy and procedures.

Security Officer

Assigned security responsibility is the second administrative safeguard standard that is detailed in 45 CFR§164.308(a)(2). This standard requires CEs to "Identify the security official who is responsible for the development and implementation of the policies and procedures required by this subpart [the Security Rule] for the entity" (45 CFR §164.308(a)(2)). CEs must establish who in their organization is responsible for compliance with the Security Rule requirements. This position is similar in scope and responsibility to that of the privacy officer required by the HIPAA Privacy Rule. CEs may (but are not required to) appoint the same individual to fill the role of both the privacy and security officer.

Workforce Security Standard

Workforce security (45 CFR §164.308(a)(3)) is the third administrative safeguard standard and has three associated addressable implementation specifications. This standard requires the organization to ensure that those with a legitimate need to access information are able to do so while at the same time ensuring that those workforce members that do not have a legitimate need to that information are prevented from gaining access.

The first implementation specification for this standard is authorization and supervision, which speaks to the unique needs of an organization based on size, function, and structure and spells out how each organization must determine each workforce member's level of access. Workforce clearance procedures is the second implementation specification and states that the CE must "Implement procedures to determine that the access of a workforce member to electronic protected health information is appropriate" (45 CFR §164.308(a)(3)). The third implementation specification in this section is termination procedures, which challenges CEs to implement appropriate methods to ensure workforce members access privileges are removed when they terminate employment (willingly or unwillingly). This implementation specification also outlines the need to ensure changes in employee scope and function be addressed by policy and procedures that facilitate timely revisions to access level as indicated by position changes.

Information Access Management Standard

The fourth administrative safeguard standard is named the information access management standard (45 CFR §164.308(a)(4)). This standard works in tandem with 45 CFR §164.308(a)(3) to uphold the basic security tenet of restricting access to only those that need it to perform their jobs. However, this standard specifically calls out a required implementation specification for isolating healthcare clearinghouse functions to ensure that clearinghouses that are part of a larger organization have their own policies and procedures to segregate ePHI access from unauthorized access by the larger organization.

Two addressable implementation specifications for access authorization and access establishment and modification are also included in the information access management standard. In terms of access authorization, the previous workforce security standards established workforce member rights to access information; the access authorization implementation specification addresses the policies and procedures for granting access to ePHI. Parallels are also drawn between the workforce security implementation specifications and the authorization and access establishment and modification implementation specification. This implementation specification is "Implement policies and procedures that, based upon the entity's access authorization policies, establish, document, review, and modify a user's right of access to a workstation, transaction, program, or process" (45 CFR §164.308(a)(4)).

Security Awareness and Training Standard

The fifth administrative safeguard standard requires CEs to "Implement a security awareness and training program for all members of its workforce (including management)" (45 CFR §164.308(a)(5)). Four addressable implementation specifications support this standard and provide ample flexibility for CEs to meet both the intent and spirit of this standard. This standard requires all existing workforce members to receive security training prior to the Security Rule compliance date. In addition, periodic retraining as indicated by changing conditions and training for new staff are required.

Security reminders, protection from malicious software, log-in monitoring, and password management are the four addressable implementation specifications. Each of these addressable implementation specifications have a single requirement (if reasonable and appropriate for the CE), but allow the CE to choose from many options to meet the requirement. For example, in the security reminder implementation specification, the requirement mandates the CE to implement periodic security updates. The organization can choose from a variety of methods including print, electronic, or face-to-face reminders as the way to achieve this mandate. Security awareness and training specific to a workforce member's role in protecting the CE's information assets from potential damage resulting from malicious software is addressable. Readers of this text are probably familiar with the concept of log-in monitoring. This addressable implementation specification is used to help detect and prevent unauthorized access to information and includes such techniques as locking out users who enter their log-in name incorrectly more than once. In the password protection implementation specification, CEs must have appropriate policies and procedures in place to create, change, and safeguard passwords.

Security Incident Procedures Standard

The security incident procedures standard states that CEs must "Implement policies and procedures to address security incidents" (45 CFR§164.308(a)(6)). Clearly, the numerous preceding standards are all foundational supports that enable the achievement of this standard. Response and reporting is the single required implementation specification that states CEs must "Identify and respond to suspected or known security incidents; mitigate, to the extent practicable, harmful effects of security incidents that are known to the covered entity; and document security incidents and their outcomes" (45 CFR §164.308(a)(6)). Among others, some examples of security incidents include such things as lost or stolen passwords, information system virus attacks, and theft of electronic media storage devices.

Contingency Plan Standard

The contingency plan standard is central to being able to ensure availability of data. This standard requires CEs to "Establish (and implement as needed) policies and procedures for responding to an emergency or other occurrence (for example, fire, vandalism, system failure, and natural disaster) that damages systems that contain electronic protected health information" (45 CFR §164.308(a)(7)).

This standard is supported by three required and two addressable implementation specifications. The required data back up plan implementation specification requires CEs to "Establish and implement procedures to create and maintain retrievable exact copies of electronic protected health information" (45 CFR §164.308 (a)(7)). To meet this implementation specification, organizations not only have to document what data needs to be backed up, but also must understand the sources of all of that data. The disaster recovery plan implementation specification is also required and mandates CEs to "Establish (and implement as needed) procedures to restore any loss of data" (45 CFR §164.308 (a)(7)). For the development of such a plan, a facility must determine the potential means of loss for their specific facility and location. Fire, water, and system destruction losses might be common among most organizations but loss due to tornadoes and hurricanes would be more specific to the geographic area. The required emergency mode operation plan implementation specification demands that CEs "Establish (and implement as needed) procedures to enable continuation of critical business processes for protection of the security of electronic protected health information while operating in emergency mode" (45 CFR 164.308(a)(7)). Prior to developing these procedures, the critical business processes must be identified as a first step before the procedures can be developed.

Testing and revisions procedures is the first of the two addressable implementation specifications in this section. Where this implementation specification is reasonable and appropriate for a CE it must "Implement procedures for periodic testing and revision of contingency plans" (45 CFR 164.308(a)(7)). This implementation specification applies to data back up plans, disaster recovery plans, and emergency mode operations. Many factors may influence the frequency and comprehensiveness of the testing and revisions procedures. Some of these factors include the organization's size as well as the availability of financial and human resources. Application and data criticality analysis is the second addressable implementation specification falling under this standard. When this implementation specification is deemed reasonable and appropriate for the specific CE, then it must "Assess the relative criticality of specific applications and data in support of other contingency plan components" (45 CFR 164.308(a)(7)). In essence, this specification compels organizations to truly understand the value of their systems and to balance recovery and management efforts to the criticality level of each system in the organization. Procedures must also be in place for assessing the systems as new ones are added or any other changes made in the normal operations of the systems.

Evaluation Standard

The eighth standard of the administrative safeguards is referred to as the "evaluation" standard (45 CFR §164.308(a)(8)). This standard is singular in requirement and has no supporting implementation specifications. It requires CEs to

> Perform a periodic technical and nontechnical evaluation, based initially upon the standards implemented under this rule and subsequently, in response to environmental or operations changes affecting the security of electronic protected health information, that establishes the extent to which an entity's security policies and procedures meet the requirements of this subpart of the Security Rule (45 CFR 164.308(a)(8)).

The constant advances in technology and the growing use of new technologies are just two reasons demonstrating the need for this standard. An ongoing evaluation process is most likely to meet the spirit of this regulation, but the complexity of integrated health information technology often limits such an approach. The evaluation standard recognizes the limitations organizations may face in using an ongoing evaluation tool and supports alternative approaches provided they meet the intent of this standard.

Business Associate Contracts and Other Arrangements Standard

45 CFR §164.308(b)(1) is the final standard in the administrative safeguards section of the Security Rule; it addresses BAs. By definition, a business associate is, according to the HIPAA Privacy Rule, (1) an individual (or group) who is not a member of a CE's workforce but who helps the CE in the performance of various functions involving the use or disclosure of individually identifiable health information, or (2) a person or organization other than a member of a CE's workforce that performs functions or activities on behalf of or affecting a CE

that involve the use or disclosure of individually identifiable health information (AHIMA 2012, 54).

In January 2013 a final omnibus rule went into effect to provide greater protections for patient information than were in the original Health Insurance Portability and Accountability Act (HIPAA) of 1996 (OCR 2013a). The changes were, in part, to address items from the American Recovery and Reinvestment Act (ARRA) of 2009 and the Genetic Information Nondiscrimination Act (GINA) of 2008. One of the four final rules was to "make business associates of covered entities directly liable for compliance with certain of the HIPAA Privacy and Security Rules' requirements" (OCR 2013a). The final rule modified business associate to include health information organizations (HIO), e-prescribing gateways, and other persons that facilitate data transmissions, as well as vendors of personal health records.

Specific items that were addressed included that BAs

- Follow the Security Rule for ePHI.
- Have business associate agreements (BAAs) with their subcontractors who must also follow the security rule for ePHI. CEs do not have BAAs with these subcontractors.
- Obtain authorization prior to marketing (AHIMA 2013).

There is much implied under the first item regarding following the Security Rule. This means that the BA must follow all of the requirements of the rule just as the CEs do. They will need to have their security procedures in place, assess them, have BAAs with their subcontractors, and report breaches or potential breaches of information, to name a few of their new responsibilities.

Check Your Understanding 11.1

Instructions: Choose the best answer.

1. An inherent weakness or absence of a safeguard that could be exploited by a threat is a
   a. Security incident
   b. Breach
   c. Vulnerability
   d. Threat

2. The Security Rule safeguards are
   a. Administrative
   b. Physical
   c. Technical
   d. All of the above
   e. b and c only

3. Which one of the following is an administrative safeguard action?
   a. Facility access control
   b. Documentation retention guidelines
   c. Maintenance record
   d. Media reuse

4. The data backup plan requires that organizations
   a. Know what data needs to be backed up and sources of that data
   b. Create nightly data backup procedures
   c. Utilize offsite storage
   d. Act in accordance with the contingency plan

Instructions: Indicate whether the following statements are true or false (T or F).

5. The Security Rule specifies the methods for conducting the required risk analysis.

6. The required implementation specification for the security incident procedures standard is response and reporting.

⊙ Physical Safeguards Standards

The Security Rule defines **physical safeguards** as "physical measures, policies, and procedures to protect a covered entity's electronic information systems and related buildings and equipment, from natural and environmental hazards, and unauthorized intrusion" (45 CFR §164.310; HIPAA Security Series 2007b). These standards are far reaching as they require CEs to consider all physical access to the organization's ePHI. Like the administrative safeguards standards, the physical safeguards standards also have addressable and required implementation specifications. Where a CE deems an implementation specification to be reasonable and appropriate for their organization, they must then fulfill the addressable or required specifications.

Facility Access Control Standard

The facility access control standard requires CEs to "Implement policies and procedures to limit physical access to its electronic housed, information systems and the facility or facilities in which they are housed, while ensuring that properly authorized access is allowed" (45 CFR §164.310(a)(1)). Important to this discussion is an understanding of what the term facility means. For the purposes of the Security Rule, the definition of facility is "the physical premises and the interior and exterior of a building" (45 CFR §164.310(a)(1)). The four addressable implementation specifications for this section of the Rule are: contingency operations, security plan, access control and validation procedures, and maintenance records.

The contingency operation addressable implementation specification requires CEs to "Establish (and implement as needed) procedures that allow facility access in support of restoration of lost data under the disaster recovery plan and emergency mode operations plan in the event of an emergency" (45 CFR §164.310(a) (1)). Contingency operations are complex and will vary from organization to organization with the intent being that CEs have the flexibility to determine the best approach for their given situation.

The facility security plan is the second addressable implementation specification under this standard. The intent of this implementation specification is that the facility security plan is to document the use of access controls. The CE is required to "Implement policies and procedures to safeguard the facility and the equipment therein from unauthorized physical access, tampering, and theft" (45 CFR §164.310(a)(1)) To meet this implementation specification, organizations should consider methods such as lock and key controls, security tagging equipment, using video cameras for surveillance, monitoring identification badges, and the use of human workforce to perform facility security checks.

The third addressable implementation specification associated with this standard is access controls and validation procedures. This specification indicates that CEs must "Implement procedures to control and validate a person's access to facilities based on their role or function, including visitor control, and control of access to software programs for testing or revision" (45 CFR §164.310(a)(1)). The characteristics of the CE (that is, size) may influence some of the decisions made in regard to this specification. For example, in large facilities badge access may be visually confirmed for every workforce member every day. In smaller organizations where the staff is small, identification badge access confirmation may not be a daily activity since, presumably, everyone knows the workforce members by face. In addition to workforce members, CEs must evaluate practices to control and limit visitor access to information. This implementation specification requires CEs to document the rationale for how they reach their security decisions.

Maintenance records are the final implementation specification in this section. This specification states that CEs must "Implement policies and procedures to document repairs and modifications to the physical components of a facility which are related to security (for example, hardware, walls, doors and locks)" (45 CFR §164.310(a)(1)). Again, environmental (that is, facility size, location, and so on) factors may influence how an organization makes it decisions for this specification. Manual logs may be appropriate in some cases and more sophisticated controls may be appropriate in other cases.

Workstation Use Standard

The workstation use standard stands alone without additional implementation specifications. To meet this standard the CE must

> Implement policies and procedures that specify the proper functions to be performed, the manner in which those functions are to be performed, and the physical attributes of the surroundings of a specific workstation or class of workstation that can access electronic protected health information (45 CFR §164.310(b)).

An important note is that this standard applies not only to workstations located physically in the facility. It applies at a much broader level to workforce members using workstations offsite to complete their work activities. At a minimum, any safeguards that are required in the office must also be required offsite. An example of this kind of safeguard is timeouts or logouts that break the system connection if the workstation remains idle for a specified period of time.

Workstation Security Standard

The workstation security standard requires CEs to "Implement physical safeguards for all workstations that access electronic protected health information, to restrict access to authorized users" (45 CFR§164.310(c)). This standard differs from the previous workstation use standard that addresses policies and procedures for how workstations should be used and protected. The workstation security standard addresses how workstations are to be physically protected from unauthorized access.

Device and Media Controls Standard

The device and media controls standard states that CEs are to "Implement policies and procedures that govern the receipt and removal of hardware and electronic media that contain electronic protected health information, into and out of a facility, and the movement of these items within the facility" (45 CFR §164.310(d)(1)). The Security Rule defines electronic media as "electronic storage media including memory devices in computers (hard drives) and any removable/ transportable digital memory medium, such as magnetic tape or disk, optical disk, or digital memory card." A major consideration for organizations trying to meet this standard is the need to understand what all of their information resources are and where they all lie. This often leads to the need for establishing an effective method for inventorying systems. Not only do organizations need to document their existing and new systems, they must also track movement of components of each system as well as track system and system component obsolescence and replacement. Two addressable and two required implementation specifications support this standard. The two addressable specifications are accountability and data backup and storage. The required specifications are disposal and media reuse.

The required disposal implementation specification states that CEs must "Implement policies and procedures to address the final disposition of electronic protected health information, and/or the hardware or electronic media on which it is stored" (45 CFR §164.310(d)(1)). There are multiple methods that can be used to make ePHI unusable or unreadable. The Security Rule specifically mentions degaussing as one of those methods, but stops short of requiring degaussing as the preferred method for rendering data unreadable or unusable when a CE wishes to dispose of electronic media that contains ePHI.

The required media reuse implementation specification states that CEs must "Implement procedures for removal of electronic protected health information from electronic media before the media are made available for re-use" (45 CFR §164.310(d)(1)). This implementation specification is applicable to both internal and external reuse of media scenarios and requires organizations to develop policies and procedures to address media reuse.

The addressable accountability implementation specification states that the CE must "Maintain a record of the movements of hardware and electronic media and any person responsible therefore" (45 CFR §164.310(d)(1)). This implementation specification presents a growing challenge in many healthcare organizations where mobile technology is increasing in use, increasing in cost, increasing in data storage, and decreasing in size. The decreasing size factor creates an increased risk due to the opportunity for concealment and theft. The flipside to this discussion is the value it offers in terms of convenience to the user. Like so many concepts addressed by HIPAA, organizations must devise methods to ensure an appropriate balance of protection and access or use. This addressable implementation specification speaks again to the need for inventorying and tracking of electronic media.

Data backup and storage is the final addressable implementation specification for this standard. Under this implementation specification the CE must "Create a retrievable, exact copy of electronic protected health information, when needed, before movement of equipment" (45 CFR §164.310(d)(1)). This implementation specification parallels the data backup plan for the contingency plan standard in the administrative safeguards section of the Rule. As such, both components of the rule are often fulfilled with a combined policy and procedure that meets the requirements of both sections.

⊙ Technical Safeguards Standards

As technological advances occur they often bring with them new security challenges. The conundrum of duality of interests again presents itself here. Advancing technology leads to great opportunity, but at the same time increases organizational risk. Balancing these two facets to capitalize on the benefits and reduce the risks is often at the center of both the HIPAA Privacy and Security Rules.

The Security Rule defines **technical safeguards** as "the technology and the policy and procedures for its use that protect electronic protected health information and control access to it" (45 CFR §164.308). In keeping with the flexibility, scalability, and technological neutrality concepts of meeting the Security Rule requirements, CEs must determine which security measures and technologies are reasonable and appropriate for implementation in its organization (HIPAA Security Series 2007c).

Access Control Standard

The access control standard directs CEs to "implement technical policies and procedures for electronic information systems that maintain electronic protected health information to allow access only to those persons or software programs that have been granted access rights as specified in §164.308(a)(4)[information access management]" (45 CFR §164.312 (a)(1)). Of importance here is the concept that access controls should be appropriate for the role and function of the workforce member. Two required and two addressable implementation specifications are included in this standard.

The required unique user identification implementation specification states that CEs must "Assign a unique name and/or number for identifying and tracking user identity" (45 CFR §164.312(a)(1)). Unique identification methods allow for the user's actions to be monitored and serve as the method of enforcing accountability of user actions.

The second required implementation specification is referred to as the emergency access procedure. This specification states that CEs must "Establish (and implement as needed) procedures for obtaining necessary electronic protected health information during an emergency" (45 CFR §164.312(a)(1)). This description, at face value, conveys the import of ensuring availability of information as needed to perform one's role in emergency situations. From a technology standpoint, many systems have a "**break the glass**" method that allows users to access data that they may not otherwise be allowed to access. The users are alerted in advance that their actions are being monitored giving them an opportunity to halt their actions, if inappropriate.

Automatic logoff is the first addressable implementation specification, which states that CEs must "implement electronic procedures that terminate an electronic session after a predetermined time of inactivity" (45 CFR §164.312(a)(1)). This concept is probably not foreign to readers as it is commonly used in many types of information systems, healthcare and otherwise.

Encryption and decryption is the final addressable implementation specification. Where this implementation specification is a reasonable and appropriate safeguard for a CE, the CE must "Implement a mechanism to encrypt and decrypt electronic protected health information" (45 CFR §164.312(a)(1)). **Encryption** is a technical method that reduces access and viewing of ePHI by unauthorized users. Encryption is defined as the process of transforming text into an unintelligible string of characters that can be transmitted via communications media with a high degree of security and then decrypted when it reaches a secure destination (AHIMA 2012, 153).

Audit Controls Standard

The audit control standard is singular in focus and requires CEs to "Implement hardware, software, and/or procedural mechanisms that record and examine activity in information systems that contain or use electronic protected health information" (45 CFR §164.312(b)). This standard recognizes that regardless of the controls put into place to prevent unauthorized access, there must be a way to track and record user activities in the system. Such tracking can be used to monitor intentional and unintentional actions taken by users to access ePHI.

Integrity Standard

The integrity standard is supported by one addressable implementation specification. The integrity standard states that CEs must "implement policies and procedures to protect electronic protected health information from improper alteration or destruction" (45 CFR §164.312(c)(1)). This standard is intended to ensure data integrity, which is defined as the extent to which healthcare data are complete, accurate, consistent, and timely; it is a security principle that keeps information from being modified or otherwise corrupted either maliciously or accidentally (AHIMA 2012, 120). Ultimately, data integrity supports high-quality clinical care and the effect of compromised data integrity can be significant. For these reasons, organizations must take steps to ensure data are not improperly altered or destroyed. The addressable implementation specification mechanisms to authenticate ePHI requires CEs to "implement electronic mechanisms to corroborate that electronic protected health information has not been altered or destroyed in an unauthorized manner" (45 CFR §164.312(c)(1)).

Person or Entity Authentication Standard

The person or entity authentication standard requires CEs to "Implement procedures to verify that a person or entity seeking access to electronic protected health information is the one claimed" (45 CFR §164.312(d)). Simply put, this standard seeks to ensure that organizations put methods in place to verify that users are who they claim they are. Passwords, smart cards, tokens, fobs, and biometrics are some of the many methods used in healthcare settings to confirm user identity.

Transmission Security

The transmission security standard recognizes the potential risk involved with data in transit and requires CEs to "implement technical security measures to guard against unauthorized access to electronic protected health information that is being transmitted over an electronic communications network" (45 CFR §164.312(e)(1)). Two addressable implementation specifications are associated with this standard. The integrity controls implementation specification directs CEs to "implement security measures to ensure that electronically transmitted electronic protected health information is not improperly modified without detection until disposed of" (45 CFR §164.312(e)(1)). Specifically covered in this implementation specification is the assurance that ePHI is not improperly modified during transmission. The encryption addressable implementation specification states that CEs must "implement a mechanism to encrypt electronic protected health information whenever deemed appropriate" (45 CFR §164.312(e)(1)). Encryption converts the original message into encoded or unreadable text. When decrypted, the message returns to its original state and can be read by the recipient. Senders and receivers must use compatible technology tools in order to encrypt and decrypt messages.

⊙ Confidentiality, Integrity, and Availability

The HIPAA Security Rule seeks to uphold confidentiality, integrity, and availability of data. The previously discussed administrative, physical, and technical safeguards also require and recommend methods to ensure confidentiality, integrity, and availability of data.

Confidentiality

Confidentiality is a legal and ethical concept that establishes the healthcare provider's responsibility for protecting health records and other personal and private information from unauthorized use or disclosure (LaTour et al. 2013, 904). In the context of the Security Rule, confidentiality means that ePHI is accessible only by authorized people and processes.

Integrity

Maintaining data integrity is central to the Security Rule. Under the Rule, **integrity** means that e-PHI is not altered or destroyed in an unauthorized manner. With continuing advancements in technology and electronic data management come additional legal obligations for ensuring data integrity. In addition to Security Rule requirements, concepts such as e-discovery that implore organizations to establish and follow methods to ensure integrity are becoming commonplace in healthcare organizations.

Availability

Equally as important as protecting ePHI from unauthorized users is the concept of ensuring that it can be accessed as needed by authorized users. **Availability** is the veritable "flip side of the coin" in the discussion of protecting information from inappropriate access. Encompassed in the concept of availability are many of the previously discussed safeguards such as the data backup and storage specification.

⊙ Penalties and Enforcement

Penalties and enforcement were addressed in the original HIPAA bill but have changed over time. The determination of penalties is complex depending on the kind of violation; whether it was an inadvertent release of information, neglectful, or done knowingly; whether it was a primary or subsequent violation; and whether there was negligence in correcting known policies and procedures that led to violations. The history of the enforcement is complex due to the numerous changes of the agencies responsible; however, the duplication of efforts has been recognized and responsibility streamlined as a result.

The Office for Civil Rights

The **Office for Civil Rights (OCR)** is currently the enforcement agency for the HIPAA Privacy and Security Rule. Since April 14, 2003, the Privacy Rule has been enforced by the OCR. The Security Rule was enforced by the Centers for Medicare and Medicaid Services (CMS) from its effective date of April 20, 2005 through July 26, 2009. Since that time, the Security Rule has been enforced by the OCR as well. While the Privacy and Security Rules were enforced by separate enforcement agencies, lack of clarity and duplication of efforts were noted. For these reasons, the OCR became the single enforcement agency for both Rules. The OCR must investigate all reported violations and appropriately initiate investigations for cause in absence of a reported violation.

Civil Penalties

The Privacy and Security Rules both outline various penalties for violations. **Civil penalties** are generally fines or money damages used to sanction violators. The Final Rule for HIPAA modified civil penalty enforcement language in both the Privacy and Security Rules by outlining a tiered structure of enforcement guidelines. The tiered method specifies a minimum to maximum penalty range based on the specific category of violation. The four main categories of civil violations are escalating in nature and start at the bottom rung with violations where the individual did not know (or through reasonable diligence would not have known) that he or she violated HIPAA and range to the fourth and final category, which is reserved for those that violate HIPAA through willful neglect and do not correct the violation pattern. The civil money penalties listed below first list those penalties that were in effect prior to February 18, 2009 and then what was in effect on or after February 18, 2009.

Civil money penalties prior to February 18, 2009, may not impose

- More than $100 per violation, or
- In excess of $25,000 for identical violations during a calendar year

The amount of civil money penalties imposed on or after February 18, 2009 is subject to the following limitations:

- For a violation in which it is established that the CE did not know and, by exercising reasonable diligence, would not have known that the CE violated such provision,
  - In the amount of less than $100 or more than $50,000 for each violation, or
  - In excess of $1,500,000 for identical violations during a calendar year (January 1 though the following December 31)
- For a violation in which it is established that the violation was due to reasonable cause and not to willful neglect,
  - In the amount of less than $1,000 or more than $50,000 for each violation, or
  - In excess of $1,500,000 for identical violations during a calendar year
- For a violation in which it is established that violation was due to willful neglect and was corrected during the 30-day period beginning on the first date the CE liable for the penalty knew, or, by exercising reasonable diligence would have known that the violation occurred,
  - In the amount of less than $10,000 or more than $50,000 for each violation, or
  - In excess of $1,500,000 for identical violations during a calendar year
- For a violation in which it is established that the violation was due to willful neglect and was not corrected during the 30-day period beginning on the

first date the CE liable for the penalty knew, or, by exercising reasonable diligence, would have known that the violation occurred,

o In the amount of less than $50,000 for each violation, or

o In excess of $1,500,000 for identical violations during a calendar year (45 CFR §160.404)

Criminal Penalties

If the OCR reviews a complaint and determines that it qualifies as a criminal violation the case is referred to the Department of Justice (DOJ). In 2005, the DOJ clarified that criminal violation enforcement is applicable to both individuals and CEs. When **criminal penalties** are appropriate, the OCR works in conjunction with the DOJ to pursue possible violators. Criminal penalties can be a fine or imprisonment, whether suspended or not.

Enforcement Activities to Date

The **HIPAA Enforcement Rule** is found at 45 CFR §160, subparts C, D, and E. This Rule spells out the authority of the OCR as previously described. The complaint process is fully outlined on the OCR website and presents the process from initial complaint through referral, investigation, and resolution. After investigation, resolutions range from the OCR finding no violation to obtaining corrective action to the issuance of formal findings of violation. In addition, reported violations may be found unenforceable due to technical issues such as not filing the complaint within the required time frame, the entity not being considered a CE, or the incident as described not violating the Rules.

Since 2003, over 77,866 complaints have been filed with the OCR for HIPAA privacy violations with 91 percent of those complaints having been resolved at the time of this writing. Privacy Rule enforcement data reveals that approximately 24 percent of the reported violations have required changes in privacy practices or other corrective actions. Approximately 12 percent of the reported violations were investigated and found to be without merit and were resolved as nonviolations. Of the remaining complaints, approximately 55 percent were closed due to not being enforceable under the Rule. Security Rule enforcement activities have been less structured than their privacy rule counterparts. This may be partly due to the methods by which security violations are found. Security violations are more insulated within the organization and may not be found without external review. For this reason, the OCR initiated compliance reviews in 2008. CMS initiated these reviews based on complaints filed against the entities, identification of potential Security Rule violations through the media, or recommendations from HHS and OCR (HIPAA Compliance Review Analysis 2008). With transitioning of enforcement activities to the OCR in 2009, more routine complaint reporting is anticipated due to increased efforts to educate consumers about how to file security complaints. Since OCR began reporting its Security Rule enforcement results in October 2009, approximately 645 complaints have been received alleging a violation of the Security Rule. Seventy-five percent of the complaints have been closed after investigation and appropriate corrective action. At the last reporting, OCR had 238 open complaints and compliance reviews (OCR 2013b).

Breach Notification

In January 2013 the Final Rule modifications went into effect. These modification are related to various parts of HIPAA, including breach notification rules. They updated preceding HIPAA rules and those changes that had been made previously under the HITECH Act and GINA Act. The final rule on breach notification for unsecured protected health information under the HITECH Act replaces the breach notification rule's "harm" threshold with a more objective standard and supplants an interim final rule published in August 2009.

The rule requires CEs and BAs to report breaches of unsecured protected health information. Unsecured protected health information is protected health information that has not been rendered unusable, unreadable, or indecipherable to unauthorized individuals through the use of a technology or methodology (13402(h) (2) of Public Law 111-5). Encryption and destruction are the technologies and methodologies for rendering protected health information unusable, unreadable, or indecipherable to unauthorized individuals. The National Institute for Standards and Technology of the United States Department of Commerce (NIST) has issued a series of special publications that address encryption of data at rest and in motion as well as destruction of both electronic and nonelectronic media. These special publications are numbered in the 800 series and can be located at the NIST website.

A **breach** is defined under the 2013 final rule as "the acquisition, access, use, or disclosure of protected health information in a manner not permitted….which compromises the security or privacy of the protected health information" (45 CFR§ 164.402). Reporting requirements mandate notification to the individual whose information was breached, and in the case of breaches of more than 500 individuals' information, to the media and Secretary of HHS. Three exceptions to this definition exist with the first being when a workforce member unintentionally acquires, uses, or discloses PHI while acting under the authority of a CE or BA. The second exception is applicable when an authorized workforce member inadvertently discloses protected health information to another authorized workforce member within the same CE or BA setting. The final exception is applicable when the CE or BA who made an inadvertent disclosure has reason to believe that the recipient of the PHI would not have been able to retain the information. For example, if the provider called a patient with a common name to discuss laboratory results they might dial the wrong phone number. Although they might discuss "John Smith's" lab results, as long as no hard copy results were sent to the wrong patient, it is reasonable to believe that the wrong John Smith could not "keep" the information.

Risk Assessment

Covered entities and business associates must have procedures in place to conduct a risk analysis. This is done to assess the potential risks and areas of vulnerability to the security of the protected health information just as is required for the privacy aspect of HIPAA. It is important to identify and correct those things that might threaten the confidentiality, integrity, and availability of the information. Failure to conduct such an audit could be detrimental in the event of an audit or investigation of a complaint.

Check Your Understanding 11.2

Instructions: Choose the best answer.

1. Inventorying systems includes
   a. Existing and new systems
   b. Movement of components of each system
   c. Tracking system and system component obsolescence
   d. All of the above

2. The technology and the policies and procedures for its use that protects electronic protected health information and control access to it is
   a. Administrative Safeguards
   b. Technical Safeguards
   c. Physical Safeguards
   d. Integrity Controls

3. The integrity standard protects
   a. From unauthorized access
   b. From unauthorized use
   c. From improper transmission of data
   d. Improper alteration or destruction

Instructions: Indicate whether the following statements are true or false (T or F).

4. Small mobile devices are at greater risk due to the potential for concealment and theft.

5. When encrypted information is decrypted, it is in a different format than the original state.

6. Maintaining access to ePHI is less important than the protection of ePHI.

7. The difference between the levels of civil penalties has to do with whether the CE knew or should have known that a violation occurred.

8. Requirements for breach notification for business associates are the same as for CEs.

⊙ Medical Identity Theft and Disaster Preparedness

Health information serves many functions, the most important of which is patient care. However, health information serves many other functions. The legal considerations for health information extend beyond privacy, security, and the legal electronic health record (EHR). The legal considerations now include the responsibility of providers to protect against medical identity theft, consider legal liability related to medical malpractice in light of EHR use, and disaster planning and preparedness. The first two issues are relatively new and the third requires new and different ways of thinking, but they are vitally important in the evolving world of health information technology and EHRs. This section will discuss the challenges of each in turn and include recommendations for addressing each.

Medical Identity Theft

Medical identity theft is defined as the assumption of

> a person's name and sometimes other parts of his or her identity—such as insurance information or Social Security Number—without the victim's knowledge or consent to obtain medical services or goods, or when someone uses the person's identity to obtain money by falsifying claims for medical services and falsifying medical records to support those claims (Springer 2009).

Instances that would not be considered identify theft are where health information on the wrong patient was inadvertently put in the incorrect record. When the financial information on a patient is used to purchase nonmedical items and services, this is not considered medical identify theft. The key factors for a situation to be medical identify theft are that a form of a patient's identification is taken without the patient's knowledge and the identification is then used to acquire some sort of medical services. Some may question why anyone would want to steal one's medical identification. This theft is almost always done to then use the medical identification for the purpose of fraudulently obtaining medical goods and services.

In addition to the obvious financial implications of medical identity theft, medical identity theft carries the very real possibility that the incorrect information could be used to deliver patient care, putting patients at risk. This can occur if critical medical conditions, procedures, medications, allergies, and other information are either omitted from the record or wrongfully included (Rhinehart-Thompson 2008). Unfortunately, victims of identity theft can find themselves unable to access their records because some providers will refuse to release the records containing another patient's information—even if the other patient broke the law. Figure 11.2 illustrates how medical identity theft can affect an individual from the initial theft to the integrity of the health information.

A recent study was conducted to determine whether patient identity was confirmed during the admission and registration processes, as well as the methods used to establish patient identity at admission and registration (Mancilla and Moczygemba 2009). Using a combination of online surveys, telephone interviews and onsite observation, these HIM researchers learned that the majority (91.9 percent) of healthcare providers established identity with a driver's license, while just over 20 percent of the respondents indicated they were not aware of how their organizations handled exceptions to standard practices. Other interesting information was that the majority of medical identity theft cases arose in the

Figure 11.2　The cascading effect of medical identity theft

| The Cascading Effect of Medical Identity Theft |

Medical identity theft begins with the theft of individually identifiable health information. ⟷ Individually identifiable health information elements come from multiple sources.

The information can also be used inappropriately and without authorization outside the healthcare continuum. ← The information is then used inappropriately and without authorization within the healthcare continuum.

Primary healthcare continuum market players include patients, providers, payers/plans, sponsors, and support vendors.

Data Integrity of Health Information

Internal Controls for Privacy and Security Policies and Practices to Prevent, Detect, and Mitigate Medical Identity Theft

The misrepresented information within the healthcare continuum results in false claims, theft of health services from plan sponsors, false research, and false public health reports.

Secondary healthcare continuum market players include reporting agencies, research, public health, law enforcement, and support vendors

This can lead to identity theft.

The corrupted health records lead to health risks for the victim of the medical identity theft.

The effects of medical identity theft cascade throughout the healthcare continuum. Beyond being used to submit false claims, false data make their way into oversight agency databases, skewing public health findings. Ultimately, corrupted data in the victim's medical record may place the individual at risk in future treatment.

Source: AHIMA 2008.

emergency room, time constraints or demands placed on admissions personnel may result in noncompliance with policies and procedures, biometrics are not widely used, and the widespread use of the Social Security number helps contribute to medical identity theft (Mancilla and Moczygemba 2009). The study concluded that healthcare organizations face multiple regulations from many oversight agencies when attempting to detect and prevent medical identity theft (Mancilla and Moczygemba 2009).

Medical identity theft is an ongoing issue that healthcare organizations will have to address as healthcare organizations expand their use of information technology and expand that use to include the widespread transfer of data. New methods will need to be developed to prevent medical identity theft.

Red Flag Rules

In response to increasing identity theft, often used for financial gain, the Federal Trade Commission (FTC), Department of the Treasury, Federal Reserve System, Federal Deposit Insurance Corporation, and the National Credit Union Administration simultaneously issued regulations known as the "Red Flag Rules" in November 2007 (King and Williams 2008). These rules require creditor and financial institutions to implement an Identity Theft Prevention Program

(King and Williams 2008). The portion of these rules that apply to healthcare organizations are contained in 16 CFR § 681, under the enforcement authority of the FTC (Springer 2009). The **red flags** that are addressed in the rules are suspicious documents, information, or behaviors that indicate the possibility of identity theft (AHIMA 2012, 355). Examples of red flags include inconsistencies in documents (driver's license and insurance card), documents that appear to be altered, and not having more than one form of ID (insurance card but no other form of ID)

First, healthcare organizations must understand whether they are subject to the Red Flag Rules. Healthcare providers may be subject to the Red Flag Rules if they (1) meet the definition of creditor under the Fair Credit Reporting Act; or (2) use consumer credit reports, subjecting them to the Address Discrepancy Rule (Springer 2009). A healthcare creditor would include any organization that allows for payment on medical services provided to a patient after those services were provided or over a period of installment payments (King and Williams 2008). This includes most healthcare organizations, especially hospitals. Fortunately, the Red Flag Rules include guidelines to assist in the development of an Identity Theft Prevention Program.

1. Identify Covered Accounts: Most patient accounts and billing records qualify as covered accounts since they contain information sufficient to enable identity theft if lost or stolen.

2. Identify Relevant Red Flags: A red flag is a pattern or practice of specific activity that indicates the possible existence of identity theft. Red flags can include alerts, notifications, or other warnings that might be received from consumer report agencies or other service providers; suspicious documents such as identification cards or other documents which are inconsistent or appear to be falsified; other suspicious information such as odd changes of address; or other unusual use of or other suspicious activity related to a given account.

3. Detect Red Flags: Organizations must develop reasonable approaches for detecting potential red flags. This requires that organizations determine what information and documentation will be required of patients. Many now require both an insurance card, as well as a photo identification card such as a driver's license. Additionally, organizations must establish policies and procedures. This is quite important since liability increases if the workforce either cannot or does not follow the policies and procedures. Thus, the policies and procedures should support the detection of red flags in a feasible way.

4. Respond to Red Flags: An adequate response to red flags includes prevention and mitigation via monitoring covered accounts; contacting patients or consumers if needed; changing passwords and security codes; handling accounts carefully; or notifying law enforcement. These responses will, of necessity, be context-dependent and often require judgment on the part of the healthcare organizations. For example, what will the organization do if the patient cannot produce all of the identification required or the identification presented has discrepancies?

5. Oversee the Program: As with all operations, the Identity Theft Prevention Program falls under the purview of the board of directors, trustees, or the designated member of management.

6. Train Employees: The workforce, especially those responsible for creating, maintaining, and administering patient accounts, must be trained in all aspects of identity theft prevention.

7. Oversee Service Provider Arrangements: The healthcare organization must take steps to ensure that any service providers granted access to covered accounts carries out the Identity Theft Prevention Program.

8. Approve the Identity Theft Prevention Program: The board of directors or appropriate committee must review and approve the Identity Theft Prevention Program.

9. Provide Reports and Periodic Updates to the Identity Theft Prevention Program: A written report on the status of the program, service provider arrangements, any significant incidents, and recommendations for any needed changes should be included in the annual report (King and Williams 2008).

Organizations that have already implemented the Red Flag Rules report finding increases in attempted and successful identity theft (Keith 2010). Unfortunately, they report that it is difficult to detect red flags at the time it is being perpetrated though they do try. Some have implemented special designations in their registration pathways so that all employees can identify records of victims, perpetrators, or those with suspicious activity. Yet, most medical identity theft is still detected when the bill is issued (Keith 2010).

Operational Recommendations

The obligations of health informatics and HIM professionals related to medical identity theft fall into three general areas. The first is to urge and educate consumers to adopt preventive measures such as

- Exercising caution when sharing personal and health information with providers
- Monitoring the Explanation of Benefits (EOB) they receive from insurance companies
- Maintaining copies of healthcare records
- Monitoring credit reports and history documents for unexpected medical charges or liens
- Protecting all health insurance and financial information (AHIMA 2008)

The second area is establishing organizational methods to prevent and detect medical identity theft. Some of these methods include

- Conducting and acting upon an information security risk analysis on an annual basis

- Ensuring background checks are performed for employees and BAs when hiring, especially for work in high-risk areas
- Establishing patient identification verification processes that are compliant with the HIPAA Security Rule, but are also feasible for high-throughput areas with significant time demands
- Minimizing the use of Social Security numbers for identification, suppressing it when possible and when not, displaying only the last four or six digits of the number
- Implementing policies and procedures that safeguard the privacy and security of individually identifiable health information, in compliance with applicable HIPAA and other federal and state regulations
- Creating an alerting and identity theft response plan if any suspicious activity is discovered
- Implementing ongoing staff training programs to ensure all employees with access to identifiable patient information can assist in preventing identity theft (AHIMA 2008)

The third medical identity theft area where HIM professionals have an obligation to assist is related to the data in the patient record and is particularly important. The steps an HIM professional can help with include

- Drafting policies and procedures to ensure victims of medical identity theft are not denied access to their patient records
- Establishing mechanisms to correct inaccurate information in patient records, which includes assisting victims in identifying those who may possess inaccurate records by providing a full accounting of disclosures
- Staying abreast of medical identity theft–related legislation and regulations
- Providing victims of medical identity theft with the checklist of actions and resources found in figure 11.3.

Figure 11.3   Medical identity theft response checklist and resources for consumers

Task	✓ When Complete
1. Explore the resource "Tools for Victims" provided by Federal Trade Commission (available online at www.ftc gov/bcp/edu/microsites/idtheft/tools.html). Consider completing the universal affidavit to submit to creditors.	
2. Review credit reports, correct them, and place a "Fraud Alert" on them.	

(*Continued*)

Figure 11.3 Medical identity theft response checklist and resources for consumers (*Continued*)

Task	✓ When Complete
3. If a Social Security number is suspected of being used inappropriately, contact the Social Security Administration's fraud hotline at (800) 269-0721.	
4. In the case of stolen or misdirected mail, contact the US postal Service at (800) 275-8777 to obtain the number of the local US postal Inspector.	
5. For stolen passports, contact the US Department of State at (877) 487-2776 or http://travel.state.gov.	
6. If the thief has stolen checks, contact both check verification companies: Telecheck ([800] 366-2425) and the international Check Services Company ([800] 526-5380) to place a fraud alert on the account to ensure that counterfeit checks will be refused.	
7. Contact the health information manager or the privacy officer at the provider organization or the antifraud hotline at the health plan where the medical identity theft appears to have occurred.	
8. Request an accounting of disclosures. If the provider or plan refuses access to medical records, file a complaint with the Office for Civil Rights at Health and Human Services at (866) 627-7748 or www.hhs.gov/ocr/privacyhawtofile.htm.	
9. Take detailed notes of all conversations related to the medical identity theft. Write down the date, name, and contact information of everyone contacted, as well as the content of the conversation.	
10. Make copies of any letters, reports, documents, and e-mail sent or received regarding the identity theft.	
11. Work with the organization where the medical identity theft occurred to stop the flow of the incorrect information, correct the existing inaccurate health record entries, and determine where incorrect information was sent.	
12. File a police report and send copies with correct information to insurers, providers, and credit bureaus once the identity theft has been confirmed.	
13. File a complaint with the attorney general in the state where the identity theft occurred. The National Association of Attorneys General provides state-by-state information at www.naag.org/attorneys_general.php.	

Task	✓ When Complete
14. Check with state authorities for resources. Many states provide consumer protection and education related to insurance and accept online complaints. To determine if a state has a state insurance department for online complaints, visit the National Association of Insurance Commissioners at www.naic.org and file a complaint as appropriate.	
15. File a complaint with the Identity Theft Data Clearinghouse, operated by the Federal Trade Commission and the Internet Crime Complaint Center. Information available for filing a complaint can be found at https://m.ftc.gov/pls/dod/widlpubl$.startup?Z_ORG_CODE=PU03.	
16. Contact the Department of Health and Human Services at (800) 366-1019 or by visiting the website at www.hhs.gov/ocr for suspected Medicare or Medicaid fraud.	
17. Review health records to make sure they have been corrected prior to seeking healthcare.	
18. Change all personal identification numbers and passwords for protected accounts, sites, access points, etc. Choose unique personal identification numbers and complex passwords rather than common ones (e.g., mother's maiden name, birth date, or pet name).	

Source: AHIMA 2008.

Medical identity theft or financial identity theft causes significant problems for consumers, insurers, and providers at a minimum. It is important that all possible steps be taken to both prevent medical identity theft and mitigate or minimize the effects of medical identity theft once it occurs.

Disaster Preparedness

Health informatics and information management professionals have two very important roles related to disaster preparedness: (1) ensure the protection of the organization's information assets; and (2) ensure the information functions will continue in the event of a natural or man-made disaster affecting the entire organization. These two roles can be separated because the first can occur without the second, but are related. The first role of protecting the information assets needs to be done in all situations, including those that might not technically be termed a disaster, such as attacks by hackers or technical system failure due to network or software malfunctions. Since this role focuses largely on protecting the information assets, it is largely under the purview of the HIM and IT departments. The second role crosses all departments or functions in the organization and, while HIM and IT are expected to meet the organizational needs, it is extremely collaborative in nature.

Protecting Information Assets

Protection of organizational information assets is a part of the HIPAA Security Rule. While the technical requirements of the Security Rule seem fairly straightforward, the information security team must prepare thoroughly, thinking outside of the box, envisioning worst-case scenarios or trying to imagine how a technically savvy person could do harm to the organization via the different installed information systems. The NIST has published guides to help organizations, including the federal government, prepare contingency plans for information systems operations and systems. NIST Special Publication 800-34 Rev. 1, Contingency Planning Guide for Federal Information Systems, gives guidance and provides multiple templates for developing disaster plans for information services. NIST Special Publication 800-30, Rev. 1, Guide for Conducting Risk Assessments, can also help with information asset protection planning. These and additional NIST guidance can be found at http://csrc.nist.gov/publications. Several examples of risks follow to illustrate the possibilities, while table 11.1 provides a matrix for conducting a **business impact analysis**, which is one method for evaluating and prioritizing the risks.

Significant risks to information systems that might put the organization at risk include hackers attacking computers that control medical equipment and facilities that are on networks with weak security, or significant downtime due to a massive system failure. Both of these have occurred in recent years and have been publicized. The first situation occurred in Texas where the heating, ventilation, and air conditioning system for a medical center had been set up to be accessed remotely by an outside company that managed the system (Gupta 2011). Hackers attempted to use this poorly secured computer to gain access to other systems. Upon investigation by law enforcement, it was discovered that the system had been attacked previously more than 10 times (Gupta 2011). In that same vein, another healthcare system experienced a worst-case scenario when the geographical area where their data system was located suffered a massive loss of power (Conn 2012). Since it was not where the organization itself was located, operations in the organization needed to continue unimpeded. Unfortunately, the backup generators only worked for a short time (Conn 2012).

Information technology and health information management personnel must prepare for these and other potential threats to their systems with the initial step of a business impact analysis (BIA). Concepts important to a BIA are the **recovery point objective (RPO)** and the **recovery time objective (RTO)** (Ranajee 2012). RPO represents the length of time which you can operate without a particular application. RTO is the maximum amount of time tolerable for data loss and capture (Ranajee 2012). The goal of the BIA is to identify any gaps in your current recovery capability and to develop a strategy for meeting the identified RTO and RPO. The following steps should be taken and the following questions should be asked:

1. Identify the minimal resources required to maintain business operations. What are essential operations and what is required to keep them running? What might be out of sight downstream that needs to be considered?

2. Determine the business recovery objectives and assumptions. How much downtime and loss of data can each department sustain? How is the data received and processed by each department?

3. Establish order of priority for restoration of business functions. What are the key patient care departments? What are the IT applications that support these critical operations?

4. Estimate the operational, financial, and reputational impact due to loss of data. While IT and HIM can provide data and information regarding these impacts, it is more appropriate for executives with input from the board of directors or trustees to make the final estimations and decisions. (Ranajee 2012)

Table 11.1, the impact analysis matrix, can be used to help make prioritization decisions. Items that fall into the red or orange quadrants should be handled first, not implying that those which fall in the yellow and green quadrants should not be addressed, only that they are a lower priority.

Once the BIA and prioritization have been accomplished many decisions remain to be made such as the type and location of backup data facilities. There are usually three different types of facilities:

1. **Hot site**: for critical applications and operations, which can be online within hours. This option is the most expensive.

2. **Warm site**: provides basic infrastructure, but takes time, possibly a week, to activate. Obviously, this is less expensive.

3. **Cold site**: equipment must be brought in, but the site is powered and secure. Much less expensive, but this could take up to a month to operationalize (Ranajee 2012).

Requirements such as HIPAA security regulations, BAAs, and so forth continue to pertain. Additionally, the backup data center should be located in a low-risk geographical location, that is, not in an earthquake or tornado zone; and should have multiple layers of physical security such as biometrics, mantraps, video monitoring and so on; expansion capabilities; and an established history of uptime and redundancy (Ranajee 2012).

Protecting the various patient care and other information systems, some of which might not have been considered, such as HVAC systems, is the first step to health information disaster preparedness. These systems can be attacked or

Table 11.1 Information security threat analysis quadrant

	Low Risk to Operations	**High Risk to Operations**
Low Probability of Occurring	Green	Orange
High Probability of Occurring	Yellow	Red

compromised in situations that do not necessarily include natural or man-made larger disasters and must be planned for accordingly.

Organizational Information Services Continuity during External Disasters

Hurricanes, tornadoes, flooding, earthquakes, and man-made disasters such as terrorist attacks and shooting sprees cannot, unfortunately, be ignored by health information professionals. Keeping operations going during an external disaster, whether an act of nature or man-made, is required. While disasters often result in some type of gap in services, a significant failure to plan could be considered negligence in certain circumstances. This section will explore different models and include recommendations for organization-wide information services **disaster recovery planning (DRP)**. For the purposes of this book, DRP for organizational information services is focused upon the recovery of physical disasters, including some elements usually included as a part of **business continuity planning (BCP)**. BCP includes the recovery and use of the technology as in DRP as well as the ability of the organization to continue the processes required for ongoing business operations. Sometimes BCP requires operational procedures in the absence of information technology.

Overview of Disaster Planning

Disaster planning can occur at many different levels, especially in a healthcare organization. Obviously, it can occur for the entire organization; however, departments can also plan for disaster, as can the entire community, which may be dependent upon that healthcare organization. In conjunction with many different levels of planning are the different components of preparedness, planning, response and recovery involved in disaster planning. Figure 11.4 is a graphical representation of how the different levels and different phases may interact.

One of the strategies learned after major disasters in the United States is that the workplace should help its workforce with their individual disaster planning. A 2004 Centers for Disease Control (CDC) study revealed that almost half of Florida residents had not created a personal evacuation plan prior to the very busy 2004 hurricane season (Beaton et al. 2008). Given that the disaster plan for any organization often rests with the workforce, the organization may want to ensure that its "essential" personnel have a personal disaster plan in place. For example, if in an earthquake zone, do the different family members know how they are supposed to communicate if an earthquake occurs? If in a hurricane or flood zone has the employee thought through when, where, and how his or her family would evacuate? If power is lost does the employee have a generator or a backup plan? One study reported that persons who feel their family might be at risk would be less likely to report to work (Beaton et al. 2008).

Naturally, healthcare organizations must have a disaster plan; however, within the organization the plans may exist at different levels. In the model included in figure 11.4, hospitals are considered a special case of workplace. Unfortunately, even the best planning does not make hospitals immune from significant problems. During Hurricane Katrina several hospitals were incapacitated. Ochsner Hospital

Figure 11.4   Model with Disaster Planning Levels and Steps

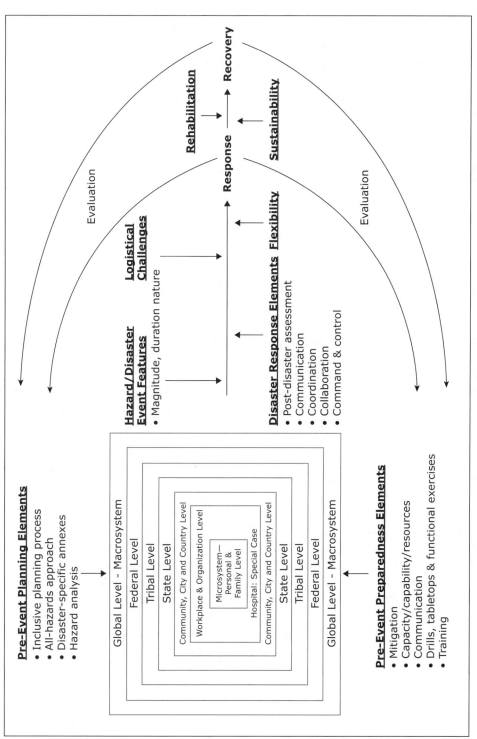

Reprinted with permission from SLACK Incorporated: Beaton, R., Bridges, E., Salazar, M.K., Oberle, M.W., Stergachis, A., Thompson, J., Butterfield, P. (2008). Ecological model of disaster management. AAOHN Journal, 56(11), 471–478.

reported difficulties contacting employees because the hurricane hit on a weekend, while East Jefferson General Hospital had not planned for the depth and breadth of the emergency, which resulted in the loss of backup generators and Internet (Harrison et al. 2008). Likewise, Mercy Hospital in Joplin, MO, was unprepared for the total destruction of their facility during the 2011 tornado (Braun 2012). The bottom line from an organizational perspective on planning is that it is almost impossible to truly envision the worst case unless it is total destruction. Therefore, the planning must be comprehensive and cannot presume continued electricity, operating generators, or other "niceties."

Community-level planning, at the town, city, county, state, or national level, relies heavily on the quality of the planning done at the lower levels, especially for hospitals and healthcare organizations. It is imperative that those doing the planning and carrying out the plan remember that the nature of disasters is dynamic and in flux, requiring constant adjustment and, ultimately, learning from previous disasters (Beaton et al. 2008).

Considerations for Disaster Planning

This section will explore the different components of disaster planning, especially related to information system and information process continuity. The four generally accepted components are planning (or mitigation or prevention), preparedness, response, and recovery (Beaton et al. 2008; Reynolds and Tamanaha 2010; Smith and Macdonald 2006; Gibson et al. 2012). The first two components must be accomplished prior to the disaster, with the third constituting the response to the disaster and the fourth including an analysis of how well the organization was served during the disaster. Each will be examined in turn.

Planning

Sometimes called planning or mitigation or prevention, the first step in the process is to involve all stakeholders so that understanding, agreement, and consensus can be reached regarding the goals for the disaster plan under development (Beaton et al. 2008). In the hospital this would include the executives, but also the front-line workers and key representative from all business units or functional areas. A good place to start is with the goal of the disaster plan. The BIA is an excellent tool to understand what is needed to achieve the goals. For example, continuing full operations with admissions still being accepted is quite a different goal than the orderly shutdown of operations. Neither is better or worse than the other, but will be dependent upon the mission or business focus of the healthcare organization. Generally, acute-care hospitals with emergency rooms must usually continue operations, while a clinic or specialty hospital might be able to discontinue clinical operations.

The second step for the planning process is to conduct a risk assessment or hazard vulnerability assessment (HVA) (Herzig 2010). This involves identifying persons, situations, or events that pose a particular danger or are particularly vulnerable (Beaton et al. 2008). For example, newborns and the elderly are more vulnerable to environmental changes or extremes. Thus, it would be important to consider the needs of special populations such as these in the disaster plan.

These two steps are really the prework for the disaster plan, ensuring that all of the necessary parties are involved and special situations that might change the plan are identified.

Preparedness

The next step is preparedness. This largely entails determining how the different risks that have been identified will be handled. Risks can be removed, reduced, assigned, or accepted (Nelson 2008). The preparedness component includes

1. Development of the plan
2. Organizing to carry out the plan
3. Training
4. Equipment acquisition
5. Testing or disaster drills
6. Evaluation
7. Improvement

The development of the plan requires significant input from information technology or systems since the success of the healthcare organization's disaster plan will be dependent upon communication during the disaster. The plan should be concise, well-written, easy-to-read, use generic job titles instead of names, and define the command structure and responsibilities (Herzig 2010).

There are recommendations to include in the organization of the plan that have been learned and shared by organizations that have survived other disasters. First and foremost is the importance of communication. Specifically, many organizations will have a telephone tree in place for contacting employees in case of emergency. However, those who have tried to communicate via telephone have found that it often does not work. Fortunately, texting often does work because it requires much less bandwidth than maintaining an open line for a call (Herzig 2010; Harrison et al. 2008). In one disaster report, a flood severely displaced staff. The organization put information including emergency contact information on its website; however, this had not been a part of the communication plan so people did not know to check there (Anon. 2011). Another important part of the plan organization is to ensure that roles and responsibilities are clear. Everyone should understand at least their initial tasks when disaster strikes (Beaton et al. 2008).

Training is a very essential part of preparedness. As was shared in the previous paragraph, staff had not been trained for the ultimate communication method rendering it somewhat ineffective. One reference maintains that all staff should know

⊙ Where the disaster plan is located
⊙ Which staff members are essential and should be contacted
⊙ Emergency contact details for all staff members
⊙ Evacuation procedures for their department or work location

⊙ The location of any disaster records in the hospital

⊙ How to access any electronic lists of patient details that exist (Smith and Macdonald 2006)

Equipment acquisition for preparedness can include everything including determining where, when, and how a hot backup of the EHR will operate; ensuring that adequate emergency documents are available in selected storage sites; ensuring solar-powered batteries are purchased and available for cell phones or other communication devices if necessary; and ensuring adequate water and food is available for patients and essential staff in an emergency (Beaton et al. 2008). Since these decisions for additional equipment or supply acquisition may involve considerable expense they are usually made at the executive or above level.

Healthcare facilities are required to conduct training, disaster drills, and other exercises to maintain their accreditation (Beaton et al. 2008). These exercises and drills often reveal weaknesses or other deficiencies that can then be addressed in the disaster plan. Any backup systems or remote storage or anything not used day-to-day should be tested to ensure it works as planned.

Ongoing evaluation of the disaster plan is essential. At a minimum the plan should be reviewed annually or sooner if significant changes to operations or information systems are made. Changes, including new clinical processes or equipment, are easy to implement without consideration given to disaster preparedness. Of course, the main reason for evaluation is to continue to improve the disaster plan and preparedness.

Although organizations must go through the planning and preparedness components, they do it in the hopes that they will never have to experience the next two, response and recovery.

Response and Recovery

The worst has happened and disaster has struck. It is time to activate the disaster plan. A dogmatic insistence on following the plan in every detail is not recommended. Instead, the response needs to be flexible, with imagination and ingenuity helping the workforce implement an effective disaster response (Beaton et al. 2008). In the instance of Mercy Hospital in Joplin, MO, this entailed contacting the OCR within the Department of Health and Human Services because paper records have been scattered throughout the area (Braun 2012).

Once past the response crisis, it is important to use recovery to learn from the experience. It is also important to pay attention to the psychosocial effects of a disaster on the workforce. Once the adrenaline and worst of the crisis passes people can experience posttraumatic stress or depression as they learn how to cope with changed circumstances, sometimes in both their personal and work lives.

Check Your Understanding 11.3

Instructions: Indicate whether the following statements are true or false (T or F).

1. Hospitals are not required to create and test a disaster plan for accreditation purposes.

2. Text messaging is preferred over cell phone calling during a disaster.

3. The Security Risk Assessment, as required by HIPAA, should not be considered part of the disaster plan.

4. Health informatics and information management professionals really have no obligations to consumers when it comes to medical identity theft.

5. Other than the fact that it occurs in the a healthcare facility, medical identity theft is identical to financial identity theft.

6. The Red Flag Rules were only issued by the Federal Trade Commission.

⊙ Summary

The HIPAA Security Rule demands compliance with a compendium of standards. The standards and implementation specifications allow for the flexibility to design an information security plan that meets the specific needs of the CE and BA. The Security Risk Analysis serves as the guidepost for development and implementation of the security plan. The administrative, technical, and physical safeguards standards provide the framework to ensure confidentiality, integrity, and availability of ePHI. As the health informatics field continues to develop there will, most assuredly, be new challenges to be faced in the realm of information security. HIPAA and the like will be the baseline protective measures upon which future regulations will be built. Disaster preparedness is both to protect information assets and to help organizations maintain their communication and information services in adverse situations. Thorough planning and preparation are essential and the responsibility of health informatics and information management professionals. Failure can place patients and organizations at risk. Health informatics and information management professionals are often well versed in the privacy and security aspects of using and managing health information. The additional issues of medical identity theft, liability and medical malpractice related to EHRs, and disaster preparedness require attention if widespread adoption and use of EHRs is to be successful.

REFERENCES

45 CFR 160.404: Amount of a civil money penalty. 2013.

45 CFR 164.304: Definitions. 2013.

45 CFR 164.308(a): Administrative safeguards. 2013.

45 CFR 164.308(a)(1): Administrative safeguards. 2013.

45 CFR 164.308(a)(2): Administrative safeguards. 2013.

45 CFR 164.308(a)(3): Administrative safeguards. 2013.

45 CFR 164.308(a)(4): Administrative safeguards. 2013.

45 CFR 164.308(a)(5): Administrative safeguards. 2013.

45 CFR 164.308(a)(6): Administrative safeguards. 2013.

45 CFR 164.308(a)(7): Administrative safeguards. 2013.

45 CFR 164.308(a)(8): Administrative safeguards. 2013.

45 CFR 164.308(b)(1): Administrative safeguards. 2013.

45 CFR 164.310: Physical safeguards. 2013.

45 CFR 164.310(a)(1): Physical safeguards. 2013.

45 CFR 164.310(b): Physical safeguards. 2013.

45 CFR 164.310(c): Physical safeguards. 2013.

45 CFR 164.310(d)(1): Physical safeguards. 2013.

45 CFR 164.312(a)(1): Technical safeguards. 2013.

45 CFR 164.312(b): Technical safeguards. 2013.

45 CFR 164.312(c)(1): Technical safeguards. 2013.

45 CFR 164.312(d): Technical safeguards. 2013.

45 CFR 164.312(e)(1): Technical safeguards. 2013.

45 CFR 164.402: Definitions. 2013.

AHIMA. 2012. *Pocket Glossary for Health Information Management and Technology.* 3rd ed. Chicago: AHIMA Press.

AHIMA. 2013. Analysis of Modifications to the HIPAA Privacy, Security, Enforcement, and Breach Notification Rules under the Health Information Technology for Economic and Clinical Health Act and the Genetic Information Nondiscrimination Act: Other Modifications to the HIPAA Rules. http://library.ahima.org/xpedio/groups/public/documents/ahima/bok1_050067.pdf.

AHIMA e-HIM Work Group on Medical Identity Theft. 2008. Mitigating medical identity. *Journal of AHIMA* 79(7):63–69.

Anon. 2011. All IRBs should prepare for possible disaster interruptions. *IRB Advisor* 11(11):109–111.

Beaton, R., E. Bridges, M.K. Salazar, M.W. Oberle, A. Stergachis, J. Thompson, and P. Butterfield. 2008. Ecological model of disaster management. *AAOHN Journal* 56(11):471–478.

Belfort, R. 2009. HITECH raises the stakes on HIPAA compliance. http://www.manatt.com/news.aspx?id=8912.

Braun, J. 2012. HIPAA rules stay in place during disaster—Address privacy and security issues in plans. *Hospital Access Management* (August 2):1–2.

Brodnik, M., M. McCain, L. Rinehart-Thompson, and R. Reynolds. 2009. *Fundamentals of Law for Health Informatics and Information Management.* Chicago: AHIMA.

Conn, J. 2012. Bracing for a crash. *Modern Healthcare* 42(20):32–33.

Guidance on Risk Analysis Requirements under the HIPAA Security Rule. 2010. http://www.hhs.gov/ocr/privacy/hipaa/administrative/securityrule/rafinalguidancepdf.pdf.

Gupta, A. 2011. Hackers, breaches, and other threats to elect. *Health Data Management* 19(9):3.

Harrison, J.P., R.A. Harrison, and M. Smith. 2008. Role of information technology in disaster medical response. *Health Care Manager* 27(4):307–313.

Health Information Technology for Economic and Clinical Health (HITECH) Act. Public Law 111-5.

Herzig, T.W, ed. 2010. *Information Security in Healthcare: Managing Risk.* Chicago: HIMSS.

HIPAA Administrative Simplification Statute and Rules. http://www.hhs.gov/ocr/privacy/hipaa/administrative/index.html.

HIPAA Compliance Review Analysis and Summary of Results. 2008. http://www.hhs.gov/ocr/privacy/hipaa/enforcement/cmscompliancerev08.pdf.

HIPAA Security Rule. 2003. http://www.hhs.gov/ocr/privacy/hipaa/administrative/securityrule/securityrulepdf.pdf

HIPAA Security Series. 2007a Security Standards: Administrative Safeguards. http://www.hhs.gov/ocr/privacy/hipaa/administrative/securityrule/adminsafeguards.pdf.

HIPAA Security Series. 2007b. Security Standards: Physical Safeguards. http://www.hhs.gov/ocr/privacy/hipaa/administrative/securityrule/physsafeguards.pdf.

HIPAA Security Series. 2007c. Security Standards: Technical Safeguards. http://www.hhs.gov/ocr/privacy/hipaa/administrative/securityrule/techsafeguards.pdf.

Hoffman, S. and A. Podgurski. 2009. E-health hazards: Provider liability and electronic health record systems. *Berekeley Technology Law Journal* 24(4):1523–1582.

Keith, B. 2010. Catch fraud upfront: Medical identity theft is on the rise: It's time to revamp your processes. *Hospital Access Management* 29(5):49–51.

King, P. and R.L. Williams. 2008. *Red Flag Compliance for Healthcare Providers: Protecting Ourselves and Our Patients from Identity Theft.* Chicago: American Health Lawyers Association and HIMSS.

LaTour, K., S. Eichewald-Maki, and P. Oachs. 2013. *Health Information: Management Concepts, Principles, and Practice,* 4th ed. Chicago: AHIMA.

Mancilla, D. and J. Moczygemba. 2009. Exploring medical identity theft. *Perspectives in Health Information Management* 6:1–11.

MindTools. 2013. The Risk Impact/Probability Chart. http://www.mindtools.com/pages/article/newPPM_78.htm.

National Institute of Standards and Technology Special Publication 800-66. 2008. http://csrc.nist.gov/publications/nistpubs/800-66-Rev1/SP-800-66-Revision1.pdf.

Nelson, S.B. 2008. Information management during mass casualty events … Includes discussion. *Respiratory Care* 53(2):232–238.

Office of Civil Rights, Department of Health and Human Services. 2013a. Modifications to the HIPAA Privacy, Security, Enforcement, and Breach Notification Rules under the Health Information Technology for Economic and Clinical Health Act and the Genetic Information Nondiscrimination Act; Other Modifications to the HIPAA Rules. *Federal Register* 78(17):5566–5702.

Office for Civil Rights, Department of Health and Human Services. 2013b. Enforcement Highlights. http://www.hhs.gov/ocr/privacy/hipaa/enforcement/highlights/index.html.

Ranajee, N. 2012. Best practices in healthcare disaster recovery planning. *Health Management Technology* 33(5):22–24.

Reynolds, P. and I. Tamanaha. 2010. Disaster Information Specialist Pilot Project: NLM/DIMRC. *Medical Reference Services Quarterly* 29(4):394–404. doi:10.1080/02763869.2010.518929.

Rhinehart-Thompson, L.A. 2008. Raising awareness of medical identity theft: For consumers, prevention starts with guarding, monitoring health information. *Journal of AHIMA* 79 (10)74–75, 81.

Schiff, G.D. and D.W. Bates. 2010. Can electronic clinical documentation help prevent diagnostic errors? *New England Journal of Medicine* 362(12):1066–1069. doi:10.1056/NEJMp0911734.

Smith, E. and R. Macdonald. 2006. Managing health information during disasters. *Health Information Management Journal* 35(2):8–13.

Springer, R. 2009. Medical identity theft—Red flag and address discrepancy requirements. *Plastic Surgical Nursing* 29(2):131–134. doi:10.1097/01.PSN.0000356874.56338.2c.

Sullivan, J. 2004. *HIPAA: A Practical Guide to the Privacy and Security of Health Data.* Chicago: American Bar Association.

RESOURCES

Brocato, L., S. Emery, and J. McDavid. 2011. Keeping compliant: Managing rising risk in physician practices. *Journal of AHIMA* 82(11):32–35.

Dinh, A. 2008. HIPAA security compliance – what comes next? *Journal of Health Care Compliance* 10(3):37–39.

Gibson, P., F. Theadore, and J. Jellison. 2012. The common ground preparedness framework: A comprehensive description of public health emergency preparedness. *American Journal of Public Health* 102(4):633–642. doi:10.2105/AJPH.2011.300546.

Neal, D. 2011. Choosing an electronic health records system: Professional liability considerations. *Innovations in Clinical Neuroscience* 8(6):43.

Scott, R.L. 2006. Physicians' reliance on electronic health records. University of Houston.

United States Congress. 2009. Health Information Technology for Economic and Clinical Health (HITECH) Act. *Code of Federal Regulations.* http://edocket.access.gpo.gov/2010/pdf/2010-17210.pdf.

Vigoda, M. 2008. e-Record, e-Liability: Addressing medico-legal Issues in electronic records. *Journal of AHIMA/American Health Information Management Association* 79(10):48–52.

Virapongse, A., D.W. Bates, P. Shi, C.A. Jenter, L.A. Volk, K. Kleinman, L. Sato, and S.R Simon. 2008. Electronic health records and malpractice claims in office practice. *Archives of Internal Medicine* 168(21):2362–2367. doi:10.1001/archinte.168.21.2362.

12

The Legal Electronic Health Record

By Kelly McClendon

Learning Objectives

- Define the legal health record for disclosure
- Compare and contrast a paper-based legal health record, a hybrid legal health record, and a legal electronic health record
- Identify the stakeholders and their roles for legal electronic health record definition projects
- Explain the steps involved in defining the legal health record
- Describe the importance of developing a legal health record policy
- Become acquainted with electronic record e-discovery
- Appropriately interpret the various attributes that can impact the legal health record definition and e-discovery
- Analyze patient record documentation regulations for correct utilization within legal health record policies and procedures

KEY TERMS

Accounting of disclosures
Any and all records
Audit logging
Data
Disclosure
Document and data nonrepudiation
e-discovery
Federal Rules of Civil Procedure (FRCP)
Federal Rules of Evidence (FRE)
Hybrid health records

Legal health records
Legal hold
Litigation response
Metadata
Protected health information (PHI)
Record custodians
Rendition
Spoliation
Uniform Rules for e-discovery

⊙ Introducing Legal Health Records

The goal of this chapter is to provide readers with a thorough understanding of the concepts surrounding **legal health records** (LHRs), which are a foundational element of informatics. Informatics is based upon electronic health data and the use of this data within the legal system is guided by the concepts surrounding LHRs. The concept of LHRs was created to describe the data, documents, reports, and information that comprise the formal business record(s) of any healthcare organization that are to be utilized during legal proceedings. Understanding LHRs requires knowledge of not only what comprises business records used as LHRs but also the processes as well as the physical and electronic systems used to manage these records.

While it has been recognized for years that patient safety is positively impacted by the technological advantages of electronic health records (EHRs), there has been fragmented and sporadic migration toward these electronic systems throughout the past two decades. The Health Information Technology for Economic and Clinical Health (HITECH) Act (part of the American Recovery and Reinvestment Act of 2009 (ARRA), also known as the Stimulus Plan) has incentive payment funding for the meaningful use of certified EHRs (ARRA 2009). These tightly focused requirements for vendors and providers include a time frame that requires concerted action to significantly migrate many, if not most, providers of healthcare away from a paper-based to a much more EHR. While this migration from paper and hybrid health records to electronic records offers unparalleled opportunities for patient safety and care improvement, it also raises risks and challenges to everyone involved with the access, use, and overall management of these records, including those who use the records for legal purposes.

Another dimension of change that opens realms of opportunity for cost reduction, quality, and effectiveness of care and patient safety are the health information exchanges (HIEs) moving information beyond the original, single health record and provider of care. Ideally, these data exchanges and their facilitating infrastructures, such as Health Information Organizations (HIOs) and the Nationwide Health Information Network (NwHIN), are all working to achieve the grand EHR goal of fully interoperable healthcare, where previous test results, medications, and treatments are available for each new provider's use.

As if these previous changes were not enough, there is one more expansion evolving within the industry: personal health records (PHRs). These records are very different in that patients, not the providers, store and retain their healthcare data either in paper or electronic form. This is a significant change that must be addressed in the LHR equation as these PHRs are more fully developed, used by patients, and then incorporated into provider EHRs. Many times the incorporation of PHR data into an EHR may be solely for historical reference. Between data exchange and PHRs, the idea that health records are static, paper-bound entities is rapidly becoming obsolete. There will in fact be paper records for at least a another decade or two, until the older records gradually age out of the retention time frames so that they may be destroyed. The retention period can range from 7 to 75 years, dependent upon state, federal, and other rules, regulations, statutes, and typical practices.

Therefore, any LHR planning must encompass the newly evolving electronic record, the PHR, and the older paper environment for the foreseeable future.

There are few, if any, instances where any type of legal records are called out by name within EHR standards. The net result of this failure to define LHRs is that there is not a standard terminology for these records, and the wide audience of record users and creators do not understand exactly what is meant when the term legal health record is used. However, because there are an increasing number of parties actually undertaking projects to define their own legal health records, this term is becoming de facto acceptable parlance in the healthcare industry, even without a real standards-based definition. Given that there is legitimacy in the concept of LHRs, we will illustrate and clarify these concepts, along with describing the best practices commonly found on the subject from an introductory perspective. There are other publications that explore these concepts in greater depth. This chapter is intended to define the foundations and preliminary elements for the reader in a fashion that creates a good starting point for understanding the issues surrounding LHRs.

Many within the healthcare industry believe that well-recognized health information, including the documentation of care at the point of care and the provision of patient histories for care delivery, are almost exclusively the driving forces for creating and maintaining health records. This tends to be the point of view of the providers of care; one that is not incorrect but is somewhat limited in scope. In reality, there are many more reasons for creating and maintaining sound health records. Health records have many uses, most obviously for continued treatment but also for payment, operations, quality management, research, public health reporting, and compliance with myriad rules, regulations, and laws that guide healthcare delivery in the United States.

There have been objections to the term legal health record because it might indicate that some records are more legal or useable in litigation than others. This is not the intended meaning of the term. Nearly all healthcare records and related electronic data (except those that are privileged or otherwise excluded) are admissible into evidence in court if they are kept according to widely accepted legal practice standards. Rather, the term legal health record is related to a larger conceptual framework. Great care has been taken within this text to avoid confusion and to clarify the use of the word legal including precise definitions such as the *LHR defined for disclosure* as opposed to simply naming the concepts *legal records*. Watch carefully for the use of the exact term *legal record*. It is a bit misleading and should be avoided whether in this text or within the healthcare industry. Modifiers such as "for disclosure" create a more accurate view of the definition and concept. Wherever in this text you see *legal health record* or *LHR*, be aware that it is describing the concept surrounding the health record defined for disclosure or its accompanying attributes and not its legal admissibility. It is also worth noting that the LHR for disclosure is distinct from the HIPAA Designated Record Set. Any set of health records that are maintained with individually identifiable information or protected health information (PHI) are a HIPAA Designated Record Set. However, that does not mean the record set will be a part of the LHR for disclosure. For example, the data maintained in EHR feeder systems such as a pharmacy system or laboratory information system, though using PHI, will not usually be included in the LHR for disclosure.

The concepts surrounding LHRs have been coalescing for a period of years and will continue to evolve for the foreseeable future. EHRs and the legal environment are complex. Therefore, judicial decisions, laws, rules, regulations, and precedence will continue to refine the concepts and tenets of this subject. These are not static environments. Be aware of and track the pertinent changes stemming from these judicial decisions, laws, rules, and regulations on a continual basis.

The most common legal processes and usually the most coherent for our purposes are the federal rules, laws, decisions, and guidance issued by the US Supreme Court, especially in reference to e-discovery (the discovery of electronic records for legal proceedings). These apply across the United States and often take precedence over other guidance. There is also work from a group called the Uniform Commissioners from which state laws and rules may be derived that are very similar to the **Federal Rules of Civil Procedure (FRCP)** for rules of both civil procedure and evidence. The FRCP, the guidelines that govern the procedures for civil trials, were amended in 2006 to include electronic records and continue to be very important as benchmarks for how electronic data and information can be used in both federal and state courts. State laws and rules are certainly important to many if not most legal actions and are so widely variable that no single book can account for all of them. Be sure to research your own state laws and rules for subpoenas, court orders, discovery, and similar legal processes. It is highly recommended that all LHR strategies, policies, and procedures (P&Ps) be vetted with legal counsel for advice and guidance.

⊙ Setting the Stage for LHRs

Perhaps one of the most important concepts to remember during the discussion of health records from a legal system standpoint and other perspectives is that formal health record management is actually enterprise-wide in nature as opposed to solely departmental.

No matter whether they are paper, electronic, or a hybrid mixture of multiple record formats, the basic principles of record management have not changed. Having a basis in statutes, regulations such as the **Federal Rules of Evidence (FRE)**, which govern what and how electronic records may be used and the roles of record custodianship for purposes of evidence in a trial, the FRCP, Medicare regulations, HIPAA, and various state requirements, record management in general remains the same as it has been for decades. What has changed is a vast expansion of the specific requirements related to electronic records from the requirements of paper records.

Carefully planned, organized, and efficient work processes providing high-quality record keeping are still a requirement for healthcare providers. Now the requirements for managing all the disparate components of information comprising the dozens of types of **data** including dates, numbers, images, symbols, letters, and words that represent basic facts and observations about people, processes, measurements, and conditions have come together to form health records, taking these core principles to new depths of complexity. The same basic concepts remain unchanged, but the scope and depth to which they must be utilized in daily operations are indeed expanded.

Stakeholders for LHR Definition Projects

The stakeholders in any LHR definition project and the processes that surround both the legal and healthcare processes to manage these records are enterprise-wide and diverse. Any LHR definition project should include stakeholders from as many levels of the organization as possible. While all opinions are welcome, be sure to vet prospective stakeholders to ensure they have the organization's best interest at heart. Recommended stakeholders are listed in table 12.1.

Paper, Electronic, and Hybrid Health Records

Paper health records have prevailed for more than a century, are mostly self-evident in their content and practices, and can be easily described. Paper records permanently record health information through the use of handwriting, transcription, or printouts. They are stored in paper folders or similar hard copy files and are maintained in this form until destruction. At some point in their life cycle, healthcare entities may convert and replace their paper records with archival scanning into electronic document management systems or EHR systems, at which point the paper record becomes a hybrid health record.

There are myriads of federal, state, and other statutes, rules, and regulations that guide what must comprise a health record and to date, these have largely been promulgated for paper records. Electronic records can and should utilize

Table 12.1 Recommended stakeholders

Stakeholder	Role
C-suite and practice managers	In general, the more supporting C-suite (chief executive officer, chief operating officer, chief information officer, and others) and practice manager–type stakeholders brought into the project the better, as they will support development of project materials and strategies that must be institutionalized.
HIM professionals	Lead the LHR definition project as much as possible. The strategies decided upon are typically carried out in large part by HIM staff, who ensure the accessibility, completeness, accuracy, reliability, and archiving of the EHR and paper-based medical record information. HIM staff also typically manage the subpoena disclosure and release-of-information processes for medical records.
Information technology staff	From the CIO to HIM and EHR analysts, IT also has key roles. Management and direct custodians of the various EHR and source systems that feed the EHRs are absolutely crucial to the success of an LHR project. IT staff are responsible for the hardware and software applications that manage electronic records contained within EHR systems. They have invaluable information about the granular level of details on how the software should operate and how it is implemented to work within the organization.

(Continued)

Table 12.1 Recommended stakeholders (*Continued*)

Stakeholder	Role
Record custodians	These staff, who are from patient accounts, diagnostic imaging, and physician practice areas, along with secondary custodians such as source system (for example, laboratory, radiology, and transcription) managers, are also valuable to the project. Record or data stewards are titles also related to record custodians; however, their scope of responsibility may be somewhat wider than record custodians.
Privacy, compliance, and security officers; risk managers; and quality managers	All have key roles to play in these projects because the decisions arrived at directly affect their daily work processes. Risk managers are many times an important HIM ally in LHR definition projects as they understand the liabilities and embrace strategies to reduce them.
Clinicians (including physicians, nurses, and ancillary clinical staff)	These staff who develop, create, input, modify, update, and use the data contained inside EHR systems as part of their daily practice bring unique and vital information to the project team. Clinical informatics professionals, especially nursing clinical informaticists, are extremely valuable in guiding legal aspects of documentation procedures that factor into LHR definition and organization projects.
Legal counsel	Whether internal or external, legal counsel and risk managers both play roles in subpoena disclosure, litigation response, and discovery (or e-discovery) processes. Vetting of LHR P&Ps is also required.

these requirements, combined with current paper health record documents, to help create the LHR defined for disclosure. Defining EHRs in the sense of what is to be disclosed for legal requests is more difficult than defining disclosure from paper records.

Hybrid health records are increasingly seen as the most common transition points between fully paper and completely electronic records. Transitioning from paper to electronic records is costly, very time consuming, and hugely reliant on vendor applications that may not be as well conceived as their users would like for them to be (as is often discovered during system implementation). Hybrid records may be a mixture of paper and electronic or multiple electronic systems that do not communicate or are not logically architected for record management.

Health **record custodians**, also known as record stewards, are typically within the HIM workgroup or department, and are commonly charged with leading multidisciplinary definition projects for both the HIPAA-required Designated Record Set and the LHR. They are also expected to develop proper organization, management, guidelines, and processes related to the use of business records as a protective legal defense tool. Most of the time, this effort is performed in conjunction with other stakeholders such as IT, compliance, and risk management.

Check Your Understanding 12.1

Instructions: Indicate whether the following statements are true or false (T or F).

1. The term legal health record has the same meaning across all settings.

2. Maintenance and protection of a healthcare organization's legal health record is solely the responsibility of the record custodian.

3. E-discovery refers to a process within legal proceedings that utilizes electronic records.

4. The HIPAA Designated Record Set is the same as the legal health record.

Instructions: Choose the best answer.

5. Of the following, the most important use of health records is
   a. Patient care
   b. Research
   c. Quality management
   d. Public health reporting

⊙ Why Define a Legal Health Record?

LHR definitions provide formal recognition of which record sets, components, data, and documents comprise the official business records denoted as medical or health records. These defined LHRs may be purely paper, electronic, or a hybrid combination. Creating sound LHR definitions clarifies the roles of all records and their uses and sets foundational policy for record management operations. Note that these definitions must be formal and published in-house. However, definitions will change as documents and data migrate from paper or other electronic systems, so they must be continually reviewed and updated as their constituent record components evolve.

LHR Definition Project Steps

Several high-level activities comprise LHR definition projects. Adequate time should be allocated to define the LHR for an organization (see table 12.2). At each step in the process, there are requirements for learning new concepts and in researching the literature as well as best practices from others who have solved similar problems. Be sure the project team has access to knowledgeable experts and resources to perform these steps. There is much to consider when creating an organization-wide LHR definition project. If the LHR definition project is part of a larger EHR implementation, it is recommended that the LHR project timeline be embedded within the critical path of the organization's overall implementation of an EHR. The following LHR definition steps are based upon common and standard best practices.

Table 12.2 LHR definition project steps

Date Completed	Step	LHR Definition Process
MM/DD/YYYY	*Step 1*	Determine the LHR stakeholder team.
MM/DD/YYYY	*Step 2*	Determine strategy and plan for an LHR definition project. Get executive sponsorship and empowerment.
MM/DD/YYYY	*Step 3*	Gather LHR-related knowledge and investigate your state electronic medical record requirements, including retention. Review other related statutes, rules, and regulations, including any federal guidelines. Gain an understanding of electronic record disclosure and e-discovery principles.
MM/DD/YYYY	*Step 4*	Develop a master source system matrix or list that organizes data related to the various systems that create medical record documents, data, and reports.
MM/DD/YYYY	*Step 5*	Create a document matrix of LHR component documents, data, and reports, at least at the major record section level.
MM/DD/YYYY	*Step 6*	Assess and catalog EHR systems for their LHR attributes within your organization for e-discovery purposes.
MM/DD/YYYY	*Step 7*	Determine and revise affected policies and procedures, including e-discovery and litigation response. Vet these policies and procedures with your legal counsel.
MM/DD/YYYY	*Step 8*	Determine guidelines for LHR maintenance going forward. Continue to maintain and refine your LHR P&Ps on an ongoing basis. Establish a process for regular review and revision of processes and procedures related to LHR.
MM/DD/YYYY	*Step 9*	Create a slide presentation for education and training for appropriate workforce members.
MM/DD/YYYY	*Step 10*	Conduct necessary training for appropriate parties who will change, affect, use, or provide critical information for the LHR.

Step 1: Determine the LHR Stakeholder Team

The stakeholder team will drive the creation of the LHR documentation, undertake the LHR definition project, and be responsible for its continued maintenance. Refer to table 12.1 for a list of recommended stakeholders. It is highly recommended that the record custodian be in charge or included as a member of the team. In addition to the C-suite described below, HIM professionals, information technology staff, record custodians from related areas, privacy and security officers, risk management, clinicians, and legal counsel should all be included on the team.

In the first step of undertaking an LHR definition, create a process to move the project along according to formal rules adopted by the enterprise. Creating a definition in a small, physicians practice office is usually simple enough. The stakeholders are all nearby and there may be few of them. But in the larger organization with a more complex electronic record environment, it is harder to achieve consensus regarding an LHR definition. Therefore, using formal project methodology is highly recommended. It is up to record custodians, risk management, and legal staff to facilitate the project with carefully selected project team members.

Step 2: Determine Strategy and Plan for the LHR Definition Project, and Get Executive Sponsorship and Empowerment

Project governance and leadership is another important aspect of an LHR project. The executive or senior management must sponsor and empower the team to make the difficult decisions related to the LHR. Often the HIM department primary record custodian manages the LHR definition processes and other times, risk management, compliance, or legal staff may lead the initiative. Regardless of which staff members provide the leadership, it is crucial that LHR definition projects be managed as formal projects, with an explicit strategy and plan, until they are completed. The C-suite or executives are vital to help determine strategies, sign off on them, and help make them operational. There are good reasons to have some powerful stakeholders to get the respect and attention these projects require.

Step 3: Gather LHR-related Knowledge

The next step of the process is to become familiar with existing guidance and resources. The resources listed at the end of this chapter represent guidance on LHRs. Reading, continuing education, networking, keeping up with American Health Information Management Association (AHIMA) resources, and questioning experts are all excellent learning methods. The mission is to become one of the facility's experts on legal records. Additionally, most healthcare providers should have access to some type of legal counsel, whether it is in-house or external to the organization. Establishing and maintaining that relationship is key. One needs to understand federal, state, and local record retention requirements and evidentiary and civil procedure requirements that are applicable to each organization.

Step 4: Develop a Master Source System Matrix

Regardless of its title, the first deliverable from an LHR definition project should be a master list of all clinical, financial, and administrative EHR systems (referred to as EHR modules under the 2010 meaningful use rules) that manage or contribute to the health record as well as patient accounts and diagnostic imaging records, if they are a focus of the project. If fortunate enough to already have such a list from the IT department, examine it to confirm that it is current and add any other systems necessary to move the project forward. If starting from scratch, involve IT staff as they manage the hardware platforms and software applications that comprise the EHR systems.

Step 5: Create a Document Matrix of LHR Components

Once an EHR source system matrix is created, the next step is to develop a list of documents, data, and reports that comprise the LHR as defined for disclosure. The matrix of LHR components will vary from organization to organization. A small physician practice may only have a few applications, while a large integrated health system may have thousands of applications. In fact, the larger system may have an application to help manage IT resources, such as applications, which may make maintaining the list of LHR components easier. However accomplished, it is essential to know exactly what comprises the LHR.

Step 6: Assess and Catalog EHR Systems for Their LHR Attributes

Next, create evaluation criteria in the form of questions to be posed and a space for recording answers. Such criteria will facilitate the assessment of EHR systems for their attributes that may be important during e-discovery. These questions might be related to attributes such as the ease of producing a single, readable electronic record upon request, the ability of the system to segregate sensitive data subject to separate regulations, or functionality employed when a patient requests an amendment to the EHR. The key to this assessment is not just asking the suggested questions but asking everything necessary to ensure the EHR and its functionalities and limitations related to record management are clearly understood.

Step 7: Determine the Need for New and Revised Related Policies and Procedures

It is necessary to create new P&Ps related to the LHR definition project. There may also exist P&Ps that need to be updated, so take care to review any existing P&Ps that may be impacted.

Step 8: Determine the LHR Maintenance Plan

Be sure to include regular reviews and updates of related P&Ps to ensure the organization is always in compliance with the latest rules and trends in LHRs. It is also a good idea to utilize actual P&P documents to train workforce members.

As IT projects are added or updated, be sure to document where data is located and how it fits into litigation response, legal hold, and other potential legal responses. Update the source system matrix to include new applications, pertinent data stored therein, and the custodians for each system.

Steps 9 and 10: Create a Presentation and Conduct Education and Training for Appropriate Workforce Members

Educate as many staff as possible so they will understand and have guidance in following defined LHR P&Ps. These educational sessions should include administrative, departmental, nursing, medical, and IT staff. It is crucial to educate not only the project stakeholders but also key members from across the enterprise on the realities and processes used to create highly defensible health records, regardless of their format.

Check Your Understanding 12.2

Instructions: Indicate whether the following statements are true or false (T or F).

1. It is only important for HIM department staff to understand and abide by the LHR policies and procedures.

2. Once the legal health record is defined, the healthcare organization will need to regularly review the policies and procedures.

3. It is not necessary to have organizational legal counsel review and approve the LHR policies and procedures.

4. A matrix of all LHR components is not needed.

5. Appropriate sponsorship of an LHR project is required.

⊙ Defining the Components of a LHR

Each organization may have different components that serve to define their LHR. It is not reasonable to expect a solo primary care practitioner to have the same components in their LHR as a tertiary care academic medical center. The problem with failing to define the components adequately is that the organization has little reasonable defense should they receive a request for a component in the absence of a definition. For example, if the clinicians use e-mail to communicate regarding patients and e-mail is not explicitly excluded from the LHR, attorneys can legitimately request any e-mail related to a particular patient's care and the organization will have to produce them. Thus, following the guidance below to define what is and is not included in the LHR is essential.

Creating a Tailored LHR Definition for Disclosure

The first task to be accomplished after the identification of stakeholders and project structure is to request a list of all clinical information EHR systems. These may be referred to as clinical EHR modules or source systems. The list should include the names of the systems as well as additional data fields such as the resident system expert, vendor name, data format, and others listed in table 12.3.

The next task is to create a document matrix, which is a list of all documents and data that comprise the current LHR utilized for routine disclosure. This may

Table 12.3   Source system matrix

List EHR systems that contain data		Basic e-Discovery Information								
Provider Site Name of System	Application Name from Vendor	Vendor Company Name and Contact Information	Responsible Department	Department Primary Contact / Custodian	IT Primary Contact	List and Description of Data / Documents	Does system contain PHI; Designated Record Set	How to Access Data or Documents	Reasonably Accessible or Not Reasonably Accessible	Time / Cost to Obtain
Main/ EHR	Powerchart	Cerner	Health Information Management	Jill Jones	John Smith	History and Physical; MD Orders	Yes, both	Request via HIM	Dependent upon type of request	10 business days; $80

actually be a list or simply point to the master document table within an electronic document management system (EDMS). This typically comprises a list of hundreds of documents and can become unwieldy. Therefore, it is recommended that a list of chapters (sometimes known as index tabs) be created of what is included in the paper or hybrid health record. A spreadsheet-based matrix can be used to manage these data (see table 12.4). It is a good idea to create a single spreadsheet-based workbook (using Microsoft Excel or a comparable program) and to have these lists of source systems and LHR data and documents on separate worksheets within the workbook.

It is important to keep in mind the reason for creating a document matrix as a part of the LHR definition. The record custodian has the responsibility to

Table 12.4 Document matrix for documents, data, and reports defined as *included* in an LHR (with examples)

Facility			
Document Name Data Set Report Name	**EHR or Hybrid**	**Source System**	**Comments**
Approved for LHR and Routine Disclosure			
Advanced Directives	EDM	Paper	
Consents	EDM	Paper	
Emergency Department Report	EDM	ED System	
Continuity of Care Documents	Clinical Repository	HIE, Clinical EHR	
Diagnostic Imaging Reports	PACS	RIS	
EKG & EEG Reports	EDM	Paper	
Laboratory Reports	EDM	Lab	
MAR	Clinical Repository	Medication Mgmt	Different system than the Inpatient EHR
Multidisciplinary Notes	Clinical Repository	Inpatient EHR	
Nursing Documentation	Clinical Repository	Inpatient EHR	

(Continued)

Table 12.4 Document matrix for documents, data, and reports defined as *included* in an LHR (with examples) (*Continued*)

Facility			
Document Name Data Set Report Name	**EHR or Hybrid**	**Source System**	**Comments**
Operative, Recovery Room, Anesthesia Notes	EDM	Paper	Will be scanned into EDM soon
CPOE—Orders	Clinical Repository	Inpatient EHR	
Problem List	Ambulatory EHR	Ambulatory	
Psychological Assessment Document	Paper	Paper	Soon will be scanned into EDM
Physician Progress Notes	Clinical Repository	Inpatient EHR	
Physician Orders	Clinical Repository	Inpatient & Ambulatory EHR	Can be related to either Inpatient or Ambulatory encounters
Transcription	Paper	Paper	
Patient Billing Documents	Billing System	Billing System	
Remits	Paper	Paper	Soon to be electronically captured
Patient ID Photo and Documents	EDM	EDM	
Use to catalog your documents, data, and reports included in your defined LHR.			

determine what business records or components of these records they will release upon legal request and to also determine which records actually fulfill the content of the record request as stated in the request document.

Typically, a document matrix (such as table 12.4) is created in a spreadsheet with details about the documents and data included in the LHR defined for disclosure. Excluded documents and data that are commonly used or filed and stored with LHR components should be listed as well (see table 12.5). Common documents from the

Table 12.5 Document matrix for documents, data, and reports defined as *excluded* from an LHR.

Facility			
Document Name Data Set Report Name	**EHR or Hybrid**	**Source System**	**Comments**
Excluded for LHR and Routine Disclosure			
Administrative Documents, Data, or Reports			
Abbreviation Lists			
Audit Logs			
Coding Query Forms			
Derived Data (that is, Accreditation Reports, Best Practice Guidelines, Clinical Paths, Statistical Reports)			
Indexes			
Metadata (that is, not otherwise viewable within medical record documentation reports or printouts)			
Operational Documents, Data, or Reports			
Physician Task Lists			
Privileged Legal Information			
Worksheets			
Use to catalogue your documents, data, and reports excluded from your defined LHR.			

previous or current paper-based health record are nearly always included; therefore, paper records are typically a good starting point for populating the matrix.

The organization may already have completed projects that generated lists of documents that could serve as the basis of a document matrix. Such projects include forms redesign projects, especially for an EDMS, or forms-on-demand projects. In other cases, healthcare organizations have found that the HIPAA Designated Record Set (DRS) may be a useful starting point for an LHR defined for disclosure if the DRS has been cataloged. Check this DRS list of components and documents for concurrence with the LHR defined for disclosure, as they might be very similar. Be sure that the formal definition of the DRS expands well beyond that of the LHR. The DRS applies to any information within a healthcare organization that is used to make a decision about patient care and includes nearly all documentation with any **protected health information (PHI)**. PHI is individually identifiable health data or information, maintained or used by a covered entity (CE) or business associate (BA). This is usually a much wider set than the LHR defined for disclosure, even though the LHR is a subset of the DRS. If already cataloged, the DRS may be a great place to derive documents and data for the document matrix.

The LHR Policy Imperative

Creating a LHR defined for disclosure is very important for a healthcare organization. The LHR policy determines what data and information can or should be released pursuant to a request from a third party. Without the LHR policy, a healthcare organization is at risk related to requests for data and information that the organization is not prepared to release. For example, if the organization does not determine how e-mail will be treated, a third-party requester could request any e-mails related to patient care and the organization would have no standing for refusing the request. Typically, this policy is created within an organization's defined template and filed in an appropriate filing system, which increasingly is maintained online for all authorized users to access. In fact, all policies should be accessible and readily useable by the entire authorized workforce. The policies should be used as training tools for regularly scheduled review.

Figure 12.1 shows an example of a few sections taken from a well-written LHR policy. This policy was created in conjunction with source system and document matrixes. The length and complexity of an LHR policy will depend upon the needs of the healthcare organization.

Figure 12.1   Sections from an LHR policy created in conjunction with source system and document matrixes

SCOPE: All organization workforce members.

PURPOSE:
The business record documenting the delivery of healthcare rendered at **<insert site name>** is defined as the *Legal Health Record* (otherwise referred to as the LHR). This LHR will be disclosed upon routine legal or administrative record disclosure requests, such as subpoenas. Other routine record (PHI) disclosures will also be based on this defined LHR, such as the subset of the HIPAA defined Designated Record Set for individual inspection, copies, amendment of PHI, and other release of information requests. Minimum necessary provisions under HIPAA will apply to all disclosure requests.

This LHR Defined for Disclosure is a hybrid record **(if indeed your record is a hybrid, if not modify this language)** created from the paper medical record and **<insert EHR system(s) name(s)>** documents.

The scope of this policy is for **<insert site name>** HIM managed records. Other **<insert site name>** medical record types (that is, medical practices and certain other Outpatient Services records) are not currently addressed by this policy.

The LHR at **<insert site name>** includes the documentation of healthcare services provided to an individual in all delivery settings by our clinical and professional staff. The LHR consists of individually identifiable data in any medium, collected, processed, stored, displayed, and directly used in documenting healthcare delivery or health status.

The LHR at **<insert site name>** is a hybrid record **<modify as necessary to reflect your environment>** utilizing both paper-based and electronic documents, which are captured both manually and via electronic processes; see the LHR Source System Matrix and Document Matrix worksheet for details of the LHR component documents. Each encounter is maintained under a unit record number and includes subsequent patient visits. Only individuals authorized to do so by hospital or medical staff policies and procedures make entries into the LHR. Standardized formats are used for documenting all care, treatment, and services provided to patients.

The LHR contains sufficient information to identify the patient, support the diagnosis, justify the treatment and services, document the course and results of care, and promote the continuity of care among health providers.

The LHR will include records from *other healthcare providers* as the result of tests and exams when they were utilized for the evaluation of the patient and subsequent treatment.

The Federal Rules for Civil Procedure (FRCP) instituted December 1, 2006, expand the process of discovery and provide guidelines for electronic records utilized as evidence and this policy is in accordance with the guidance provided by these rules.

It is important to define the location of the documents (in either paper or **<insert EHR system(s) name(s)>**) within the **<insert site name>** Legal Health Record (LHR) for timely access, use, and disclosure as necessary for patient care and other requirements, such as disclosure requests. As **<insert site name>** transitions from a paper-based record to hybrid records, and then

(Continued)

Figure 12.1 Sections from an LHR policy created in conjunction with source system and document matrixes (*Continued*)

> to a more complete EHR, the location and management of the **<insert site name>** LHR must be evaluated, monitored, and kept updated for medicolegal purposes.
>
> The Document Matrix will serve as a dynamic tool used to define the LHR components in their present form. As **<insert site name>** implements new EHR systems, the matrix will be reviewed and updated. It will serve as the guideline for the legal location of our medical record from which we disclose protected health information.
>
> **Related Materials:**
>
> - Source System Matrix
> - Document Matrix

Litigation Response Policy and Procedures for Record Custodians

The most common meaning of the term disclosure in healthcare is the act of releasing, upon proper authorization, copies of business or health records. Healthcare providers must take great care to recognize any release of information request that may become involved in litigation. **Litigation response** is typically the term used to describe the processes invoked if the potential for lawsuits or litigation is detected. Litigation response is not only triggered by atypical record disclosure requests but by any sign or action that shows a potential for a lawsuit. Litigation response should result in protective measures being taken by the provider to ensure maximum defensive posture, including appropriate responses to subpoenas and court orders, and protecting against **spoliation** (the malicious alteration, concealment, or destruction of evidence) or other acts that later can be questioned and even sanctioned by the courts and opposing counsel.

Upon any legal request for disclosure of health information, the appropriate healthcare staff members or contractors will examine the request and determine what is to be disclosed according to predefined policies. A well-defined LHR will assist in appropriately determining exactly which record components are to be disclosed upon routine legal request. If the request is in any way unusual or meets the criteria to invoke litigation response as set by each organization, different procedures must immediately be instituted. Staff training and well-written P&Ps are key to maximizing the use of healthcare business records as tools in legal defense. Litigation response is simply a set of procedures that, when instituted, protects the records, whether they are health records, billing records, administrative, or metadata, whenever litigation is involved.

Within the FRCP and **Uniform Rules for e-Discovery** (amendments to the FRCP specifically designed for electronically stored information), once litigation is suspected or known to be occurring, a specific litigation response, including record protection, must be established. The Uniform Rules apply to federal but not state courts. However, they are appropriate guidance to follow since state courts are generally less proscriptive in these areas. State laws and regulations must be considered when creating litigation response P&Ps.

Creating Litigation Response Policies and Procedures

Typically, the larger and more complex an organization's healthcare delivery system, the more likely it is to have formalized P&Ps to guide actions when litigation is known or suspected. But experience has shown that even these organizations may not have codified their litigation response into clearly defined procedures used to train staff and ensure all parties act accordingly. Failure to have well-defined processes can increase liability and financial risk. All healthcare entities, from the very largest to the smallest, should examine their litigation response P&Ps to prevent potentially costly lapses during legal actions. Litigation response may or may not be the responsibility of a single department or staff member.

Development of litigation response P&Ps starts with documentation of the steps and personnel already performing these tasks. Once the current practices are assessed, formalization into more model processes can occur. The best practices guidelines presented in the next section have been drawn from actual practice settings. As always, customize these practices to fit your specific requirements.

Check Your Understanding 12.3

Instructions: Indicate whether the following statements are true or false (T or F).

1. Healthcare providers must be concerned about policies and procedures to guide formal litigation response.

2. There is little need to organize the small amount of data defining legal records into tables or spreadsheets.

3. Litigation response is simply a set of procedures that, when instituted, protects the records.

Instructions: Match the terms with the appropriate descriptions.

   a. Any healthcare data used to make clinical decisions.
   b. The processes invoked if the potential for lawsuits or litigation is detected
   c. Federal rules governing how litigation proceeds
   d. The malicious alteration, concealment, or destruction of evidence

4. _____ Spoliation

5. _____ Protected health information

6. _____ Uniform Rules for e-Discovery

7. _____ Litigation response

⊙ EHR System Attributes That Impact LHR Definitions and e-Discovery

It is crucial to understand each installed EHR system, its purpose in the normal course of daily business, and it functionality from a legal process perspective. This functionality will come into play at many points within litigation or routine legal proceedings. This is especially true as related to questions of accuracy, trustworthiness, and reliability.

When responding to a legal request relating to the EHR, there is not a great deal of time to put together lists of all the important system attributes, functionalities, and user experiences within an EHR system that works to create and manage health records. Therefore, it is advisable to catalog these attributes during the LHR definition project. If not performed in advance, the cataloging must be performed during the course of litigation. If performed during litigation, all answers to specific questions in reference to functionality and system record management attributes should be kept on a permanent basis for future reference.

The following functionalities are important to assess and use in practice to demonstrate that important and mandated attributes are met by your EHR system for optimal defensive legal purposes. It is recommended that these questions be logged into spreadsheets for permanent access and future usage.

Audit Logs

Audit logging refers to metadata kept on each transaction or event that occurs within an EHR system. Not all audit logs are the same. There is wide variability between products and vendors. Audit logs are key records that are expected to be producible if required in legal cases involving health records. Audits logs are essential to successfully execute many required operations such as reporting on who accessed and used data within an EHR. Certification of EHR products includes a requirement (45 CFR §170.302) to have audit logs with a minimum capability to generate an audit log, record the actions of users, and have the ability to be sorted. In order to meet these criteria, the audit log must contain the following for all transactions (or "uses") of an EHR:

- ⊙ Date
- ⊙ Time
- ⊙ Patient identification
- ⊙ User identification (including name, not just an assigned user number)
- ⊙ Brief description of the actions taken by the user (for example, create, print, view, update, and so on) (45 CFR § 170)

Audit logs should be managed as an important component of the organization's "content" (another term for data), documents, and various electronic record sets. Managing audit logs is an important part of the organization's business records that imposes retention and storage issues. The audit logs should be maintained for a retention period of at least six years for HIPAA and longer if required by other regulations.

Authorship and Authentication of Entries and Electronic Signatures

An author is a person or system who originates or creates information that becomes part of the record. Each author must be granted permission by the healthcare entity to make such entries. Not all users will be granted authorship rights into all areas of the EHR. The individual must have the credentials required by state and federal laws to be granted the right to document observations and facts related to the provision of healthcare services. Through medical staff bylaws, rules and regulations, or through documentation guidelines, a provider will indicate the type and frequency of entries to be made in the health record. Often, the bylaws, rules and regulations, or guidelines are based on the documentation requirements published by various government and regulatory agencies.

How clinical documentation and documents are authenticated or electronically signed by the author can have significant ramifications in legal definitions and proceedings. Authentication is a process by which a user (a person or entity) who authored an EHR entry or document is seeking to validate that they are responsible for data contained within it. Authentication can be performed manually with a pen or it can be performed with electronic (and digital) technology. If performed with electronic technology, it is usually called an electronic signature.

Business Continuity

Backups, disaster recovery, and business continuity in the face of failure from routine to catastrophic is important to understand from an LHR perspective. Determining backups and disaster recovery is a product of performing Security Risk Analysis as required by HIPAA as well as part of meaningful use compliance. There are many guidance documents published by the National Institute of Standards and Technology (NIST) and AHIMA to guide the creation of the systems and processes to ensure continuity of business in the face of disaster or any kind of downtime.

Business Rules

The rules and triggers that create work lists, workflows, and other automated processes including clinical decision support alerts and reminders within an EHR are called "business rules" and should be well documented to ensure the best legal defensibility. There can be a large number of these rules. If they are not well documented and are called into e-discovery or court with a limited time frame for production, the organization may find it difficult to put together the details of these rules and their impact on work processes.

Data, Document Management, and Nonrepudiation

The integrity of each piece of data, including any document, must be ensured to maintain highly defensible business records. **Document and data nonrepudiation**, characteristics that defend against charges questioning the integrity of data or documents, delineate the methods by which the data are maintained in an accurate form after their creation, free of unauthorized changes, modifications, updates or similar changes. All EHRs have features to provide for this integrity but with varying combinations of technologies and recommended business processes. How each user organization decides to utilize and continually maintain the highest level of integrity are variables that need to be addressed during each EHR system implementation and operation.

Accuracy, trustworthiness, and reliability are key legal tests of any EHR; however, they are conceptual in nature, defined generally for use in the law but more specifically in each instance based on the needs of the legal proceeding. There are many ways to ensure EHR data accuracy, trustworthiness, and reliability. As EHRs are being developed and implemented, the combination of technological features and means with which the users apply them determine the overall capabilities in these areas.

Retention, Data Permanence, and Migration Plans

Planning for the eventual obsolescence of a technology is often not given a high priority. Record managers need to understand how data would be migrated to ensure compliance with the long retention periods (years to decades) required for EHR systems. There are no standardized guidelines for this type of planning except generally to adopt standards-based sources of EHR data and record management as much as possible. Technology continues to advance and will for decades to come. Migration of data of all kinds needs to be established as systems are expanded and changed. Standards-based technology is essential to continued operational efficiency and integrity of older, but still useful, data and documents. Use of open formats, such as XML, PDF, and formatted continuity-of-care content such as Clinical Continuity Documents (CCD) and Clinical Continuity Records (CCRs), are already providing some guarantee of portability and permanence and making obsolescence less of an issue. More standards will continue to emerge to address these needs.

Interfaces

Typically, most EHR systems import and export documents and data in some fashion via interfaces. As with most other attributes of EHR systems, there are few mandated standards, although Health Level 7 (HL7) has become ubiquitous for some types of interfaces due to industry adoption rather than a mandate (HL7 Record Management 2007). As for LHR ramifications, there are not many with interfaces directly. It is necessary to catalogue the interfaced data or documents for inclusion within the defined LHR and make them a part of the receiving facility's records. Once a record is received and made a part of a legal record set, it becomes a part of the record to be redisclosed upon appropriate request. The receiving facility cannot attest to accuracy, but if used, or even possibly used for care delivery, the record becomes a part of the receiving facility's legal record.

How interfaces are actually executed and reconciled (checked for quality and appropriate placement of data record) is important for record custodians.

Their processes should strive to ensure the procedures for managing interfaced data are well thought out and documented so that they do not become problematic during court proceedings.

Legal Hold

There is a concept of **legal hold** in the healthcare environment. The legal hold requires special, tracked handling of patient records to ensure no changes can be made to a record involved in litigation. Common in the paper record environment to substantiate the integrity of the record, this is less common in the electronic environment where audit logs are the standard. This presupposes that the audit logs have been secured as previously discussed. Record managers need to address the use of legal hold for patient records in any information mode or medium. Very often, consultation with legal counsel will be required.

Metadata

Metadata are data about data and are sometimes very hard to quantify. Litigation is highly dependent upon metadata, and metadata is sure to be an issue in e-discovery. Advanced assessment of these characteristics is important to meet short court clocks. Record custodians need to list all reasonably accessible (per FRCP rules) metadata within the source system. They also need to consider the following:

- ⊙ What data elements are kept for each system document, data, or report within the database, not necessarily within the audit log? Are the following included?
  - o Patient or user identification information
  - o User name or user ID
  - o Name or number of computer (dependant upon system capabilities) used to create the data or document
  - o Date and time created, modified, accessed, or printed, and file or network path location
  - o Revision history, if any changes were made to the data
  - o Patient identification number
  - o What data, documents, or reports were created, modified, accessed, or printed

Electronic Health Record Output

Maintaining control of PHI has always been a challenge. In the paper world, records could be copied and even carried out of the facility. These challenges have evolved and increased in the electronic environment. Output can now take the form of printed documents, or electronic documents that can be attached to e-mails, texted, downloaded to portable storage such as flash drives, captured as screenshots, and sent to social media sites, along with other as yet unidentified output mechanisms. It is essential for the organizational health information manager, privacy officer, security officer, and legal counsel to carefully consider the different types of potential output and how those can be controlled. For example, audit logs can track output to a printer. The printed copies could have annotations indicating that they are not full copies of the record. Likewise, many organizations have decided to disable the USB ports on many or all of the computers in the organization to prevent unauthorized downloads of PHI. The goal with controlling output is not to hinder patient care or any authorized access to PHI but rather to prevent any unauthorized release of PHI.

Another intersection of meaningful use and the LHR defined for disclosure is being sure to catalog all mandatory EHR output as a part of the LHR defined for disclosure. Discharge instructions, copies of records including summaries, and HIE data need to be cataloged within the list of document types that are to be disclosed as appropriate. They may be a part of a hybrid record or all contained within a single EHR. It is most important to keep these cataloges current as the EHR system is increasingly widely adopted.

Rendition

Rendition is the act of rendering data into documents, usually in report form. Report writers are the most common form of rendering, but there are others such as the creation of documents for continuity of care based on preprogrammed routines as required by meaningful use. Production of an LHR may be required in paper or other standard formats. It is important to take this into account when creating policies, procedures, and a litigation response plan.

Snapshots and Screen Views

Snapshots of data, or how screens are populated and what they looked like at discrete points in time, is increasingly being asked for in legal proceedings but are rarely provided in a satisfactory manner within EHR systems. Snapshots and screen views are difficult to create due to a lack of vendor capability.

Privacy Attributes

Given that HIPAA has strengthened privacy rules and increased enforcement, the following EHR system attributes take on elevated importance in determining privacy violations and breach notification:

- Does the EHR system create secured or unsecured PHI by HIPAA definition?
- How are patient's requests for access, viewing, and copying accomplished for this source system?
- In what format are electronic copies given to patients upon requests for access to their own records?
- How are requests for restrictions (out-of-pocket and other) accomplished?
- How is **accounting of disclosures** (AOD) tracked? AOD is a HIPAA requirement to list, upon patient request, all disclosures made outside of the entity holding the information.
- Is the audit log work detailed enough for privacy and access audits?

Version Controls

The LHR must be the record as created during the course of business. In some respects, EHR technology is still evolving. For example, a record may have been printed for an attorney or the software was upgraded and the record as viewed is different than the original record view. When changes, new data, or documents are added to the EHR, how are the old versions managed? Are they available or overwritten? Each EHR system typically has its own version management and also contains flexibility in implementation.

Check Your Understanding 12.4

Instructions: Choose the best answer.

1. Which of the statements below is an accepted authentication factor?
   a. Something you know, that is, a password or personal identification number
   b. Something you have, that is, an ATM card or other security token
   c. Something you are, that is, biometrics, such as a retinal scan or fingerprint
   d. All of the above

2. Which of the following is not a key legal test for the EHR?
   a. Legibility
   b. Reliability
   c. Trustworthiness
   d. Accuracy

3. It is important to get data and information out of EHRs. Which of the following are considerations for EHR output?
   a. Version controls
   b. Screen snapshots
   c. Audit logs
   d. All of the above

Indicate whether the following statements are true or false (T or F).

4. The formats for electronic copies given to patients upon request is a privacy attribute.

5. Rendition converts documents into data.

◉ Patient Record Documentation Considerations

All healthcare providers must establish P&Ps to maintain the health record in a way that establishes its validity, preserves its integrity, and facilitates efficient and timely response to legally permissible requests. Some record management considerations to factor into your LHR P&Ps are included in this section.

Accuracy

Accurate documentation in a health record should reflect the true, correct, and exact description of the care delivered for both content and timing. The accuracy and the completeness of the entries in the health record are the responsibility of the author(s) and are governed by the organization's P&Ps. The P&Ps should include documentation standards based on the regulations, standards, and other sources noted in this chapter. Any decision regarding the inclusion or exclusion of information in the content of the LHR should be noted in the P&P documentation.

Amendments, Corrections, Deletion, and Other Documentation Issues

Providers must have a process in place for handling amendments, corrections, and deletions in health record documentation. Other concerning documentation issues are copy and paste forward, unexpected late entries and the use of canned text, boilerplates, or other mechanisms that limit documentation. When healthcare providers determine that patient care documentation is inaccurate or incomplete, they must follow the established P&Ps to ensure the integrity of the record.

Patient-Requested Amendments

Healthcare organizations need policies to address how patients and their representatives can request amendments to their health records. An amendment is an alteration of the health information by modification, correction, addition, or deletion (AHIMA 2012b). HIPAA standards require that specific procedures and time frames be followed for processing a patient's request for changes or additions to the patient record. A separate entry, such as a progress note, form, or typed letter, can be used for patient amendment documentation. The amendment should

- Refer back to the information questioned, by type of document or information, and the date and time of the original entry
- Document the information believed to be inaccurate and the information the patient or legal representative believes to be correct

The documentation in question must not be removed from the health record or obliterated in any way. The patient cannot require that the documentation be removed or deleted, and the provider of care is not required to perform record amendments. However, if they do not allow the amendment, they must advise the patient of this and there are complex rules to follow in order to document this refusal.

Corrections

Proper procedures must be followed when correcting documentation problems or mistakes. A correction is a change in the information meant to clarify inaccuracies after the original electronic document has been signed or rendered complete

(AHIMA 2012a). The system must have the ability to track corrections or changes to the entry once the entry has been entered or authenticated. An individual viewing the record should see an indicator that a new or additional entry has resulted and should also be able to see the new information. It must be clear to the user that there are additional versions of the data being viewed. Additional information related to error corrections can be found in AHIMA Practice Brief: Maintaining a Legally Sound Health Record—Paper and Electronic (AHIMA 2005).

Deletions

Deletion and retraction are closely related concepts, sometimes used synonymously. Both refer to totally eliminating or hiding from view information that was determined to be incorrect or invalid. A deletion is the action of permanently eliminating information that is not tracked in a previous version. A retraction is the action of correcting information that was incorrect, invalid, or made in error, and preventing its display or hiding the entry or documentation from further general views (AHIMA 2012a). Any record documentation policies must address the occasional need to delete or retract information from a patient record without a visible record. An example of when this might be utilized is when information is filed or saved to the wrong patient's record. This might happen when two patient names are very similar. Another example might be when the clinician hears the patient say they have an allergy when they do not. The incorrect information needs to be hidden from view so that it is not used for future decision making. At the same time, the audit logs for the system should retain a record of the deletion or retraction and who completed the action. Additionally, it is important that the organizational policies strictly control deletion and retraction functionality, as it should be used sparingly.

Copy and Paste Forward

The technology used to support the EHR can provide many enhancements over the paper record (for example, multiple simultaneous access and audit trails). Technology also presents the potential for weakening the integrity of the information. One such risk occurs with the copy-and-paste-forward functionality present in many operating system and software programs. This functionality allows a user to highlight all or a portion of a document or screen display and then copy and paste the portion into a different or new document, potentially overwriting the original text. How they are implemented and used by the provider is usually a differentiator in system functionality. Regardless of the technology used, there are certain foundational concepts to be addressed about whether data can be copied and pasted. The appropriate use of these functions can prevent billing compliance and clinical data trustworthiness issues.

Fundamentally, the underlying concern of copy functionality is that it can damage the trustworthiness and integrity of the record for medicolegal purposes. A compelling reason for cautionary use of the copy functionality is patient care. From a clinical point of view, to copy information into records that is not current, accurate, or applicable to the particular patient visit may have a direct impact on patient care. If indiscriminate use of copy functionality results in the copy forward of health conditions that were resolved, physical findings and symptoms may be inconsistent within the healthcare record. Other providers and organizational staff may become confused by the inconsistent documentation.

If provider documentation functionality such as copy is used appropriately, the functionality can assist providers in working efficiently while maintaining optimal care and compliant documentation. In that regard, copy functionalities may be appropriate when copied information is

- Based on external and independently verifiable sources, such as basic demographic information that is stable over time
- Clearly and easily distinguished from original information, such as automatic summaries that populate data fields that are clearly identified as nonoriginal and cannot be mistaken for original information
- Not actually rendered as part of the record until after a reauthentication process and is auditable for identifying actual origination

There can be many appropriate uses of copy forward functionality. For example, while copy forward is inappropriate for addressing a patient's health history and physical examination findings, it may offer a benefit in bringing forward a patient's problem or medication list.

Late Entries

Late entries occur when a pertinent entry is missed or is not written in a timely manner (AHIMA 2012b). When a late entry is documented, it should be clearly identified as a late entry. The author of the entry needs to record the current date and time as well as the date of the event that is the subject of the late entry. The author should also refer to counsel or any sources of information or circumstances surrounding the late entry. The longer the time period between the occurrence of the event and the recording of the late entry, the less reliable the information entered becomes.

Resequencing and Reassignment

The action of resequencing involves moving a notation or document within the same episode of care for the same patient (AHIMA 2012a). It does not require tracking or any special action. Reassignment of documentation is defined as moving a document or notation between episodes of care within the record of a single patient (AHIMA 2012a). It is recommended that a notation be left at the original location so clinicians can consult the documentation if necessary.

Templates, Boilerplates, Canned Text, and Structured Input

Care must be taken that devices such as templates, boilerplates, canned text, and structured input support clinical care and accurate documentation and are not used simply to expedite the documentation process. Creation and periodic review of these tools should be based on clinically appropriate, standards-based protocols for common or routine information. Documentation by these methods should require an active choice by the provider of care. When a clinician reviews and authenticates an entry in a patient's health record, the author is indicating that he or she reviewed and completed the documentation and accepts its accuracy as his or her own.

⊙ e-Discovery Overview

There are two main legal processes that custodians of records need to be concerned about related to defined electronic or hybrid LHRs: disclosure and e-discovery. Legal counsel will be concerned with both of these processes as well as more traditional legal process issues such as waivers, timing, and strategies. **Disclosure** is the output and release upon request of appropriate health record documents. **E-discovery** is the process of discovering what parts of the patient's records may be used for litigation or further legal proceedings and is an opportunity for opposing counsel to obtain *relevant* information. E-discovery is named to reflect an emphasis on electronic records; however paper–electronic hybrids may also be included. E-discovery can be required from a single or a mix of EHR systems and may also require hybrid portions.

The FRCP distinguishes between reasonably accessible records and those that are not. This is the key that allows healthcare providers to define exactly what the defined LHR will consist of that will be released upon typical, appropriate requests.

LHR information derived from organizations' business records are admissible into evidence through an exception to the hearsay rule contained within FRE 803(6) and the Uniform Business and Public Records Act, which most states have adopted. The records must be kept in the normal course of daily business, authenticated, and identified prior to admission into legal proceedings. The legal and regulatory acceptance of electronic records is predicated on these records meeting certain well-established legal requirements. The basic requirement is that records are authentic and can be deemed to be reliable, trustworthy, and accurate. Tests of these requirements show through various means that the electronic record must have been captured at or near the time of the event or transaction and is complete and available for retrieval.

Amended FRCP amendments took effect December 1, 2006, to more consistently conform to the current LHR environment. These rules are very likely to be adopted by state and local jurisdictions. Adopting them as standards for your facility is prudent. The federal rules continue to mandate formal record custodianship as evidenced by the FRCP for electronic records. The record custodian is charged with the ability to certify exact copies of the original record components; supervise all record inspections by third parties; copy or duplicate records for external release for admission into evidence; and attest to the admissibility, timeliness, and management of the day-to-day record-keeping environment.

Output can be admitted into evidence if it meets the criteria required by the Uniform Photographic Copies of Business and Public Records as Evidence Act (there are both federal and state versions). This act states that a reproduction made by any process that accurately reproduces or forms a durable medium for reproducing the original is as admissible in evidence as the original itself.

The FRCP for e-discovery is responsible for widespread updates and modifications of record management for evidentiary purposes. There are rules addressing legal holds, spoliation, and the e-discovery process, which may take place at the beginning of litigation. Electronic systems must not only securely store data and documents for your defined retention period, but record custodians must also protect them from unauthorized alternation or destruction and be able to secure them from changes during litigation, especially upon court order.

E-discovery is not a "fishing expedition" that grants plaintiffs' counsel the ability to comb through all the patient's records looking for issues to litigate. The concept of **any and all records** can be limited in e-discovery. The term "any and all records" has the expected meaning of all available records. A more focused approach on what is deemed relevant for the case is necessary. Counsels may not agree on these points, and the judge or court officer may be forced to make the determination. Requests stating "any and all records" will be difficult to respond to given the extensive nature of multiple electronic records. If such requests are received, work with your counsel to limit the scope of the request based on relevance to the claim.

Check Your Understanding 12.5

Instructions: Match the terms with the appropriate descriptions.

    a. EHR functionality that allows a user to highlight all or a portion of a document or screen display and move or re-use the documentation.
    b. Changes to the entry once the entry has been entered or authenticated.
    c. An entry made after a pertinent entry is missed or is not written in a timely manner.
    d. A patient's request for changes or additions to the patient record.
    e. The true, correct, and exact description of the care delivered for both content and timing.

1. _____ Accurate documentation

2. _____ Late entries

3. _____ Cut, paste, and copy forward

4. _____ Patient-requested amendments

5. _____ Corrections

Instructions: Indicate whether the following statements are true or false (T or F).

    6. e-Discovery rules are mostly patterned after the Federal Rules of Civil Procedure.

    7. e-Discovery is not an important concept in LHR management by healthcare providers.

    8. Patients have a right to receive amendments at all times.

    9. Copy and paste forward must be a well-controlled activity with defined policies and procedures.

⊙ Summary

The movement of the healthcare business record into a primarily electronic format has raised new and challenging questions for health informatics and health information management professionals. These stakeholders must consider federal and state laws and regulations regarding record content and maintenance, legal process, as well as accreditation and other requirements. This topic will be constantly changing as the technology continues to evolve. Regular monitoring and care must be exercised. The materials in this chapter cover a wide range of subjects from the creation of a project team to define LHRs through reference table and policy creation. Each of these steps is key to preparing healthcare providers for the current state of hybrid paper and electronic records combined with extensive rules governing electronic record use in court.

REFERENCES

45 CFR 170. Health Information Technology: Initial Set of Standards, Implementation Specifications, and Certification Criteria for Electronic Health Record Technology; Interim Rule.

AHIMA. 2012a. *Amendments in the Electronic Health Record Toolkit*. Chicago: AHIMA Press.

AHIMA. 2012b. *Pocket Glossary for Health Information Management and Technology*. 3rd ed. Chicago: AHIMA Press

AHIMA e-HIM Work Group on Maintaining the Legal EHR. 2005. Practice brief: Maintaining a legally sound health record—Paper and electronic. *Journal of AHIMA* 76(10):64A–L.

American Recovery and Reinvestment Act (ARRA) of 2009. Public Law 111-5.

Federal Rules of Civil Procedure (FRCP). Revisions and additions to Rules 16, 26, 33, 34, 37, and 45, as well as Form 35; effective Dec. 1, 2006

Federal Rules of Evidence (FRE). Article VIII, Rule 803(6), Rule 901(a).

HL7 Record Management and Evidentiary Standards. 2007. http://www.hl7.org.

Uniform Photographic Copies of Business and Public Records as Evidence Act.

RESOURCES

AHIMA. 2008. Copy Functionality Toolkit. Chicago: AHIMA.

AHIMA. 2009. e-HIM Workgroup on Best Practices for Electronic Signature, Attestation, and Authentication.

AHIMA e-HIM Work Group on the Legal Health Record. 2005. Guidelines for defining the legal health record for disclosure purposes. *Journal of AHIMA* 76(8):64A–G.

AHIMA e-HIM Work Group: Guidelines for EHR Documentation Practice. 2007. Guidelines for EHR documentation to prevent fraud. *Journal of AHIMA* 78(1):65–68.

AHIMA e-HIM Work Group on e-Discovery. 2006. The new electronic discovery civil rule. *Journal of AHIMA* 77(8):68A–H.

AHIMA EHR Practice Council. 2007. Developing a legal health record policy. *Journal of AHIMA* 78(9):93–97

Burrington-Brown, J. 2007. Legal EHR FAQs. *Journal of AHIMA* 78(9):77, 80.

California Hospital Association. 2007. State of California Consent Manual.

Dougherty, M. 2005. Practice brief: Understanding the EHR system functional model standard. *Journal of AHIMA* 76(2):64A–D.

Federal Rules of Civil Procedure (FRCP). 2006. Rule 17, Appendix A, chapter 2.

Health Insurance Portability and Accountability Act of 1996 (HIPAA). http://www.hipaa.org/

Klein, S.R. 2007. Legal perspective: Welcome to the digital age. *Journal of Healthcare Information Management* 21(4). 6–7.

McLean, T.R. 2009. Authenticating EHR metadata. *Journal of AHIMA* 80(2):40–41, 50.

McLendon, K. 2006. LHRs in the electronic record age: What we know so far. AHIMA's 78th National Convention and Exhibit Proceedings.

McLendon, K. 2007. Record disclosure and the EHR: Defining and managing the subset of data disclosed upon request. *Journal of AHIMA* 78(2):58–59.

McLendon, K. 2010. *The Legal Health Record: Regulations, Policies, and Guidance*, 2nd ed. Chicago: AHIMA Press.

McLendon, K. 2010. Copy that? Meeting the Meaningful Use objectives for electronic copies, parts 1 and 2. *Journal of AHIMA* 81(4):42–43.

National Conference of Commissioners on Uniform State Laws. 2007. Uniform Rules Relating to Discovery of Electronically Stored Information.

Reich, K.B. 2007. Developing a litigation response plan. *Journal of AHIMA* 78(9):76–78, 86.

Roach, W.H., R.G. Hoban, and B.M. Broccolo. 2006. *Medical Records and the Law*. Sudbury, MA: Jones & Bartlett.

Sarbanes-Oxley Act of 2002. www.soxlaw.com/

The Society of American Archivists - A Glossary of Archival and Records Terminology. http://www.archivists.org/glossary/index.asp.

United States Government. Drug Enforcement Administration. 2010. Electronic Prescriptions for Controlled Substances; Final Rule. *Federal Register*, 75(61): 16236–16319.

Consumer Health Informatics

By Juliana J. Brixey

Learning Objectives

- Define consumer health informatics
- Describe characteristics of the online health information consumer
- Identify current and past consumer health informatics technology
- Discuss ubiquitous computing
- Characterize the differences between validity and reliability
- Explain privacy and security issues for online health information

KEY TERMS

Blue Button
Computer literate
Consumer
Digital immigrant
Digital native
eHealth literacy
Health
Health literacy
Informatics

Literacy
Numeric (computational) literacy
Online diagnoser
Patient portal
Personal health record (PHR)
Reliability
Technology literacy
Validity
Visual literacy

⊙ Introduction

It is important for healthcare consumers to be involved in their own care and help healthcare providers maintain the best health possible. Getting consumers involved in their healthcare and the healthcare of their loved ones is a focus of the Office of the National Coordinator for Health Information Technology (ONC 2013). The widespread use of computers and the Internet have made this a reasonable and achieveable goal for most healthcare consumers. A 2012 Pew survey of Internet users revealed that 72 percent had looked online for health information within the past year. That number continues to increase along with those that are classified as **online diagnosers**. These individuals use the Internet to determine a diagnosis or identify a medical condition (Fox and Duggan 2013, 2–6). Today, the general public can search for health information anytime and anywhere using computers and wireless mobile devices such as tablet computers and smart phones. As part of Meaningful Use Stage 2 clinicians are expected to provide patients with secure access to information in their electronic health record (EHR) via a patient portal, as well as exchange secure e-mail with them (CMS 2013a). A **patient portal** is "a secure method of communication between the healthcare provider and the patient" (AHIMA 2012). This is all part of the efforts to engage patients in their care. This chapter will provide an overview to consumer health informatics focusing on the use of technology and information to empower the consumer to achieve better health.

⊙ Consumer Health Informatics: A Standardized Definition?

Definitions are inherently important in the discussion of any domain. Failure to have a standardized definition results in ambiguity, uncertainty, and an overall lack of precision regarding the examination, analysis, evaluation, discussion, or consideration of consumer health information (CHI). For example, CHI combines three concepts: consumers, health, and informatics.

A general definition is provided for each concept before reviewing definitions of CHI.

- ⊙ A **consumer** is defined as a person who purchases goods and services for personal use.
- ⊙ **Health** is defined as the state of being free from illness or injury.
- ⊙ **Informatics** is defined as the study of collecting, organizing, storing, and using electronic information (Oxford 2012).

The above definitions should provide the underpinnings in forming a universal definition for CHI. However, a review of the literature indicates a lack of consensus in defining CHI. As CHI was emerging, the United States Government Accountability Office Accounting and Information Management Division (GOA) defined CHI as "the union of health care content with the speed and ease of technology" (US GOA 1996).

Consumer health informatics has also been defined as a branch of medical informatics that "analyzes consumers' needs for information, studies and implements methods of making information accessible to consumers, and models and integrates consumers' preferences into medical information systems" (Eysenbach 2000, 1713).

The Agency for Healthcare Research and Quality (AHRQ) defines CHI applications "as any electronic tool, technology, or system that is: 1) primarily designed to interact with health information users or consumers (anyone who seeks or uses health care information for nonprofessional work) and 2) interacts directly with the consumer who provides personal health information to the CHI system and receives personalized health information from the tool application or system; and 3) is one in which the data, information, recommendations or other benefits provided to the consumer, may be used with a healthcare professional, but is not dependent on a healthcare professional" (AHRQ 2012).

The American Medical Informatics Association (AMIA) Consumer Health Informatics Working Group (CHIWG) defines CHI as

> .... the field devoted to informatics from multiple consumer or patient views. These include patient-focused informatics, health literacy and consumer education. The focus is on information structures and processes that empower consumers to manage their own health—for example health information literacy, consumer-friendly language, personal health records, and Internet-based strategies and resources. The shift in this view of informatics analyses consumers' needs for information; studies and implements methods for making information accessible to consumers; and models and integrates consumers' preferences into health information systems. Consumer informatics stands at the crossroads of other disciplines, such as nursing informatics, public health, health promotion, health education, library science, and communication science (AMIA, 2012).

Analysis of the definitions reveals both explicit and implicit themes. The themes are depicted in a Mindmap (figure 13.1). The explicit themes that emerged include

- Types of consumers
- The term health as opposed to disease or illness
- Tools and applications
- Rationale for CHI
- Nondependency on a healthcare professional for health information
- Intersection with other disciplines

The implicit themes that emerge from the definitions include

- Content is created by experts.
- Information is available in a searchable repository.
- The acquisition of health information is a solitary and personal activity.
- Consumers do not seek health information from other consumers.

Figure 13.1   Mindmap

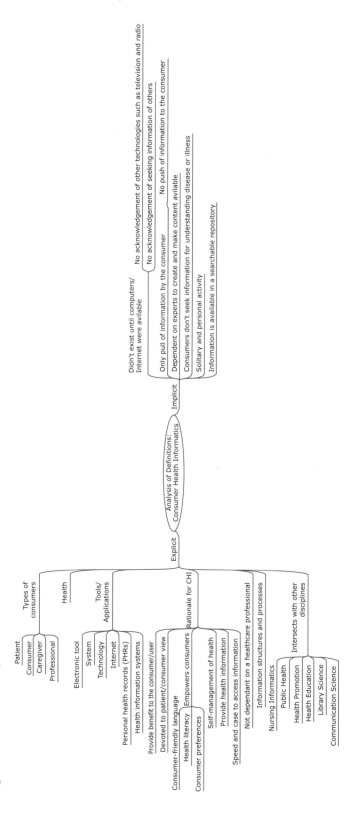

⊙ The desired information is pulled or retrieved by the consumer.

⊙ There is no push of information to the consumer.

⊙ Limited to staying healthy; not about finding information about disease or illness.

In summary, a review of the literature suggests an absence of a standard definition for CHI. Unique and diverse definitions hinder the examination, analysis, evaluation, discussion, and consideration of CHI. It is imperative that all stakeholders (consumers, clinicians, informaticians, health educators, and developers of consumer of health information products) work together to formulate a standard definition.

Literacy: A Fundamental Skill

In order to access and use health information effectively, an individual must possess different literacy skills. **Literacy** is broadly defined as "the ability to read and write" (Oxford Dictionaries 2013) or "using printed and written information to function in society, to achieve one's goals, and to develop one's knowledge and potential" (Kirsch et al. 2002, 2). Health literacy was introduced as a concept in the mid-1970s. **Health literacy** is defined as "the degree to which individuals have the capacity to obtain, process, and understand basic health information and services needed to make appropriate health decisions" (Simonds 1974; Ratzan and Parker 2000, 2). Health literacy can make a difference in patient care, especially when a consumer understands enough to question instructions or to know when they and their support system lack the capabilities to adhere to recommendations. Visual and numeric literacy should be considered as part of health literacy. **Visual literacy** is defined as the "ability to understand graphs or other visual information" (NNLM 2012). For example, the consumer may need to understand a graph trend line of laboratory results. Whereas **numeric or computational literacy** is defined as the "ability to calculate or reason numerically" (NNLM 2012). An example of the need for this can be found in an understanding of body-mass index calculations or if drug dosing may call for calculations. Today, an individual must have **eHealth literacy** skills, which entails "the ability to seek, find, understand, and appraise health information from electronic sources and apply the knowledge gained to addressing or solving a health problem" (Norman and Skinner 2006). Given the reliance on the Internet for health information and knowledge, this skill is especially important. The first source that pops up for a selected search may also be the most unreliable. It is important to know whether a source can be trusted or not. Additionally, an individual must be **computer literate**. Precisely, this is defined as "having sufficient knowledge and skill to be able to use computers, familiar with the operations of a computer" (Oxford Dictionaries 2013). While consumer informatics may not totally rely on computers, the use of computers has made health information much more accessible to consumers. **Technology literacy** is related to computer literacy and entails "having some basic knowledge about technology, some basic technical capabilities, and [the ability to] think critically about technological issues and act accordingly" (Gamire and Pearson 2006, 21). It is reasonable to expect that new literacies will be required as new technologies are introduced.

It is an expectation of The Office of the National Coordinator for Health Information Technology (ONC) that in coming years the use of health IT will support patients to become more engaged and informed regarding their health (Mostashari 2012). However, in order for this to occur, healthcare consumers will not only have to be literate, they will have to have minimal skills in the areas mentioned previously. Unfortunately, in a national literacy survey, many individuals have limited literacy skills and few have high literacy skills (Kirsch et al. 2002, 16, 18, 19). Lower literacy skills were attributed to such factors as English as a second language; years of education completed; ethnicity or race; physical, mental, and health conditions; and age over 65. Millions of people have low health literacy, struggling to understand and take actions based on health information, and even people with strong literacy skills may have trouble obtaining, understanding, and using health information (Nielsen-Bohlman et al. 2004, 1–2). There is agreement among healthcare professionals that many people lack the skills to find, read, listen to, analyze, understand, and use health information and access health services (Baur 2012). Because of this and similar findings, the national government initiative known as Healthy People 2020 includes a goal to improve health literacy skills for all citizens. (Healthy People 2020 2012). The task of health informaticians is to minimize the barriers of understanding and technology for consumers. As an example, instead of using terms such as myocardial infarction, the words heart attack should be used. Likewise, the use of codes and other tools (which help with automatic processing and even bill payment) should be translated for consumers into understandable words. The idea is to make health information more accessible to persons who have not spent many years studying in the healthcare field. In this way, consumers will be empowered to assist healthcare providers who are trying to improve and maintain their health.

Digital Immigrant or Digital Native

It is important to understand as much as possible about the health information consumer when designing and providing online health information. For example, is the health information consumer a **digital immigrant** or **digital native**? A digital native is a person who has only known a world of digital toys and tools (Prensky 2001). In contrast, a digital immigrant is an individual who lived before the advent of the digital age but has adapted more or less to the digital age. This is important since the majority of healthcare is used in two phases of life. Parents of young children, many of whom are now digital natives, will use technology to seek or track the care of their children. This can be for a variety of purposes, including tasks such as providing the school with a list of immunizations. At the other end of the spectrum, older citizens, including their adult children and caregivers, will need to use technology to manage the care required as they age. The technology and computer literacy of the digital native and the digital immigrant will be different, as will their preferred types of applications and communication.

⊙ Characteristics of the Online Health Consumer

A telephone survey of 3,014 adults living in the United States was conducted over a month-long period to learn how people used the Internet to locate health information. From the findings:

- ⊙ 81 percent of US adults use the Internet.
- ⊙ Of those Internet users, 72 percent say they have looked online for health information in the past year.
- ⊙ 59 percent of US adults have searched the Internet for health information in the past year in an effort to determine their own medical condition or that of another individual.
- ⊙ Demographics of those searching for health information using the Internet:
  - o Female
  - o Younger people
  - o White adults
  - o Those in a household earning $75,000 or more
  - o College or advanced degree
- ⊙ 77 percent of those seeking online health information used a search engine.
- ⊙ Those 65 and older were more likely to search the Internet on their own behalf.
- ⊙ 85 percent of US adults own a cell phone.
- ⊙ Of all cell phone users, those who are Latino or African Americans, those between the ages of 18–49, and with some college education are more likely to have used their phone to search the Internet for health information.
- ⊙ 45 percent of US adults own a smart phone.
- ⊙ Younger adults, and those with higher income and higher educational levels are more likely to own a smart phone.
- ⊙ 52 percent of smart phone users have searched for health information using their smart phone (Fox and Duggan 2013).

The findings provide important information about online health information consumers. Since a majority of those who are connected have used the Internet to search for health information, it seems to follow that this is a good option when trying to disseminate health information. For example, whether or not the consumer has some college education appears to impact whether or not they will use the Internet to search for health information. The findings also provide insight into the technologies consumers are using to search the Internet.

Health Topics of Interest for the Online Health Information Consumer

Similarly, it is important to know what health topics online health consumers are exploring. The Pew Survey group began researching consumer behaviors related to online health behaviors beginning in the early 2000s. They found online health consumers began searching for information about

- A specific disease or medical problem
- A specific medical treatment or procedure
- Doctors or other health professionals
- Hospitals or other medical facilities
- Health insurance, including private insurance, Medicare, or Medicaid
- Environmental health hazards (Fox 2011)

Presently, the online health information consumer is searching for information about

- Food safety or recalls
- Drug safety or recalls
- Pregnancy and childbirth
- Memory loss and dementia or Alzheimer's
- Medical test results
- Management of chronic pain
- Long-term care for an elderly or disabled person
- End of life decisions (Fox 2011)

These topics suggest current consumers are seeking online health information about time-sensitive topics such as recalls as well as for complex or chronic health conditions. Time-sensitive information such as recalls requires the availably of dynamically updated online factual content. In contrast, complex or chronic health conditions do not require minute-to-minute updates but incremental changes as new information becomes available. Thus, it is important for the consumer to understand what they are asking for; however, it is also essential that the information provider know the reasonable life span of the information it is posting and update or retract it in a responsible fashion.

Getting Connected to the Internet for the Online Health Information Consumer

Online health consumers require Internet access. The online dial-up services of the 1990s have largely been replaced by broadband and wireless services. "Americans believe it is a major disadvantage to lack broadband to access online health information" (Fox 2011). In 2011, about two-thirds of US homes had a broadband connection. However, many rural or low-population areas still relied on dial-up services. In these areas, it is often too expensive or too difficult to offer broadband connections, resulting in a digital divide between those with broadband services and those that do not. The widespread use of mobile phones with web-browser functionality and similar technologies may offer a solution to bridge the digital divide (Fox 2011).

Check Your Understanding 13.1

Instructions: Provide the best answer.

1. Could one expect to find information on a specific disease on a CHI site?
   a. Yes
   b. No

2. Could one expect to find information about environmental health hazards on a CHI site?
   a. Yes
   b. No

3. Currently, how many of US homes have a broadband connection?
   a. 1/10
   b. 1/4
   c. 1/2
   d. 2/3

Instructions: Answer the following questions on a separate piece of paper.

4. Would you say that people with higher incomes are more likely to use CHI than people with lower incomes?

5. How important is the spread of CHI to smart phones?

6. Which groups are less likely to search for online health information?

7. Give an example of time-sensitive information that could be found on at CHI site.

8. What is a digital divide?

9. What is a possible way to bridge the digital gap caused by lack of broadband coverage?

◉ Consumer Health Informatics Technology

The availability of CHI has been dependent on the endlessly evolving information technology. The current technologies making health information available to consumers include

- ◉ Self-help books
- ◉ Online health articles or sites
- ◉ Bulletin boards and online discussion groups
- ◉ Automated appointment reminders
- ◉ Automated systems for learning more about health conditions
- ◉ Wearable sensors, such as glucose monitors
- ◉ Social media sites such as Facebook and Twitter

There are a wide variety of interactive systems where health information consumers can communicate with other individuals using e-mail, bulletin boards, online discussion groups, and social media. The communication is recognized as not limited to healthcare professionals but includes self-help groups.

Initial technologies may seem antiquated in comparison to the myriad of technologies that today's health information consumers can choose from. Increasingly sophisticated technologies are becoming available to deliver health information to the consumers. For example, a smart toilet can document and examine weight, BMI, blood pressure, and glucose levels (Saenz 2009). Most recently, a smart bra has been developed to detect breast cancer (Quick 2012). Sensors embedded in the bra monitor the breasts to detect changes in skin temperature, which is often indicative of breast cancer. Women in the United States can expect the bra to be available in 2014 if approved by the Food and Drug Administration (FDA). Technology is expected to continue evolving, with more and more ways for consumers to monitor their health and the health of their loved ones.

⊙ Ubiquitous Computing of Online Health Information

Patients no longer have to schedule an appointment with a physician to ask a question about a disease or how to stay healthy. Today, consumers have access to anytime, anywhere information using the Internet. There is a plethora of websites on the Internet to choose from depending on the consumer's need. They range from free-standing websites designed to serve consumers to healthcare provider and professional association websites to health insurance company websites to federal, state, and local governmental websites. Consumers want, and many stakeholders are ready to provide, ubiquitous access to health information.

For example, WebMD was founded in 1996 by Jim Clark and Paven Nigam as Healthscape, later Healtheon, and then was acquired three years later by WebMD (founded by Jeff Arnold) to form Healtheon/WebMD (Funding Universe 2013). Later the name was shortened to WebMD. The WebMD homepage immediately engages the consumer with a wide variety of health, wellness, and disease-oriented content. A selection of health and illness content is available without creating a user account. The website offers the consumer the option of creating a free of charge secure account. With an account, consumers can create a personalized weight loss plan, track vaccines, or join a community that specializes in a specific health topic. There are many similar websites, such as Sharecare, proof of the potential commercial success for these technologies in healthcare.

Healthcare organizations and hospitals are making information available to consumers. For example, the Mayo Clinic (Mayo Clinic n.d.) launched its social media outreach on May 5, 2011, for patients, caregivers, and consumers. Mayo Clinic offers such applications as blogs, Facebook, Twitter, YouTube, and e-patient.net in an effort to actively engage people in managing their health.

Medical libraries provide health information to consumers. For example, MedlinePlus from the US National Library of Medicine and the National Institutes of Health (NIH) maintain numerous online information websites to provide consumers with reliable and up-to-date information (NIH n.d.b; NLM 2012b). According to MedLine Plus, consumers can find easy to understand information on more than 900 diseases, as well as prescription and nonprescription drugs, along with links to clinical trials and the option to engage in interactive tutorials. Additionally, consumers can view videos to learn more about anatomy in addition to surgical procedures. The website also provides health information in Spanish. Additionally, the website is updated daily to provide the most current information to consumers. Unlike many commercial sites, the government-sponsored website is free of advertising.

In addition, medical libraries such as The Texas Medical Center (TMC) Library provide on-site services to consumers by making two touch-screen computers available. Librarians are available to help the consumer search and retrieve health information. The library provides a number of training opportunities such as the free delivery of health information via mail, e-mail, or fax; the use of local and national consumer health databases; and in-depth health topics. Also, the library helps consumers find health information through the provision of recommending national and local websites. Additionally, the library makes information available at the TMC International Visitor's Lounge in the International Terminal of Bush Intercontinental Airport. Furthermore, the library supports consumer health outreach not only in Houston but in the surrounding counties. Likewise, The Dykes Library of Health Sciences located at the University of Kansas Medical Center makes health information available to consumers. The library website provides a link to Kansas Health Online. The website provides consumers with a wealth of information. The website informs consumers of new health topics of interest such as medical genealogy.

A number of disease societies such as the American Cancer Society (American Cancer Society [ACS] 2012) and American Diabetes Association (American Diabetes Association [ADA] 2012) have made health information available to consumers. For example on the ACS website, consumers can learn more about cancer from the provided online resources as well as learning more about volunteer efforts and campaigns. Similarly, the ADA provides consumers with information regarding the types of diabetes alongside tips for healthy eating and exercise.

Moreover, retail pharmacies, such as Walgreens, CVS, and Walmart, health insurance companies, such as Blue Cross Blue Shield and UnitedHealth Group, online news services, such as CNNHealth and Fox News, grocery stores, and a host of other organizations are making health information available to consumers. This is not an exhaustive list but examples of where consumers may find online health information. These entities make health information available to their consumer population. For instance, these websites provide health information about healthy eating, health risk assessment, surgeries and procedures, tools and trackers, women's health, immunizations, medication resources, weight management, stress management, and guidelines for drug disposal. Furthermore, employers provide health promotion information to their employees (Texas State University, n.d.; Nestlé, 2012). Additionally, the Centers for Disease Control and Prevention provides a website with information that employers can use to make CHI available to their workers (CDC 2012).

The proliferation of mobile technology is an influencing force in how consumers access health information. Although access still requires access to the Internet and a web browser, the consumer is no longer limited to desktop computing. The consumer can access the health information on their mobile devices (a smart phone or tablet computer). Along with the new technology is the explosion of health applications, more commonly called apps. The apps can help consumers maintain a personal health record (PHR), track their weight, record progress in health and wellness programs, and monitor their heart rate. These are a few examples of health apps. Consumers can expect more sophisticated apps to be developed in the future.

It should not be overlooked that consumers are seeking online health information from social networking sites such as Facebook, Twitter, YouTube, and Second Life. Second Life is a 3-D virtual world of user-created content. For example, visitors to Second Life can learn more about health, pregnancy and childbirth, cancer, or experience what is like for the schizophrenic patient to hear voices by visiting virtual clinics and hospitals. Consumers can search for health information created by both healthcare professionals as well as lay persons. As with all online health information, it is important for the consumer to carefully evaluate the information from social networking sites.

Consumers have moved from an environment where health information was sparse and difficult to retrieve to a situation of information overload due to the unlimited access and availability of health and wellness resources. Furthermore, CHI is not just accessible using desktop computing but is now available ubiquitously using mobile devices such as smart phones and tablet computers. This requires health information consumers to become educated and to evaluate the quality of information they are accessing.

Check Your Understanding 13.2

Instructions: Choose the best answer.

1. Some examples of consumer sources for consumer health informatics include (select all that apply)
   a. Social media sites
   b. Bulletin boards
   c. Online heath articles
   d. All of the above

Instructions: Answer the following questions on a separate piece of paper.

2. What could a smart toilet do for you?

3. Give a definition of ubiquitous.

4. Name two examples of libraries or professional centers that consumers can access for healthcare answers.

⊙ Personal Health Records

A **personal health record (PHR)** is "an electronic or paper health record maintained and updated by an individual for himself or herself; a tool that individuals can use to collect, track, and share past and current information about their health or the health of someone in their care" (AHIMA 2012, 320). PHRs have been promoted as one method to improve health for patients and reduce the costs of healthcare (Hillestad et al. 2005). However, the use of personal health records on a large scale has not occurred and the Meaningful Use Stage 2 requirements include portals to the EHR data versus a PHR-type capability (CMS 2013). Nevertheless, PHRs remain an important consumer tool for managing patients' health and health information and will be explored below.

The PHR can be a paper record, or health information stored on a smart card, USB drive, CD, or computer (ePHR). The electronic PHR can be a stand-alone record or tethered to an EHR maintained by a health facility, such as a hospital or health insurance organization or a system such as the US Department of Veterans Affairs, explored in the discussion of the Blue Button functionality below. The PHR is not in common usage, which brings up the question of what are the barriers to the adoption of PHRs? A panel of 50 experts with years of experience working with patients and PHRs identified the following barriers:

- ⊙ Physicians question the reliability of patient-reported data

- ⊙ The question of who would pay for the costs of the PHRs. The amount that patients would be willing to pay would not cover the licensing costs, and some patients might not use the service if they had to pay for it

- ⊙ The PHRs needed interoperability to exchange data with other health systems or the PHRs could become "information islands"

- ⊙ The interoperability issues bring up the problems of patient privacy. A stand-alone record brings up the problem of security if the record is lost

- ⊙ Encryption of the records brings up problems of authentication

- ⊙ The legal implications of a health provider relying on inaccurate patient-entered PHR data

- ⊙ Some providers voiced concern that some patients might use the electronic PHR to elicit prescriptions for narcotics by falsely claiming prior prescriptions (Tang et al. 2006)

A study from Pennsylvania indicated that patients have a mostly positive view of the PHR and linked web messaging. In general, patients are supportive of PHRs, but are very supportive of technologies that enable increased communication with providers via web portals, electronic messaging, and other methods. However, clinicians who are not reimbursed for the time spent communicating with patients using new methods and technologies are, understandably, more reluctant to adopt them extensively (Hassol et al. 2004). These findings raise important policy questions regarding the time clinicians spend interacting with PHRs to their financial detriment, as well as raising concerns regarding privacy. This is also another example of the perverse incentives in the US healthcare industry, where standard reimbursement policies penalize clinicians for using technology to improve consumer health.

Disparities in access to health information when it is tied to computer technology is also an issue for the increased use of PHRs and web portals. Patients in underserved areas or without high-speed Internet access, such as with a computer at home or via a smart phone, may find themselves unable to take advantage of the latest health information technology advances. A study in Northern California of a group of over 14,000 diabetes patients, with demographic characteristics similar to the overall population in Northern California, found that older patients were less likely to use the site and found a pervasive racial and educational disparity in use of the computer portal. The study expressed a fear that "those most at risk for poor diabetes outcomes may fall further behind as health systems increasingly rely on the Internet and limit current modes of access and communications" (Sarakar et al. 2011). Thus, while it is good to develop new uses of technology and information technology to help patients, it is important for health information professionals to consider how those who do not possess the latest technology can also improve and maintain their health using information using more traditional means.

As with all technologies, the issue of costs must be considered. A cost and benefits assessment of PHRs was performed and projected an estimated 80 percent use over a 10-year period by the US population. All types of PHRs demonstrated initial negative value with breakeven points ranging from 3 to 10 or more years. The interoperable PHRs had a breakeven point at three years. The provider PHRs did not break even in 10 years. Between $4 billion and $130 billion would be needed in initial investment and between $2 billion and $42 billion would be needed in annual support. Net benefits were estimated at $13 to $21 billion annually (Kaebler et al. 2008). What is missing from this analysis is a clear description of who has paid the costs for the PHRs and where the different benefits accrue. Too often, the benefits are calculated for the entire healthcare system while the costs are borne by individuals or healthcare providers. They have to bear the costs for the greater good. Policymakers and others are trying to develop new policies to distribute the costs and burden more equitably.

Some of the benefits of using electronic PHRs relate to the interoperability of having an electronic PHR tethered to the electronic medical record. Project Health Design is a national program, funded by grants from foundations, designed to stimulate the development of new tools for personal health management by using the PHR (Brennan et al. 2007). The plan is to create a set of prototype applications to support interoperable resources for managing health challenges. If successful, the future of the PHR is bright and vibrant. The authors note: "The current PHRs are fragmented, non-scalable, without data standards, shared terminologies or common architectures" (Brennan et al. 2007). However, focusing on usability in the design of applications promotes full realization of the benefits of healthcare and makes the PHRs more useable in the management of chronic disease.

The idea that the use of personal health records will play a key role in enabling the electronic health environment is becoming more common. The PHR has the possibility to create a more balanced and complete view of the patient, especially when the consumer has multiple physicians or is unable to care for themselves.

The patient is referred to as a consumer, rather than as a patient, to reflect this mind change and to underscore the fact that health records are no longer the sole property of the physician or hospital.

The verdict on the uses and usability of PHRs is far from final; however, especially for patients who suffer from a chronic disease or have multiple providers, they can prove to be very helpful. The American Health Information Management Association (AHIMA) and the AHIMA Foundation maintain the myphr.com website, providing an overview of PHRs, as well as guidance on how to initiate a PHR for consumers and their loved ones (AHIMA 2013). As consumers become increasingly tech-savvy and as the population continues to age, understanding and managing personal health information will become ever more important.

⊙ Blue Button: Access to Health Information

On August 2, 2010, President Barack Obama stated "For the first time ever, veterans will be able to go to the VA website, click a simple **Blue Button** and download or print your personal health records so you have them and can share with your doctor outside of the VA" (Obama 2010). An individual has the legal right to access their own health information. This right is made easier through the Blue Button initiative. The idea for the Blue Button began at the Markle Consumer Engagement Workgroup meeting in January 2010 (Nazi 2010). Agreement at the meeting was to place a big button on existing patient portals in order to give patients access to their health information. The intent of the initiative is to make access to personal health information easier for veterans, uniformed service members, and Medicare beneficiaries. The Blue Button initiative was formally launched in October 2010 (Chopra et al., 2010). In August 2012, the one millionth patient used the Blue Button to download information from a PHR (United States Department of Veterans Affairs [VA] 2013). Other federal agencies and companies are encouraging their members to use Blue Button to securely access and download their health information. Accessible information includes current medications, drug allergies, treatments, and laboratory results. Claims information can be retrieved electronically using Blue Button. The information is available to print or save. The information is saved as an ASCII text file and displays as an organized report.

Each agency administers Blue Button with its own rules. For example, to use the Blue Button for Medicare data, beneficiaries must register at medicare.gov. Veterans can use their MyHealtheVet record, which they sign up for at their local VA facility, and click the Blue Button to save or print information from their health record. In addition, veterans can use the VA Continuity of Care Document (VA CCD). This is a summary of essential health and medical care information in an XML format for easier exchange of health information between healthcare organizations and clinicians (United States Department of Veterans Affairs [VA] 2013).

From this initiative, many patients can now securely access, save, print, and exchange their health information with providers and healthcare organizations. Ultimately, using the Blue Button will not only actively engage the patient in their healthcare but will improve the quality and safety of care. While not exactly a

PHR as described above since it only contains the information from the agency or provider sponsoring the Blue Button, this application does effectively expand access to health information for a large number of citizens.

⊙ Validity and Reliability of Online Health Information

Validity and reliability of online resources are a constant concern for those retrieving information from the Internet. **Validity** is defined as "1. The extent to which data correspond to the actual state of affairs or that an instrument measures what it purports to measure. 2. A term referring to a test's ability to accurately and consistently measure what it purports to measure" (AHIMA 2013). Whereas **reliability** is defined as "A measure of consistency of data items based on their reproducibility and an estimation of their error of measurement" (AHIMA 2013).

What is more, heathcare professionals and researchers continue to question the validity and reliability of online information (Hendrick et al. 2012). Concerns about the reliability of health information on the Internet was addressed in 1995 when Health on the Net Foundation (HON), an international, nongovernmental organization, was launched (Health on the Net Foundation 2011). Based on dialog with webmasters and information providers, the initial version of the HON Code of Conduct (HONcode) for medical and health websites was published in 1996. The code was revised in 1997 and has remained unchanged. The current HONcode principles are grounded in the following tenets:

- ⊙ Authoritative—expertise of the authors
- ⊙ Complementarity—uphold the doctor-patient bond
- ⊙ Privacy—ensure the privacy and security of personal data
- ⊙ Attribution—give credit to sources of information
- ⊙ Justifiable—corroborate assertions of improvement and betterment
- ⊙ Transparency—clarity of content and inclusion of webmaster's e-mail address
- ⊙ Financial disclosure—disclosure of funding
- ⊙ Advertising policy—a clear distinction between advertising and verifiable content (HON 2011)

Website certification is offered free of charge to requesting websites. HON conducts a thorough investigation of the website to ensure the web developers adhere to ethical standards in the presentation of information and the readers can determine the source and intent of the data they are reading. If approved an HON code seal is placed on the website.

Consumers should consider learning more about how to determine the validity and reliability of online health information from such trusted sources as

- ⊙ MedlinePlus Guide to Healthy Web Surfing
- ⊙ Finding Reliable Health Information Online

- ⊙ Evaluating Health Information
- ⊙ MedlinePlus Quality Guidelines
- ⊙ Medical Library Association List of 100 Websites You can Trust

The advice offered to consumers of online health information advice by NIH is to critically scrutinize online information (NIH 2012). Furthermore, NIH recommends the use of current, unbiased evidence-based information. To a certain extent, consumers accessing health information online should use the information to become more educated about their health, while exercising caution and consulting with quality healthcare providers to ensure the information is valid.

⊙ Privacy and Security

The online health information consumer should expect the privacy and security of any disclosed personally identifiable health information to be maintained. Reputable online health information websites should include a hyperlink to a privacy policy statement. The hyperlink is typically located near the bottom of the webpage. For example, NIHSeniorHealth and MedlinePlus provide information about privacy to the online health consumer regarding the following information:

- ⊙ Type of information collected
- ⊙ Cookies
- ⊙ Personally identifiable information (PII)
- ⊙ Links to other sites
- ⊙ Security
- ⊙ Third-party websites and applications
  - o AddThis
  - o Go.USA.gov and Bit.ly
  - o Facebook
  - o GovDelivery
  - o iTunes App Store
  - o Twitter (NIH 2012 and NLM 2012b)

Presently, new challenges for managing privacy and security issues have arisen related to mobile and online health information. According to Lygeia Ricciardi, acting director for the Office of Consumer eHealth, "regulations such as HIPAA and HITECH provide some parameters for privacy guidance in this changing environment, and as health information technology evolves, additional initiatives can build on and complement those protections" (Ricciardi, 2012). The ONC, primarily through its Office of the Chief Privacy Officer, has initiated the following projects to study privacy and security issues related to mobile and online health information:

- ⊙ Mobile Devices Roundtable: Safeguarding Health Information
- ⊙ mHealth Privacy and Security Consumer Research

⊙ Survey on Privacy, Security of Medical Records

⊙ Model Privacy Notice for Consumers for Personal Health Records (PHRs)

The privacy and security of personal identifiable information collected by a website or other technology must be guaranteed to the health information consumer. The ONC is taking steps to meet the challenges of privacy and security introduced by new technology.

Check Your Understanding 13.3

Instructions: Answer the following questions on a separate piece of paper.

1. What is the difference between validity and reliability?
2. What is the Health on the Net Foundation?
3. Does Health on the Net Foundation (HON) offer certification for a website and how would you know if a site has been certified?
4. Do healthcare sites ever have a privacy policy statement?
5. Would you expect to find anything about cookies in a policy statement?
6. Is the federal government doing anything to aid the consumer in online privacy?

⊙ Summary

The online health information consumer has access to a vast amount of health information available with a few keystrokes made on a computer or smart phone. Without the Internet and personal computers, the availability of online health information would have been highly unlikely. Moreover, health information consumers have become empowered to develop and lead very successful self-help group websites without the influence of healthcare professionals, demonstrating their desire to be informed about and engaged with their healthcare. PHRs and the Blue Button initiatives, as well the Meaningful Use Stage 2 patient portal requirements will continue to make consumer engagement easier. However, there are concerns. The widespread availability of online health information results in the need to ensure the validity and reliability of the information. Consumers now have tools to help them critically evaluate online health information. Most importantly, the privacy and security of any disclosed personal health information collected on a website must be ensured. It is the expectation that consumer informatics will continue to evolve as new and more sophisticated technology is developed and embraced by consumers.

REFERENCES

Agency for Healthcare Research and Quality. 2012. Consumer health IT applications. http://healthit.ahrq.gov/portal/server.pt?open=514&objID=5554&mode=2&holder DisplayURL=http://wci-pubcontent/publish/communities/k_o/knowledge_library/ key_topics/consumer_health_it/consumer_health_it_applications.html.

American Cancer Society. 2012. Resources. http://www.cancer.org/.

American Diabetes Association. 2012. Diabetes Basics. http://www.diabetes.org/diabetes-basics/.

American Health Information Management Association. 2012. *Pocket Glossary for Health Information Management and Technology*, 3rd ed. Chicago, IL: AHIMA.

American Health Information Management Association. 2013. myPHR. Retrieved from myphr.com.

American Medical Informatics Association Consumer Health Informatics Working Group. 2012. Consumer health informatics. http://www.amia.org/applications-informatics/consumer-health-informatics.

Baur, C. 2012. Health literacy around the world [Web log]. http://blogs.cdc.gov/healthliteracy/2012/09/28/health-literacy-around-the-world/.

Blue Cross Blue Shield of Texas. 2012. Health and wellness. http://www.bcbstx.com/health/index.html;

Brennan, P.F., S. Downs, and D. Kenron. 2007. Project health design: Stimulating the next generation of personal health records. *AMIA Annual Symposium Proceedings 2007*. http://www.ncbi.nlm.nih.gov/pmc/articles/PMC2655909/

CNN. 2012. CNNHealth. http://www.cnn.com/HEALTH/

CVS 2012. Health center information. Retrieved from http://health.cvs.com/GetContent.aspx?token=f75979d3-9c7c-4b16-af56-3e122a3f19e3

Centers for Disease Control: The National Institute for Occupational Safety and Health. 2012. Total worker health. http://www.cdc.gov/niosh/twh/resources.html.

Centers for Medicare and Medicaid. 2013. Stage 2. http://www.cms.gov/regulations-and-guidance/legislation/ehrincentiveprograms/stage_2.html.

Chopra, A., T. Park, and P.L. Levin. 2010. 'Blue Button' provides access to downloadable personal health data [Web log]. http://www.whitehouse.gov/blog/2010/10/07/blue-button-provides-access-downloadable-personal-health-data.

Computer-literate. 2013. In Oxford Dictionaries. http://oxforddictionaries.com/us/definition/american_english/computer-literate

Consumer. 2013. In Oxford Dictionaries. http://oxforddictionaries.com/definition/consumer

Dykes Library 2012. Patient Health Information. http://library.kumc.edu/about/consumer.html.

Eysenbach, G. Consumer health informatics. 2000. *BMJ* 320(7251):1713-6.

Fox News. 2012. Health. http://www.foxnews.com/health/index.html.

Fox, S. 2011. The social life of health information. Pew Internet & American Life Project, May 12, 2011. http://pewinternet.org/Reports/2011/Social-Life-of-Health-Info.aspx

Fox, S. and M. Duggan. 2013. Pew Internet: Health. http://pewinternet.org/Commentary/2011/November/Pew-Internet-Health.aspx.

Funding Universe. 2013. WebMD Corporation History. Retrieved from http://www.fundinguniverse.com/company-histories/webmd-corporation-history/.

Gamire, E. and G. Pearson, eds. 2006. *Tech Tally: Approaches to Assessing Technological Literacy*. Washington, D.C.: The National Academies Press.

Hassol, A., J. Walker, D. Kidder, K. Rokita, D. Young, S. Pierdon, D. Deitz, S. Kuck, and E. Ortiz. 2004. Patient experiences and attitudes about access to a patient electronic health care record and linked web messaging. *JAMIA* 11(6):505–513.

Healthy People 2020. 2012. Health communications and health information technology. http://healthypeople.gov/2020/topicsobjectives2020/overview.aspx?topicid=18.

Hendrick, P.A., O.H. Ahmed, S.S. Bankier, S.A. Crawford, C.R. Ryder, L.J. Welsh, and A.G. Schneiders. 2012. Acute low back pain information online: An evaluation of quality, content accuracy and readability or related websites. *Man Ther* 17(40): 318–324.

Health. 2013. In Oxford Dictionaries. http://oxforddictionaries.com/definition/health?q=health

Health on the Net Foundation. 2011. Health on the Net Foundation. http://www.hon.ch/HONcode/Patients/Visitor/visitor.html.

Hillestad, R., J. Bigelow, A. Bower, F. Girosi, R. Meili, R. Scoville, and R. Taylor. 2005. Can electronic medical record systems transform healthcare? Potential health benefits, savings, and costs. *Health Affairs* 24(5):1103–1117.

Informatics. 2013. In Oxford Dictionaries. http://dictionary.cambridge.org/dictionary/business-english/information-science

Kaelber, D., and E.C. Pan. (2008). "The value of personal health record (PHR) systems." In *AMIA Annual Symposium Proceedings*, vol. 2008, p. 343. American Medical Informatics Association.

Kansas Health Online. 2012. Kansas health online. http://www.kansashealthonline.org/

Kirsch, I.S., A. Jungeblut, L. Jenkins, and A. Kolstad. 2002. *Adult literacy in America: A first look at the findings of the National Adult Literacy Survey*, 3rd ed. http://nces.ed.gov/pubs93/93275.pdf.

Literacy. 2013. In Oxford Dictionaries. http://oxforddictionaries.com/us/definition/american_english/literacy.

Markle Foundation. 2003. Americans want benefits of personal health records. http://www.markle.org/sites/default/files/phwg_survey.pdf.

Mayo Clinic. n.d. Mayo Clinic Center for Social Media. http://socialmedia.mayoclinic.org/about-3/.

Medical Library Association. 2013. List of 100 Websites You Can Trust. http://caphis.mlanet.org/index.html.

Mostashari, F. 2012, January 25. Health IT taking flight—What is in store for the year ahead [Web log comment]. http://www.healthit.gov/buzz-blog/from-the-onc-desk/healthit-year-ahead/

National Human Genome Research Institute. 2011. Finding reliable health information on online. http://www.genome.gov/11008303

National Institutes of Health. n.d.a. Health information. http://health.nih.gov/.

National Institutes of Health n.d.b.. Health and wellness resources. http://www.nih.gov/health/wellness/.

National Institutes of Health. 2012. NIHSeniorHealth. http://nihseniorhealth.gov/privacy.html.

National Library of Medicine. 2012a. NLM privacy policy. http://www.nlm.nih.gov/medlineplus/privacy.html.

National Library of Medicine. 2012b. MedlinePlus. http://www.nlm.nih.gov/medlineplus/aboutmedlineplus.html

National Library of Medicine. 2012c. Evaluating health information. http://www.nlm.nih.gov/medlineplus/evaluatinghealthinformation.html.

National Library of Medicine. 2012d. MedlinePlus guide to healthy web surfing. http://www.nlm.nih.gov/medlineplus/evaluatinghealthinformation.htmlhttp://www.nlm.nih.gov/medlineplus/healthywebsurfing.html.

National Library of Medicine. 2012e. MedlinePlus quality guidelines. http://www.nlm.nih.gov/medlineplus/criteria.html.

National Library of Medicine. 2012f. MedlinePlus statistics. http://www.nlm.nih.gov/medlineplus/usestatistics.html.

National Network of Libraries of Medicine. 2012. Health literacy. http://nnlm.gov/outreach/consumer/hlthlit.html.

Nazi, K.L. 2010, December 8. VA's Blue Button: Empowering people with their data [Web log]. http://www.blogs.va.gov/VAntage/866/vas-blue-button-empowering-people-with-their-data/

Nestlé. 2012. Employee health and wellness. http://www.nestle.com/csv/ourpeople/employeehealthandwellness/Pages/employeehealthandwellness.aspx

Nielsen-Bohlman, L., A.M. Panzer, and D.A. Kindig. 2004. *Health Literacy: A Prescription to End Confusion*. Washington, D.C.: The National Academies Press.

Norman, C.D., and H.A. Skinner. 2006. eHealth Literacy: Essential skills for consumer health in a networked world. *Journal of Medical Internet Research* 8(2):e9. doi:10.2196/jmir.8.2.e9

Obama, B.H. Speech to the Disabled Veterans of America, August 2, 2010. White House. http://www.whitehouse.gov/the-press-office/remarks-president-disabled-veterans-america-conference-atlanta-georgia.

Office of the National Coordinator for Health Information Technology. 2013. www.healthit.gov.

Patientslikeme. 2012. http://www.patientslikeme.com/about.

Prensky, M. 2001. Digital natives, digital immigrants. *On the Horizon* 9(5):1-6. http://www.marcprensky.com/writing/Prensky%20-%20Digital%20Natives,%20Digital%20Immigrants%20-%20Part1.pdf.

Quick, D. 2012, October 12. Smart bra acts as an early warning system for breast cancer. http://www.gizmag.com/bse-bra-breast-cancer-monitoring/24529/

Ratzan, S.C. and R.M. Parker. 2000. Introduction. In *National Library of Medicine Current Bibliographies in Medicine: Health Literacy*. NLM Pub. No. CBM 2000-1. Edited by

C.R. Selden, M. Zorn, S.C. Ratzan, and R.M. Parker. Bethesda, MD: National Institutes of Health, US Department of Health and Human Services.

Reliability. 2012. In *Oxford Dictionaries*. http://oxforddictionaries.com/definition/english/reliable?q=reliability#reliable__3.

Ricciardi, L. 2012, March 15. Protecting privacy of health information and building trust as mobile and online health evolve [Web log]. http://www.healthit.gov/buzz-blog/from-the-onc-desk/privacy-of-health-information/.

Robinson, T.N., L. Patrick, T.R. Eng, and D. Gustafson. 1998. An evidence-based approach to interactive health communication: A challenge to medicine in the information age. *Journal of the American Medical Assocation* 280:1264–1269.

Saenz, A. 2009, May 12. Smart toilets: Doctors in your bathroom. http://singularityhub.com/2009/05/12/smart-toilets-doctors-in-your-bathroom/.

Sarakar, U., A. Karter, J. Liu, N. Adler, R. Nguyen, A. Lopez, and D. Schillinger. 2011. Social disparities in internet patient portal use in diabetes: evidence that the digital divide extends beyond access. *JAMIA* 18(3):318–321.

Safeway. 2012. Healthy living. http://www.safeway.com/ShopStores/Wellness-Center.page?#iframetop.

Sharecare. n.d.. http://www.sharecare.com/

Simonds, S.K. 1974. Health education as social policy. *Health Education Monograph* 2:1–25.

Stat My Web. 2012. Webmd.com. http://www.statmyweb.com/site/webmd.com.

Tang, P.C., J. Ash, D.W. Bates, J.M. Overhage, and D.A. Sands. 2006. Personal health records: Definitions, benefits, and strategies for overcoming barriers to adoption. *JAMIA* 13:121–126

Texas Medical Center Library. 2012. Consumer health. http://www.library.tmc.edu/consumerhealth/

Texas State University. n.d. Tools, resources, and rewards for Healthselect participants. http://www.txstate.edu/pdevelop/Services/workshops.

United States Department of Veterans Affairs. 2013. New VA Blue Buttons features for 2013: VA Notes, and CCD and more. http://www.va.gov/bluebutton/.

United States Government Accountability Office Accounting and Information Management Division (GOA). 1996. *Consumer health informatics: Emerging issues.* Washington, DC: US Government.

UnitedHealth Group. n.d. Innovation. http://www.uhginnovation.com/.

Validity. 2012. In Oxford Dictionaries. http://oxforddictionaries.com/definition/english/validity?q=validity.

Walgreens. 2012. Health information. http://www.walgreens.com/health/health_info.jsp?tab=Health+Info.

Walmart. 2012. Health: Healthy living tools. http://health.walmart.com/health-tips/healthy-living-tools/104/?povid=cat1078664-env00000-moduleA050912-lLinkLHN RelatedTopics2HealthResources.

WebMD. n.d. Investor relations. http://investor.shareholder.com/wbmd/faq.cfm.

RESOURCES

Ball, M. J., C. Smith, and R.S. Bakalaar. 2007. Personal health records: Empowering consumers. *Journal of Healthcare Information Management*, 21(1):76-86. http://www.ncbi.nlm.nih.gov/pubmed/17299929

Calabretta, N. 2002. Consumer-driven, patient-centered healthcare in the age of electronic information. *Journal of the Medical Library Association* 90(1):32–37.

Cline, R.J., and K.M. Haynes. 2001. Consumer health information seeking on the Internet: The state of the art. *Health Education Research* 16:671–692

Detmer, D., M. Bloomrosen, B. Raymond, and P. Tang. 2008. Integrated personal health records: Transformative tools for consumer-centric care. *BMC Medical Informatics and Decision Making* 8:45. doi: 10.1186/1472-6947-8-45

Do, N.V., R. Barnhill, K.A. Heermann-Do, K.L. Salman, and R.W. Gimbel. 2011. The military health system's personal health record with Microsoft HealthVault and Google Health. *JAMIA* 18(2):188–124.

Ferguson, T. 1996. *Health Online*. Reading, MA: Addison-Wesley Publishing Company.

Fox, S. 2006. Online search 2006. Pew Internet & American Life Project, October 29, 2006. http://www.pewinternet.org/Reports/2006/Online-Health-Search-2006.aspx

Fox, S. and D. Fallows. 2003. Internet health resources. Pew Internet & Amernican Life Project, 16 July 2003. http://www.pewinternet.org/~/media//Files/Reports/2003/PIP_Health_Report_July_2003.pdf.pdf.

Fox, S., and S. Jones. 2009. The social life of health information. Pew Internet & American Life Project, June 2009. http://www.pewinternet.org/Reports/2009/8-The-Social-Life-of-Health-Information.aspx

Fox, S. and L. Rainie. 2000. The online healthcare revolution: How the web helps Americans take better care of themselves, November 26, 2000. http://www.pewinternet.org/Reports/2000/The-Online-Health-Care-Revolution.aspx

Fricton, J.R. and D. Davies. 2008. Personal health records to improve health information exchange and patient safety. In *Advances in Patient Safety: New Directions and Alternative Approaches: Vol. 4. Technology and Medication Safety*. Series edited by K. Henriksen, J. Battles, M. Keyes, and M. Grady. http://www.ncbi.nlm.nih.gov/books/NBK43760/.

Greenhalgh, T., S. Hinder, K. Stramer, T. Bratan, and J. Russell. 2010. Adoption, non-adoption, and abandonment of a personal electronic health record: case study of HealthSpace. *BMJ*. 341:c5814: doi: 10.1136/bmj.c5814.

Gustafson, D.H., F.M. McTavish, W. Stengle, D. Ballard, E. Jones, K. Julesberg, H. McDowell, G. Landucci, and R. Hawkins. 2005. Reducing the digital divide for low-income women with breast cancer: A feasibility study of a population-based intervention. *Journal Health Communications* 10 (Suppl 1):173-193.

Horan, T.A., N.E. Botts, and R.J. Burkhard. 2010. A multidimensional view of personal health systems for underserved populations. *Journal of Medical Internet Research* 12(3):e32. doi: 10.2196/jmir.1355.

Houston, T.K., B.L. Chang,, S. Brown, and R. Kukafka. 2001. Consumer health informatics: A consensus description and commentary from the American Medical Association Members. *Proceedings of the American Medical Association Symposium 2001*, 269–273.

Impicciatore, P., C. Pandolfini, N. Casella, and M. Bonit. 1997. Reliability of health information for the public on the world wide web: Systematic survey of advice on managing fever in children at home. *BMJ* 314:1875–1881. http://www.ncbi.nlm.nih.gov/pmc/articles/PMC2126984/pdf/9224132.pdf.

Kahn, J.S., J.F. Hilton, T. Van Nunnery, S. Leasure, K.M. Bryant, C.B. Hare, and D.H. Thom. 2010. Personal health records in a public hospital: Experience at the HIV/AIDS clinic at San Francisco General Hospital. *Journal of the American Medical Informatics Association* 17(2):224–228. doi: 10.1197/jamia.M3200corr1.

Ko, H., T. Turner, C. Jones, and C. Hill. 2010. Patient-held medical records for patients with chronic disease: A systematic review. *Quality Safety Health Care* 19(5):e41. doi: 10.1136/qshc.2009.037531.

Lober, W.B., B. Zierler, A. Herbaugh, S.E. Shinstrom, A. Stolyer, E.H. Kim, and Y. Kim. 2006. "Barriers to use of a personal health record by an elderly population." *AMIA 2006 Symposium Proceedings*, 514-515. http://ww.ncbi.nlm.nih.gov/pmc/articles/PMC1839577/pdf/AMIA2006_0514.pdf.

Montelius, E., B. Astrand, B. Hovstadius, and G. Petersson. 2008. Individuals appreciate having their medication record on the web: A survey of attitudes to a national pharmacy register. *Journal of Medical Internet Research* 10(4).e35. doi: 10.2196/jmir.1022.

Pletneva, N., S. Cruchet, M.A. Simmonet, M. Kajiwara, and C. Boyer. 2011. Results of the 10 HON survey on health and medical Internet use. *Stud Health Technol Inform* 169:73–77.

Seidman, J. 2011. The role of health literacy in health information technology. In *Innovations in Health Literacy: Workshop Summary*. Edited by C. Vancheri (Rappoteur), 23–26. Washington, D. C.: The National Academies Press.

Sunderman, C.L. and L. Goodwin. 2008. *Personal Health Records in the Aging U.S. Population: An Analysis of the Benefits and Issues*. Unpublished manuscript. http://www.duke.edu/~cls42/PHR%20and%20the%20Aging%20US%20Population.pdf

Tenforde, M., A. Jain, and J. Hickner. 2011. The value of personal health records for chronic disease management: What do we know? *Family Medicine* 43(5):351–354. http://www.ncbi.nlm.nih.gov/pubmed?term=The%20value%20of%20Personal%20health%20records%20for%20chronic%20disease%20management%3AWhat%20do%20we%20know%3F.

Wagner, P.J., S.M. Howard, D.R. Bentley, Y. Seol, and P. Sodoma. 2010. Incorporating patient perspectives into the personal health record: Implications for care and caring. *Perspectives in Health Information Management* 7:1e. http://www.ncbi.nlm.nih.gov/pmc/articles/PMC2966356/.

Wiljer, D., S. Urowitz, E. Apatu, C. DeLenardo, G. Eysenbach, T. Harth, and K.J. Leonard. 2008. Patient accessible electronic health records: Exploring recommendations for successful implementation strategies. *Journal of Internet Medical Research* 10(4):e34. doi: 10.2196/jmir.1061.

Wiltry, M.J., W.R. Doucette, J.M. Daly,, T.L. Barcedy, and E.A. Chrischilles. 2010.

Family physician perceptions of personal health records. *Perspective in Health Information Management.* 7:1d.

14

Trends and Emerging Technologies

By Sue Biedermann

Learning Objectives

- To consider the continued evolution of the field of health informatics
- To present potential challenges to continued development
- To consider the role of health informatics in the provision of healthcare
- To present the development of health informatics educational programs
- To introduce genomics informatics

KEY TERMS

Accountable Care Organizations (ACOs)
e-health
Genome
Genomics
Health information exchange (HIE)
Meaningful use

Point-of-care testing (POCT)
Predictive modeling
Quality improvement (QI)
Regional Extension Centers
  (RECs)
Seamless care

⊙ Introduction

The exact future of health informatics is unknown, but is generally acknowledged to be bright with many challenges along the way. Federal and state initiatives to expand the use of health information technology (HIT) to provide care and redesign payment policies have provided the impetus such that the question is no longer "When will EHRs become widely implemented?" but rather "Which technologies will be most important?" and "How can HIT be used most effectively?" This chapter will explore some of the emerging trends and technologies.

⊙ Current and Emerging Trends and Terms

In projecting future health informatics trends, a variety of topics can be found in the literature that are currently in their infancy, while there is still only conjecture on when and how others will develop and what effect they might have on the field of healthcare informatics and the provision of healthcare. What follows is a discussion of the current status of health informatics and what is projected for some of the more prevalent and impactful topics.

What seems to be paramount to the identity of health informatics is establishing the domain of knowledge content to define the profession. Standardization of commonly accepted elements of data, languages, and vocabularies will be developed consistent with the identification of knowledge and skills required for the continued development of the field. The standardization of software and hardware is of prime importance, especially when exchanging data between systems.

e-Health is a term that is used more and more frequently. It is ill-defined but consistently used to describe the information available via the Internet to support the provision of healthcare. e-Health is much more comprehensive as found in the following description:

> e-Health is an emerging field in the intersection of medical informatics, public health and business, referring to health services and information delivered or enhanced through the internet and related technologies. In a broader sense, the term characterizes not only a technical development, but also a state-of-mind, a way of thinking, an attitude, and a commitment for networked, global thinking, to improve health care locally, regionally, and worldwide by using information and communication technology (Eysenback 2001).

While the benefits of advances in health informatics are vast and well understood, there continue to be areas of concern. Patient privacy and confidentiality remain a significant challenge with the increased use of technology, exchange of data, and the use of information in new ways for decision making, planning, and policy making. Another issue of concern to many includes the cost-effectiveness of developing and implementing systems. The benefits of fully functional electronic health information systems include improvements in the quality and convenience of patient care, improved accuracy of diagnosis and health outcomes, better care coordination, and increases in efficiencies and cost savings (HHS 2001). Questions remain regarding whether the cost benefit should be a consideration when there are such significant positive benefits for patient care. Consumerism will continue to be a factor as patients and providers become accustomed to having access to more information. It is becoming more of an expectation that decisions be based on appropriate data to promote optimal results in the provision and planning of healthcare and in the strategic planning and policy making for the future.

Redefining the Health Informatics Domain

Information is pervasive throughout healthcare. Along with the technological changes come changes in the way information is used or the informatics of health.

The uses presented here are not meant to be all-inclusive but rather a sampling of the influence the health informatics movement will have on healthcare from the provision of care to continued development of new technologies to the development of policy and supporting a vast research agenda.

Quality Improvement

The incorporation of **quality improvement (QI)** activities has been in existence for quite some time and is integral in the delivery of quality healthcare. QI is a set of activities that measures the quality of a service or product through systems or process evaluation and then implements revised processes that result in better healthcare outcomes for patients, based on standards of care (AHIMA 2012, 348). QI initiatives are required throughout all aspects of the delivery of healthcare and are supported through accreditation guidelines and the development of best practices. Data from health records are a primary source document for the QI function to reflect the outcomes of care that have been provided in the organization. One example of the influence of informatics on QI is the consideration of technology and how it has been utilized in the past to support QI projects. To date, the utilization of information technology for QI has been as a tool for problem identification, data collection, data analysis, as well as overall project management. One prevailing thought is the recognition that IT can be utilized as more than a tool and suggests a future where improvement in health IT can be the result of the QI process. Specifically, the QI process would result in a technological-related outcome, a method of improvement in the management and use of information that is created to address an identified specific problem to improve care (Bates et al. 2011, 87–88). Examples of the kinds of information technology that are envisioned are alert devices that will provide forewarning as a problem is developing in a patient, addressing the issue of medication errors with more sophisticated utilization of communication tools such as bar codes at the point of care, pumps that communicate wirelessly with the electronic health record (EHR), and other means of communication between providers of care who recognize the issue and the importance of the information needed. Another tool that is expected to be more widely used in the future is **predictive modeling**, where multiple data points are analyzed utilizing sophisticated software programs to identify the one characteristic that cause a problem or provides the solution.

Another use of health informatics related to the quality of patient care is **point-of-care testing (POCT)**. POCT is where the diagnostic tests are performed at or near where the patient care is taking place. This is done primarily for the convenience and support of the patient but also improves the timeliness in performing the test and receiving the results and should result in higher quality data. While the advantages of POCT include efficient use of resources and increased benefits to the patient, there continue to be challenges of assuring point-of-care quality as well as compliance with regulatory guidelines. Improved device design with quality control checks and documentation requirements incorporated will, when available, aid in addressing some of the challenges. Data management systems that eliminated the need for manual data entry would significantly improve the data that is captured and the information that results from it.

Public Health

The need for good, comprehensive health data is imperative for the provision of care, starting with data for research to identify the need for public health programs, assessing the quality of programs, and monitoring outcomes. A lack of appropriate information can mean that insufficient data is available for the correct conclusions to be drawn regarding health needs for regions, countries, and the world. **Health information exchanges (HIEs)** are organizations that support, oversee, or govern the exchange of health-related information among organizations according to nationally recognized standards (AHIMA 2012, 193). HIE organizations can play a key role in public health by being responsible for oversight of the information. As the HIE efforts continue, policies and systems to support the data needs of public health will continue to evolve. One specific example of the role of informatics in public health is the development of optimal IT-supported surveillance systems for cancer care and management. Some of the common obstacles in the development of these systems are the required changes in culture, the required financial investment, and the logistical planning for such a system (Shortliffe and Sondik 2006, 861–869) The role of health informatics is to support HIEs so that the data can be transformed into information that can then build our public health knowledge base.

Regional Extension Centers (RECs)

The **Regional Extension Centers (RECs)** were created to provide support to physicians in the selection and subsequent implementation of EHRs. Based on the agricultural extension center model, the support for the creation of RECs came from funding from the Health Information Technology for Economic and Clinical Act (HITECH Act). Another function of the RECs was to assure that systems implemented would support the **meaningful use** of EHRs. The meaningful use of information with the appropriate use of the electronic systems supports the expected outcome of an improvement in the quality of care provided, as well as promoting efficiencies in care delivery. Over time there will be improved clinical and administrative data that will "produce the care coordination, benchmark outcomes, and cost-efficiency that current care systems have yet to complete" (Cykert and Lefebvre 2011, 237). The RECs are a significant first step in the healthcare industry learning to use health information and HIT effectively and efficiently.

Accountable Care Organizations (ACOs)

A commonly accepted definition of an **Accountable Care Organization (ACO)** is an organization of healthcare providers accountable for the quality, cost, and overall care of Medicare beneficiaries who are assigned and enrolled in the traditional fee-for-service program (AHIMA 2012, 9). ACOs are a payment reform model responsible for not only providing care in instances of illness and injury but also offering potential to improve quality and promote health and wellness while eliminating waste and improving efficiencies. To be able to do this, those involved with such an organization must have complete patient health information and truly understand the care and services they provide. Often this understanding can only be obtained with data collection and analysis supported by coordinated information technology initiatives. Interoperability and a seamless flow of information are a key issue for the ACO to meet its objectives.

Seamless Care or Care Coordination

While a specific definition of **seamless care** or coordinated care is difficult to find, words used in an attempt to explain and define it include consistent, coherent, logical, without discontinuities or disparities, and of uniform quality (Hammond 2010, 3–13). One common thought emerging in most discussions of health informatics systems to support seamless care is that much of the information needed is the same data required in direct patient care. The redesign of systems is necessary to make systems more patient-centric where all health data about a patient is aggregated to form a single EHR for the individual patient. Our current system for maintaining patient information, even when EHR systems are utilized, fails to support continuity of care due to multiple providers, lack of interoperability between systems, lack of standards for systems, and lack of standardized definitions and terminologies. All are issues that directly impact the optimal utilization of health informatics.

Development of Goals and Strategies

All of the uses discussed here are instrumental to the quality and efficiency of the care provided. Biomedical informatics can be considered to be "a key enabler both for addressing availability, access, quality, and cost, and also for supporting the work of health policy, finance, and management experts" (Greens 2009, 21). While undertaking change at this level is significant and very complex, tactical strategies must focus on the expected outcomes of various health informatics initiatives. These outcomes include the identification of best practices, having reliable standardized data available where it can be accessed and used, as well as the increased use of technology for maintaining data repositories and for clinical practice. Other factors that are very important for development of systems of the future include policy development and engagement of individuals across the continuum. Organizational goals, usually set with an eye on the future, should drive the IT strategies pursued to ensure success. A discussion of goals and strategies can become quite complex when contemplating the future and the desired transformative outcomes. The health informatics revolution has taken hold with recognized benefits but also multiple challenges and issues that will continue to be encountered. Significant advances have been made, research continues, and support is evident. The evolution will continue at an exponential rate and health informatics will continue to be a field in transition for many years.

Check Your Understanding 14.1

Instructions: Choose the best answer.

1. As the field of health informatics advances areas of concern continue to be related to
   a. Patient privacy and confidentiality
   b. Use of information in new ways for planning and policy making
   c. Cost-effectiveness
   d. All of the above

2. e-Health is
   a. A patient portal for patients to access their information
   b. The relationship of internet and technology to the provision of care
   c. Synonymous with the EHR
   d. Exchange of data from one provider to another

3. Which one of the following is an example of POCT?
   a. A patient taken to the x-ray department with the report then available in the EHR system
   b. Previous x-ray reports from other facilities sent to the hospital to be scanned and available in the patient's EHR at the time of admission
   c. Portable x-ray equipment taken to the patient's room where the x-ray is taken, with a report later available in the patient's EHR
   d. Patient referred to an outpatient radiology center to have an x-ray done at their convenience

4. The organization created to support physicians with their implementation of the EHR:
   a. Regional Extension Centers
   b. Accountable Care Organizations
   c. Health information exchanges
   d. AMIA (American Health Informatics Association)

5. Accountable care organizations
   a. Support healthcare reform and implementation of the EHR
   b. Offer care that is consistent and of uniform quality
   c. Are a group providing care at the instance of illness and injury
   d. Are a group of providers with the responsibility for improving health status, efficiencies of care, and experiences for a defined population

⊙ Education

Educational programs for health informatics have been in existence for a number of years although the curriculum varies among programs and continues to change as advancements occur in the field of health informatics. While the definitions of biomedical, clinical, nursing, and healthcare informatics, among others, continue to be debated, what the field should become is of more significance. The interests and expertise of those instrumental in program development and the curriculum necessary to prepare for the needs of the workforce as it evolves will be critical with the increased use of information and technology for the improvement of health and healthcare.

Assessment of the curriculum of degree programs has been conducted in a variety of ways in an attempt to define and ultimately provide a foundation of support for further discussion and definition of professional competencies. As was presented in Chapter 1, the definitions of health informatics, healthcare informatics, biomedical informatics, and such continue to be considered and efforts will no doubt remain in an attempt to develop and achieve consensus of such a wide and varied domain. Biomedical and health informatics has been purported to be "the most comprehensive term for all fields concerned with the optimal use of information, often aided by the use of technology to improve individual health, healthcare, public health, and biomedical research" (Hersh 2009, 9–24). Studies have been conducted to compare the curriculums of a variety of programs across the United States and to compare courses within these curricula. One extensive study was conducted at the University of North Carolina. The study included a review of courses in a variety of programs and a comparison of programs in public health, and nursing, health, medical, and biomedical informatics (Kampov-Polevoi and Hemminger 2011, 195–202). This study was successful at identifying common courses or content areas across the domains of biomedical and health informatics. The more common content areas seen across most all of the programs identified as some kind of informatics program include the computer science core, and courses related to statistics and research methods, management, and topics covering the legal, ethical, and social issues that reflect the interaction of informatics with society (Kampov-Polevoi and Hemminger 2011, 195–202). A cursory review was done of current information obtained from websites of programs currently in existence throughout the United States. The curricula and focus of these programs are as varied and diverse as the definitions used to identify the field. The majority of the degrees reviewed were at the master's and PhD level. The specific names of the programs varied with the most common found to be Health Informatics, Health Care Informatics, Medical Informatics, Medical Information Sciences, Bioinformatics, and Nursing Informatics. All of these programs were found to be fairly consistent with the more common content areas noted above, but there were unique differences that provided identity and focus to each individual program. A few of these areas that distinguished one program from another included such things as coursework that focused on applications of new technology, incorporation of biomedical informatics courses with medical school courses, policy development, incorporation of engineering with the study of biomedical informatics, advanced practice for nursing leadership, and policy development. While this is just a small sampling of the master's and PhD programs for health informatics currently in place, one can readily see that formal education programs are being developed to contribute to this continuously evolving field in a variety of ways, all using information and technology to support the delivery and advancement of quality and efficient healthcare.

The Commission on Health Informatics and Information Management Education (CAHIIM) has developed standards for the purpose of accrediting health informatics degree programs at the master's level. The CAHIIM curriculum map for the health informatics master's degree is comprised of four facets of health informatics. These facets with the curricular components are outlined in table 14.1.

Since these accreditation standards were developed by CAHIIM, it is apparent that the emphasis has been placed on the information and the associated data and information systems.

Table 14.1　CAHIIM curriculum map for health informatics master's degree

Health Informatics Master's Degree Curriculum Facets	Curricular Components
Facet I. Information Systems—concerned with such issues as information systems analysis, design, implementation, and management	1. Healthcare delivery systems, organization, governance, and workflow 2. Health information systems characteristics, strengths, and limitations 3. Health information systems assessment methods and tools 4. Quality assessment including total quality management, data quality, and identification of best practices for health information systems 5. Health IT standards 6. Use of healthcare terminologies, vocabularies, and classifications systems 7. Health information exchanges (HIEs) 8. EHRs and personal health records 9. Patient rights and associated regulations 10. Privacy and confidentiality of patient health information 11. Information security practices 12. Management of information systems including life cycle analysis, system design, planning methods, and tools 13. Evidence-based systems and tools (such as *PubMed, UpToDate*) 14. Workflow process reengineering 15. Human factor engineering, work organization, and tools 16. Strategic planning 17. Project planning and management 18. Change management 19. Finance and budgeting and cost-benefit analysis for information systems 20. Assessment of commercial vendor products and software applications 21. Policy development and documentation 22. Personnel management, negotiation, communication skills, leadership, and governance. 23. Systems thinking and theory

Health Informatics Master's Degree Curriculum Facets	Curricular Components
Facet II. Informatics—concerned with such issues as the structure, function, and transfer of information, sociotechnical aspects of health computing, and human-computer interaction.	1. History of health informatics development and health informatics literature 2. Medical decision making: principles, design, implementation 3. Development of healthcare terminologies, vocabularies, and ontologies 4. Clinical data standards theory and development 5. Clinical data and clinical process modeling (such as UML [Unified Modeling Language], UP [Unified Process]) 6. Cognitive support (that is, clinical decision support) 7. Biomedical simulations 8. Personalized medicine 9. Human-computer interface 10. Principles of health information systems data storage design, including patient-centered information 11. Principles of research and clinical literature research 12. Natural language processing 13. Knowledge discovery (such as text and data mining)
Facet III. Information Technology—concerned with such issues as computer networks, database and systems administration, security, and programming.	1. Principles of computer science 2. Programming language(s) (such as SQL, JAVA) 3. Software applications—design, development, use 4. Systems testing and evaluation 5. System integration tools 6. Networking principles, methods, design 7. Principles of data representation 8. Electronic data exchange 9. Health information technology: systems architecture, database design, data warehousing 10. Technical security applications and issues 11. Information technology (IT) system documentation 12. Business continuity and disaster recovery 13. Virtual network applications and storage (such as cloud computing)
Facet IV. Additional desired course(s) content.	Biomedical sciences (such as medical terminology, anatomy, physiology, pathophysiology) Quantitative, qualitative, and mixed methods Epidemiology (public health or clinical)

Source: CAHIIM 2013.

There are a number of healthcare informatics programs in the United States that have been developed independent of the CAHIIM accreditation guidelines. These programs tend to be developed to meet a specific need in the workforce or to meet the interests and expertise of the faculty. The majority of these degree programs are at the master's and doctoral level in biomedical or clinical informatics. In addition to meeting a particular workforce need, other critical goals of the educational programs are to promote research in the healthcare informatics domain to validate the profession and define the body of knowledge, develop best practices, and find new applications in healthcare for the potential outcomes related to the intersection of information and technology.

◉ Genomics Information

Genomics is a branch of biotechnology concerned with the genetic mapping and DNA sequencing of sets of genes or the complete genomes of selected organisms. Advanced technology high-speed methods are used to organize the results in databases. The data can then be used to support medical and biological studies and developments (Merriam-Webster 2013). A **genome** is all the genetic information present in a given organism. One can readily surmise from these definitions that the foundations of health informatics and genomics are very closely related when taking into consideration the definition of health informatics. Health informatics is "the interdisciplinary study of the design, development, adoption, and application of IT-based innovations in healthcare services delivery, management and planning" (Procter 2009).

Genomics seeks to determine the entire DNA sequence of organisms. Initially genomic studies were done for sequencing and mapping of the genes and storing the data to learn more about the roles and functions of individual genes. Today, new studies for genomics include learning the pattern of genes under certain conditions. This is known as functional genomics. The possibilities for genomics are still just being discovered, but findings in the area of molecular medicine reveal that the outcomes could include improved means of diagnosing conditions, learning an individual genetic predisposition for certain conditions, and pharmacogenomics, or personalized medicine, which is the ability to customize drugs based on the genetic makeup of the individual. The primary disadvantages related to genetic information are the misuse of the information and misunderstanding of what the tests do and do not mean. Misuse of the data could constitute discrimination based on a potential medical condition, or inability to get insurance due to a genetic predisposition. Misuse or simple misunderstanding could be a potential parent attempting to use genetic information to determine characteristics their children will inherit. Other misunderstandings can occur when consumers do not understand the interaction between genes. For example, a woman with breast cancer in her family may be genetically tested, while overlooking other types of cancers. There is still a lot for everyone to learn related to genomic medicine.

The issue of the confidential nature of the genetic information was addressed in the Genetic Information Nondiscrimination Act of 2008 (GINA). This act in general prohibits health plans from discriminating against covered individuals based on genetic information. The HIPAA Privacy Rule was amended to reflect that genetic information is health information. All aspects of developing, maintaining, and utilizing health information systems must consider genetic information that may be included in a patient's health record. Policies and procedures and system functionality must assure that this information is protected consistent with GINA.

A discussion of health informatics and genomics would not be complete without including information on the Human Genome Project, a 13-year project coordinated by the US Department of Energy and the National Institutes of Health that was completed in 2003. Although coordinated by the entity listed above, a major partner was the Wellcome Trust (United Kingdom) with contributions from the countries of Japan, France, Germany, China, and others. The goals of the Human Genome Project were to

- Identify all the approximately 20,000 to 25,000 genes in human DNA
- Determine the sequences of the 3 billion chemical base pairs that make up human DNA
- Store this information in databases
- Improve tools for data analysis
- Transfer related technologies to the private sector
- Address the ethical, legal, and social issues that may arise from the project (US Department of Energy Genome Programs 2012).

The initial stages related to the goals listed are finished. The data that has been gathered during the course of the project will continue to be analyzed over time. The outcomes and benefits will continue to be realized for many years and in many forms. Involving the private sector with technology licensing and the availability of grant funding made available for research projects has already been initiated. Much of the current biotechnology industry developments and new medical applications have been a result of the outcomes of the study.

What might the future hold for health genomics as data analysis and technological advances continue? At this time, the postgenomics era (referring to the time following the completion of the Human Genome Project) is going from interest for biologists to interest for clinicians as they try to develop new treatments. The biologists study one gene at a time, monogenic diseases, tedious genotyping, the DNA level, focus on sequences and structures. They are interested in decoding the genomes and characteristics or diseases resulting from the different combinations as a separate topic. The clinical interest, involving studying hundreds or thousands of genes simultaneously, complex diseases, high throughput genetic profiling (DNA arrays), DNA, RNA, and proteins, focuses on functional and comparative studies where health informatics includes the clinical plus genetic aspects (Martin-Sanchez et al. 2002, 25–30). The challenge will be the continued integration of the genetics aspect through all levels of information, technology, and standardization as well as the potential legal issues that permeate health informatics. There will be a continued need for a trained workforce to support these efforts, which is complicated further by the speed with which the understanding of genomics is occurring. The biomedical focus of genomics sets the foundation for an almost limitless amount of research. An outcome of this movement might result in the concept of genomic medicine.

Check Your Understanding 14.2

Matching: Match the correct term with the definition.

    a. Genomics
    b. Genome
    c. Human Genome project

    1. _____ All the genetic information present in an organism.

    2. _____ Began with the identification of the human genes and led to the development of tools for data analysis.

    3. _____ Involves genetic mapping and using the applications of the resulting data in medicine or biology.

Instructions: Answer the following questions on a separate piece of paper.

    4. What are the common content areas found in most informatics educational programs?

    5. Why is research related to health informatics needed as this profession evolves?

⊙ Summary

From the beginning of this text on the foundations of healthcare informatics through the managing of information and legal issues to this final section on trends and emerging technologies, one can see that this is a field in a significant and rapid state of transition. There is no one reason for this evolution but rather the convergence of a multitude of forces. The technology has evolved to the point of providing capabilities to support numerous clinical, administrative, and research needs. Legislation and governmental initiatives are providing the impetus to move forward with the rapid deployment of the EHR, requiring the meaningful use of information, and HIE. The emphasis on the quality of care and consumerism are also forces affecting the transition taking place with the use of information and technology in the delivery of healthcare. As evidenced in current literature, the use of healthcare informatics principles, observable and measurable results, benefits, and any unintended consequences continue to be identified and reported. Even though results of this movement in healthcare are apparent, the definition of health informatics continues to be debated and the educational domains established. Great strides have been made and the healthcare informatics field continues to evolve at a fairly rapid pace, providing a fundamental change in the delivery of healthcare as well as in the expectations of the providers and consumers alike.

REFERENCES

AHIMA. 2012. *Pocket Glossary for Health Information Management and Technology.* 3rd ed. Chicago, IL: AHIMA Press.

Bates D., D. Classen, K. Joynt, J. Lanning, and L. Van Horn. 2011. IT: More than a tool for quality improvement. *Hospital Peer Review* 36(8):87–88.

Commission on the Accreditation of Health Informatics and Information Management Education. 2013. Curriculum Map and Findings—Health Informatics Master's Degree. http://www.ahima.org/schools/FacResources/CurriculumMapHI_2010.pdf.

Cykert, S. and A. Lefebvre. 2011. Regional extension coordinators: Use of practice support and electronic health records to improve quality and efficiency. *North Carolina Medical Journal* (72)3:237–239.

Department of Health and Human Services (HHS). 2013. www.health.it.gov.

Eysenback, G. 2001. What is e-Health? *Journal of Medical Internet Research* (3)2:e20.

Figlioli, K. 2011. The transformative role of healthcare IT in accountable care. *Healthcare Financial Management* 65(7):116, 118.

Greens, R. 2009. Informatics and a health care strategy for the future–general directions. *Strategy for the Future of Health.* Edited by R. Bushko. Amsterdam, Netherlands: IOS Press. doi:10.3233/978-1-60750-00-6-21.

Hammond, W. 2010. Seamless care: What is it, what is its value; what does it require; when might we get it? In *Seamless Care-Safe Care.* Edited by B. Blobel, E.P. Hvannberg, and V. Gunnarsdottir. Amsterdam, Netherlands: IOS Press. Doi:10.3233/978-1-60750-563-1-3.

Hersh W. 2009. A stimulus to define informatics and health information technology. *BMC Medical Informatics and Decision Making* 9:24.

Kampov-Polevoi J, and B.M. Hemminger. 2011. A curricula-based comparison of biomedical and health informatics programs in the USA. *Journal of the American Medical Informatics Association* 18(2):195–202.

Martin-Sanchez F, V. Maoho, and G. Lopez-Campos. 2002. Integrating genomics into health information systems. *Methods of Information in Medicine* 41(1):25–30.

Merriam-Webster. 2013. Definition of Genomics. Retrieved from http://www.merriam-webster.com/dictionary/genomics.

Procter, R. 2009. (Editor, Health Informatics Journal, Edinburgh, United Kingdom). Definition of health informatics [Internet]. Message to: Virginia Van Horne (Content Manager, HSR Information Central, Bethesda, MD).

Shortliffe E. and E. Sondik. 2006. The public health informatics infrastructure: Anticipating its role in cancer. *Cancer Causes Control* 17(7):861–869.

US Department of Energy Genome Programs. 2012. Human Genome Project Information. http://www.ornl.gov/sci/techresources/Human_Genome/home.shtml.

RESOURCES

Bushko, R. 2009. *Strategy for the Future of Health: Goal Formation and ITicine.* IOS Press. doi: 10.3233/978-1-60750-050-6-3.

Lewandrowski, K., K. Gregory, and D. Macmillan. 2011. Assuring quality in point-of-care testing: Evolution of technologies, informatics, and program management. *Archives of Pathology & Laboratory Medicine* 135(11):1405–14.

Muller R.M. and K. Chung. 2006. Current issues in health care informatics. *Journal of Medical Systems* 30(1):1–2.

Plescia, M. and J. Engel. 2008. Into the future: Public health data needs in a changing state. *North Carolina Medical Journal* 69(2):167–9.

Wyatt J.C. and F. Sullivan 2005. eHealth, and the future: Promise or peril? *British Medical Journal* 331(7529):1391–3.

Appendix A: Study Report and Request Form

There are many factors to be considered when a client or customer asks for health data. For the analyst to gather, analyze, and report the data correctly, it is essential to understand the "who, what, where, when, and why" of the request.

One of the first questions typically asked of the requester is "What questions are you trying to answer or what do you specifically want to know?"

Understanding the question is not only essential to providing accurate and correct information but also helpful in determining the project's scope.

Although the following questions are not necessarily a complete list, getting the answers to them will help you determine how complex a project is and should provide you with enough information to pull the correct data.

1. **Which patients are to be studied?**
   a. **Time Period:** calendar year (CY), federal fiscal year (FFY)
      Examples: Jan–Dec = CY Oct03–Sep04 = FFY04
   b. **Patient Type:**
      Examples: inpatient, outpatient
      If outpatient, specify which settings are to be included: hospice, home health, hospital outpatient, physician office, freestanding ambulatory surgery center, independent laboratory
   c. **Type of Service:**
      Examples: physician, supplier, facility
      Exclude/include: independent laboratories, freestanding ambulatory care facilities, and so on. Exclude/include: nurses, chiropractors, physician assistants, psychologists
   d. **Age of Population:**
      Examples: children, working adults (that is, age 18–65), seniors (65+)
   e. **Financial Class:** Medicare only, commercial insurance only (Blue Cross and Blue Shield, Aetna, WellPoint, and so on), all payers
   f. **Data Criteria to be *included* in the study:**
      1. DRG—Diagnosis Related Group; APC—Ambulatory Patient Classification
      2. Diagnosis or procedure: principal, secondary
      3. Drug: specific route or age stratification
   g. **Data Criteria to be *excluded* from the study:**
   h. **Be clear in the use of AND and OR**
      Must two or three things all be true to qualify a patient for the study (a and b and c), or can any one of them be true (a or b or c)?
   i. **Are there subsets of patients who need to be considered?**

2. **What does the requester want to know about these patients?**
   a. Interest in counts of visits, patients, admissions, procedures?
   b. Is there a need for comparisons or trending of patient groups, time periods, or procedures?
   c. Are column and row labels needed (that is, percentage, average, counts)?
   d. Where is the cutoff for reporting—at least 5 percent?
   e. Is there a need for trimming of outliers—yes or no?
   f. Is there a need for a number of separate reports?
   g. What are the summarization levels?
      - Three-digit versus five-digit code levels
      - Group breakouts, roll-ups

3. **In what format does the requester want to see the information? (example criteria shown)**
   a. Output: hard-copy report, electronic media, both
   b. File format: Excel, Access, PDF, text file, graphic layout (chart, graph, or table)

4. **What are the requester's timeline or turnaround requirements?**

5. **What is the requester's price range or budget, if known?**

Appendix B: The RFP Process for EHR Systems

Note: This Practice Brief originally appeared in the March 2012 edition of the Journal of AHIMA by June Bronnert, RHIA, CCS, CCS-P, Michelle Dougherty, MA, RHIA, CHP, Crystal Kallem, RHIA, CPHQ.

Implementing an electronic health record (EHR) requires substantial time and money for healthcare providers of all sizes and types. Product selection is a time-intensive step that requires appropriate attention. Organizations must dedicate sufficient time and resources to evaluate their goals, information needs, functional requirements, and pending regulatory requirements in advance of reviewing available EHR products and services. This advanced planning will start the organization down the road to a successful vendor selection process.

This practice brief guides organizations through the selection process, assisting providers as they issue requests for information or requests for proposal for EHRs or component systems. It is to be used in conjunction with the RFI/RFP Template in Appendix C.

RFI versus RFP: What's the Difference?

A request for information (RFI) is often used to solicit information from vendors about their products and services. It is a fact-finding process, often used as the first step in narrowing down the field of vendors when considering future purchases (AHIMA 2011).

Most vendors have marketing materials that can provide in-depth information regarding their products. For some organizations, this packet of materials, along with a profile of the company, its history and services, standard agreements, and a cover letter, may be a sufficient response to an RFI. In other instances, an RFI may include more information focused on the specific areas of organizational need as it relates to product functionality.

The RFI is a valuable tool in assessing how existing products and services within an organization measure up to current vendor product offerings. Technology changes rapidly, and managers need to know if there are more efficient and cost-effective solutions that meet their organizations' needs. Sending an RFI to vendors is an effective way to stay current and an excellent starting point for the more formal selection process.

Unlike an RFI, a request for proposal (RFP) is a formal request sent to a vendor or group of vendors for specific responses as to how their company, products, and services can meet the organization's unique requirements. It generally includes a complete summary of related costs (hardware, software) and services (support, training, implementation, and consulting).

An RFP can become the basis for a contract, which forms a legal obligation between two parties. In this case, the two parties are the vendor and the solicitor (AHIMA 2011). For this reason, both the vendor and the solicitor should carefully consider the phrasing of the questions and corresponding responses. For instance, in seeking an EHR, the solicitor should request specific information about how the product will support the functionality needed by the healthcare organization.

This additional attention to detail usually necessitates a significant resource and time commitment and frequently involves legal counsel. Organizations should consider forming a selection committee consisting of key stakeholders and end users as a first step in preparing the RFP.

Identifying Prospective Vendors

An important initial step in the selection process is identifying and including all appropriate vendors. It can be costly to learn later that one or more key vendors were missed. To prevent this situation, there are a variety of resources to help identify the vendors that should be included in the initial list for the RFI or RFP process, including

- Lists of certified EHR products
- Published EHR software vendor guides
- Peer-to-peer reviews or suggestions
- Internet searches, including vendor websites
- Professional organizations and user groups

Likewise, it does not make sense to invest time and resources in preparing an RFP for vendors that do not identify themselves as having the needed products and services. If an organization clearly states its objectives in the RFI, it should be clear which vendors are appropriate for an RFP.

Not all vendors will be interested in submitting a response to an RFI or RFP because of costs or suitability. As a first step, organizations can ask prospective vendors to indicate their intent to participate in the response process. Typically, this can be done quickly through an e-mail or letter of intent to bid. In this step, the organization may also include its requirements for completion and delivery of the proposal, including format requirements and the contact within the soliciting organization for clarification regarding the submitted documents.

Developing and Disseminating an RFP

One of the very first steps in preparing an RFP is identifying and selecting a proposal committee composed of key stakeholders. This committee should be as inclusive as possible and include, at a minimum, a physician champion and representatives from the departments that will be using or be affected by the EHR system—for example, health information management (HIM), information technology (IT), clinical staff (for example, nursing, radiology, and so on), medical staff, compliance, privacy and security officer, legal counsel, accounting, and purchasing.

The next step, once the team is assembled, is preparing a description of the organization's priorities and functional and technical requirements. These will be identified from a current and future state workflow analysis that should have been performed before RFP development. Consideration should be given to the scope of the project by identifying any specific needs such as possible master patient index cleanup, data conversions from existing systems, modifications to current hardware and software and interfaces, regulatory requirements affecting system changes (for example, ICD-10-CM/PCS, meaningful use incentive requirements, MDS 3.0, RUGs IV), customizations done in-house, and any expected nonstandard use of the system. The identified priorities and functional requirements will become the line items to be included in the RFP.

The scope document can also be used as a sign-off document for the involved departments to ensure that demonstrated products are evaluated based on the functionality requested in the RFP, not the additional features or add-on modules that may be presented at the time of demonstration. In addition, the team should gather basic data about the organization that the vendor will need, such as facility size, current infrastructure and technology, estimated budget, timelines, strategic goals, contact information, and other pertinent data.

The Value of HIM Involvement in the RFP Process

An EHR project is often initiated and managed as an IT project. Although technology is an important component, it frequently represents the least challenging element of the implementation. Ensuring HIM workflow and external regulatory and compliance requirements are adequately addressed in the EHR cannot be completed without strong HIM leadership. The AHIMA Body of Knowledge contains a wealth of resources aimed at guiding professionals and organizations through the EHR selection and implementation process.

Because of their knowledge of accreditation and regulatory content requirements, privacy and security functionality, and principles for a legal record, HIM professionals' involvement in the RFP development process and the evaluation of vendor responses is invaluable. Any clinical application that will be part of the organization's official health record must include HIM in the assessment to evaluate records management and evidentiary support functionality and ensure the application meets the business and legal needs of the organization.

RFP Proposal Formats

A simple letter of inquiry is not a sufficient or practical method for requesting a proposal. Typically, an RFP is prepared in one of two formats or a combination: a checklist or a short answer response format.

In the checklist response format, a table is usually provided with a column designated for the question or requested feature. Adjoining columns may have titles such as Yes/No, Available/Not Available, Included/Add-on, and Future Feature/ Not a Future Feature. Responses may have a numerical value associated with them (for example, a yes response may rank higher than a no response). The vendor responds to the question or feature by indicating whether the feature or service is available and if it is included in the price of the bid.

The checklist response format provides a way for the vendor to quickly respond and for the solicitor to quickly determine whether or not the requested features are available in the bid. A limitation of this format is that it might not provide enough space for vendor clarification of the selected option associated with the functional requirement. This limitation can be overcome through the use of the narrative, short answer format.

The narrative response format is written in paragraphs, providing vendors with greater opportunity to explain in detail the products and services offered and how those products and services will best meet the needs of the organization. One inherent problem with this format is that it limits the reviewer's ability to conduct a side-by-side comparison of multiple vendor responses. In addition, narrative responses may result in vague or cryptic responses, potentially hindering the solicitor's abilities to draw conclusions from the functional system requirements.

To help ensure the optimal amount of important information is gathered while minimizing the amount of reading and reviewing, organizations often develop an RFI in a checklist response format to screen for critical functionality. Based on the RFI results, a list of prospective vendors can generally be narrowed to a select few. After this step, organizations send RFPs to a smaller list of vendors and use the short answer response format, incorporating and expanding knowledge gained through the RFI process.

Another option is to combine both the checklist and narrative formats into a single RFP. A checklist section accommodates questions that can be answered easily with a yes or no response, leaving more detailed responses for the narrative section.

Regardless of the format used, responses to the RFI or RFP often include a cover letter, an executive summary, marketing collateral, and other supporting documentation that may be helpful during the decision-making process. Organizations can also request that the proposal include these items along with the responses to the proposal format.

EHR Functional Requirement Specifications

Compiling a complete list of EHR functional requirements can be challenging. In addition to conducting a complete workflow analysis that identifies requirements specific to the organization, the proposal committee should leverage the Health Level Seven (HL7) EHR System Functional Model (EHR-S FM) and Records Management and Evidentiary Support Functional Profile to identify industry-recognized EHR requirements. The functional model is based on two axes: functions and care settings. The functional axis is a hierarchy of the essential, desirable, and optional EHR functions across all care settings, with functions organized into care setting and infrastructure categories.

Several care domains have developed accompanying profiles that define how to use each function and identify the functions specific to that domain, such as Child Health, Behavioral Health, and Long-Term Care profiles. A comprehensive list of functional profiles is available in the HL7 Functional Profile Registry, sponsored by the National Institute of Standards and Technology.

Health IT Certification

The Health Information Technology for Economic and Clinical Health (HITECH) Act, enacted on February 17, 2009, amended the Public Health Service Act

(PHSA), providing the Office of the National Coordinator for Health Information Technology (ONC) with the authority to establish a certification program for the voluntary certification of health IT. The act specifies that the "National Coordinator, in consultation with the Director of the National Institute of Standards and Technology, shall keep or recognize a program or programs for the voluntary certification of health information technology as being in compliance with applicable certification criteria adopted under this subtitle" (that is, certification criteria adopted by the HHS secretary under section 3004 of the PHSA). The certification program(s) must also "include, as appropriate, testing of the technology in accordance with section 13201(b) of the [HITECH] Act" (HHS 2010).

With the multitude of vendors to consider, a good way to limit your list is to narrow your pool of vendors to those whose EHRs have been certified by an authorized certification body. Monitor ONC's Standards and Certification website for additional information on the new health IT certification program, certification criteria, and recognized certification authorities.

Certification status provides purchasers with an assurance that the product is able to address critical components of meaningful use. However, certification criteria should be assessed in combination with key functional requirements to ensure your organization's critical goals and objectives are addressed.

Importance of the RFP Process

Carefully preparing an RFP by clearly articulating the organization's needs and evaluating vendor responses can eliminate significant cost and risk to the organization. Organizations following the proper steps during the proposal process may reap the following benefits:

- Conserve time and resources by avoiding poorly phrased questions that result in unclear or vague responses
- Give adequate consideration to stakeholder and end user needs
- Ensure products and services include required features
- Assist in defining project scope
- Advance more fully integrated products and services
- Promote efficiency, safety, and quality in patient care
- Ensure products and services meet anticipated organizational growth
- Ensure products and services address existing and impending regulatory requirements
- Serve as an objective source for documentation supporting the inclusion or exclusion of vendors, if necessary

Vendor Selection

After a workable listing of facility background data and vendor requirements is completed, the next step is narrowing the vendor pool. Some healthcare consortia offer purchasing agreements or have vendors they prefer based on performance. A search of professional journals and organizations can provide additional information. In researching vendors, factors other than software functionality must be considered. Key considerations include

- Financial stability, reputation, and history (for example, longevity)
- Ability to provide a list of current customers and references
- Percentage of research and development reinvested into the company
- Life cycle state or maturity of EHR system products (that is, the occurrence of software obsolescence)
- Frequency of software product updates
- Customer support availability
- Certification status

All of these factors can aid in selecting vendors with staying power. The proposal committee may identify additional factors as well.

Once a set of vendors is identified, the RFI/RFP template can be used as a starting point for developing a customized proposal request. A finalized RFP can be assembled by taking the basic sections outlined in the RFP template and incorporating the facility data and requirements previously gathered. After the team has signed off on the final draft, the RFP is ready for submission to the vendors identified.

Before submitting the RFP, determine the name and contact information of the person within the company to whom the RFP should be sent. A cover letter should establish expectations such as a response deadline, response format, the name and contact information of one person to whom all questions concerning the RFP should be directed and to whom the RFP should be returned, and any other specifics that require emphasis. Any questions and responses should be shared with all prospective vendors in accordance to the established RFP timeline. If the deadline is extended for one vendor, the organization should consider granting the same extension to all vendors. Granting deadline extensions can be problematic, so the proposal committee should establish a policy for extensions before disseminating the RFPs. If a vendor fails to respond to the RFP, that vendor should no longer be considered.

One person on the selection team should be assigned to lead the compilation of vendor responses so they can be reviewed and compared side by side. The lead may compile the vendor responses on his or her own or divide the work among several team members by using a standard evaluation tool. The evaluation tool should include a column for comments to document positive or negative notes related to each line item. Any functional requirements not met should be highlighted so they are obvious at review. The team may also consider incorporating weighted scoring of requirements that are critical to the organization's goals and priorities.

Organizations should contact references provided by the vendor in the RFP response and make notes in the comments column. When all data are collected, the selection committee should meet to review the entire report and document all responses. Important high-level concepts to be considered include use of technical standards that support interoperability, ICD-10-CM/PCS and Version 5010 readiness, vendor stability, certification status, and how well the RFP requirements are addressed. Look at overall cost as well, including hidden support fees, implementation fees, and any costs associated with data conversion.

The RFP is a tool to rank and evaluate vendors, but it may not be adequate for final vendor selection. The committee should evaluate the proposals to narrow the list of vendors. The selected group of vendors should then be invited for presentations and demonstrations to provide additional learning and evaluation opportunities about their products. Before final vendor selection, their installed sites should be visited to view the product in use and assess overall user satisfaction.

REFERENCES

AHIMA. 2011. *Pocket Glossary: Health Information Management and Technology*. Chicago: AHIMA Press.

Department of Health and Human Services. 2010. Proposed Establishment of Certification Programs for Health Information Technology; Proposed Rule. *Federal Register* 75(46):11327–11373. http://edocket.access.gpo.gov/2010/2010-4991.htm.

RESOURCES

AHIMA e-HIM Work Group: Guidelines for EHR Documentation Practice. 2007. Guidelines for EHR documentation to prevent fraud. *Journal of AHIMA* 78(1): 65–68.

AHIMA. 2012. Amendments in the Electronic Health Record Toolkit. http://library.ahima.org/xpedio/groups/secure/documents/ahima/bok1_049731.pdf.

AHIMA. 2012. Copy Functionality Toolkit. http://library.ahima.org/xpedio/groups/secure/documents/ahima/bok1_049706.pdf.

AHIMA. 2012. 10 security domains (updated). *Journal of AHIMA* 83(5):48–52.

AHIMA. ICD-10-CM/PCS. www.ahima.org/icd10/default.aspx.

AHIMA. 2012. Managing copy functionality and information integrity in the EHR. *Journal of AHIMA* 83(3):47–49.

AHIMA. Managing the Transition from Paper to EHRs. (Updated November 2010).

AHIMA. Meaningful Use White Paper Series. http://journal.ahima.org/category/arra/arra-white-papers/.

Amatayakul, M.K. 2007. *Electronic Health Records: A Practical Guide for Professionals and Organizations*, 3rd ed. Chicago: AHIMA. (4th edition was published in 2009)

Carpenter, J. Practice Brief: Writing an Effective Request for Proposal (RFP). July/August 1998. Available online in the AHIMA Body of Knowledge.

Certification Commission for Health Information Technology. www.cchit.org.

Dougherty, M. 2007. Linking anti-fraud and legal EHR functions. *Journal of AHIMA* 78(3):60–61.

Hagland, M. 2005. Leading from the middle. *Journal of AHIMA* 76(5):34–37.

McClendon, K. 2006. Purchasing strategies for EHR systems. *Journal of AHIMA* 77(5):64A–D.

McClendon, K. and M. Lowe. 2011. *The Legal Health Record*, 2nd ed. Chicago: AHIMA Press.

Mon, D.T. 2010. Model EHR: Status and next steps for an international standard on EHR system requirements. *Journal of AHIMA* 81(3):34–37.

National Institute of Standards and Technology (NIST) Health IT Standards and Testing Meaningful Use Test Methods Overview. http://healthcare.nist.gov/use_testing/index.html.

Office of the National Coordinator for Health Information Technology. Standards and Certification. http://healthit.hhs.gov/portal/server.pt?open=512&ob jID=1153&parentname=CommunityPage&parentid=13&mode=2&in_hi_ userid=10741&cached=true.

Quinsey, C.A. 2007. Foundational concepts of the legal EHR. *Journal of AHIMA* 78(1): 56–57.

Quinsey, C.A. 2006. Using HL7 standards to evaluate an EHR. *Journal of AHIMA* 77(4):64A–C.

Swanfeldt, M. 2006. Is it legal? 10 questions about legal functionality to include in your RFP. *Journal of AHIMA* 77(5):60.

ACKNOWLEDGMENTS

Jill Clark, MBA, RHIA

Angela Dinh, MHA, RHIA, CHPS

Colleen Goethals, MS, RHIA, FAHIMA

Julie Hatch, RHIT, CCS

Joy Kuhl, MBA, CPF

Mary Stanfill, MBI, RHIA, CCS, CCS-P, FAHIMA

Allison Viola, MBA, RHIA

Diana Warner, MS, RHIA, CHPS

Lydia Washington, MS, RHIA, CPHIMS

Lou Ann Wiedemann, MS, RHIA, CPEHR

Denise Dunyak, MS, RHIA

Karen Fabrizio, RHIA

Susan Fenton, PhD, RHIA

Bill French, MBA, RHIA, CPHQ, CPHIT

Crystal Kallem, RHIA, CPHQ

Jennifer Meinkoth, MBA, RHIA, CHP

Dale Miller

Dawn Osborne, MHS, RHIA

Dawn Penning

Carolyn Valo, MS, RHIT, FAHIMA

Adriana Van der Graaf, MBA, RHIA,
CHP, CCS

Yeva Zeltov, RHIA

Liz Allan, RHIA

Lisa Garven, RHIA, CPC

Teresa M. Hall, MHA, RHIT, CPC,
CAC

Roger Hettinger, CPC, CMC, CCS-P

Lynn Kuehn, MS, RHIA, CCS-P,
FAHIMA

Stephen R. Levinson, MD

Mary Ellen Mahoney, MS, RHIA

Donald T. Mon, PhD

Harry Rhodes, MBA, RHIA, CHPS

Helayne Sweet

Michelle Wieczorek, RN, RHIT,
CPHQ, CPUR

Margaret Williams, AM

Appendix C: RFI/RFP Template

The request for information/request for proposal (RFI/RFP) process is vital to procuring a system that meets organizational and user needs. Because of this, it is imperative that adequate time be allotted for the process.

This template is provided as a sample tool to assist healthcare providers as they issue an RFI or an RFP for electronic health record (EHR) or component systems. It is meant to be used in conjunction with the practice brief titled "The RFP Process for EHR Systems."

Healthcare providers should customize this sample template by using the components that are applicable for their needs, adding components as necessary, and deleting those that are not.

Sections 1 and 2 should be completed by the facility.

1. Introduction (introducing the facility to the vendor)

   a. Brief Description of the Facility

   b. Facility Information

      i. Complete Address

      ii. Market (acute, ambulatory, long-term care, home health)

      iii. Enterprise Information
         The organizations should provide all relevant information including whether the facility is a part of a healthcare delivery system, the facilities that are included in the project, and their locations.

      iv. Size
         The organization should provide any information that will be relevant to the product such as the number of discharges, visits, beds, and so on.

      v. General Description of Current Systems Environment
         The organization should provide general information regarding current information systems structure (that is, hardware and operating systems).

   c. Scope
      The organization should provide a brief narrative description of the project that the RFP covers and the environment sought (for example, phased approach, hybrid support).

2. Statement of Purpose

   a. Overall Business Objectives/Drivers
      The organization should list high-level business goals it is looking to achieve by implementing the software.

b. Key Desired Functionality
When requesting information for the facility-wide solution (for example, EHR), the organization should list the various features and functions of the system desired, as well as any pertinent details.

  i. Clinical Repository

  ii. Clinical Documentation

  iii. Computerized Physician Order Entry (CPOE)

  iv. Ancillary Support (for example, laboratory, radiology, pharmacy)

  v. Picture Archiving Communication System (PACS)

  vi. Electronic Document Management/Document Imaging

  vii. Customizable Workflow Management

  viii. Interoperablity (for example, health information exchange)

  ix. Patient Portals

  x. Other

c. HIM Department Operations
When requesting information for the HIM solution, the organization should list the various processes and functions of the system it is looking for, as well as any pertinent details.

  i. Chart Analysis/Deficiency Management

  ii. Coding/Abstracting

  iii. Patient Identity Management/Electronic Master Patient Index (e-MPI)

  iv. Health Record Output and Disclosure Management

  v. Release of Information

  vi. Screen Input Design

  vii. Support for Mandated Reportable Data Sets

  viii. Other

d. System Administration—Records Management and Evidentiary Support
This functionality is applicable to or used for all components or modules of an application. Facility requirements for this functionality should be specified in the detailed system requirements.

  i. User Administration

  ii. Access Privilege Control Management

  iii. Logging/Auditing Function

  iv. Digital Signature Functions

  v. Records Management Function

  vi. Archiving Functions

       vii. Continuity of Operations (for example, support for backup, recovery)

      viii. Maintenance of Standardized Vocabularies and Code Sets

   e. Future Plans

     General description of long-term plans, including identified future systems environment and projected timetables.

Sections 3 and 4 should be completed by the vendor.

  3. Requirements

     Vendors should provide availability and timelines for development of software to fulfill requirements not available at this time.

   a. User Requirements

    Each functional area is expected to have its own set of user requirements.

    Sample questions related to HIM functional user requirements and features are provided below. *This table is a sample only. Organizations must customize this RFP template to meet their needs.*

Functional User Requirements/ Features*	Available	Custom Developed	Future Development	Not Available
Chart Completion/Deficiency Analysis				
Can the organization define the intervals for aging analysis (e.g., 7-days, 14-days, 21-days)?				
Does the system allow for standard and ad hoc reporting for chart deficiency/ delinquency analysis?				
Can delinquency reports be sent to physicians/ clinicians in electronic (e.g., e-mail or fax) and paper formats (letters)?				
Does the system allow you to define or detail all deficiencies by provider, by area of deficiency, or other combinations (e.g., group practices)?				

(continued)

Functional User Requirements/ Features*	Available	Custom Developed	Future Development	Not Available
Does the system allow the organization to list all records (charts) by the deficiency type?				
Can deficiency analysis be conducted at the time the patient is prepared for discharge from the facility?				
Does the system support most industry standard dictation systems to allow transcribed reports to be easily and efficiently completed?				
Does the system allow for end user notification when information identified as incomplete/missing is completed?				
Coding Completion/Analysis				
Does the system support automation of coding work flow (e.g., computer-assisted coding)?				
Does the system support automated case assignment to work queues?				
Can the user assign cases based on special attributes (e.g., VIP, dollars, or case type such as cancer or trauma)?				

Functional User Requirements/ Features*	Available	Custom Developed	Future Development	Not Available
Does the system support online communication between employees and managers?				
Does the system support most industry standard encoders/ groupers?				
Does the system support both on-site and remote coding activities?				
Does the system support assignment of high-risk coding to supervisory staff or allow coding verification as staff complete cases?				
Does the system contain tools for monitoring and evaluating the coding process?				
Does the system support electronic query capabilities?				
Coding/Transaction Standards (see also section 4.k)				
Does the system support ICD-10-CM and/or ICD-10-PCS in addition to ICD-9-CM?				
Does the system use General Equivalence Mappings (GEMs), such as between ICD-10-CM/ PCS and ICD-9-CM or SNOMED CT and ICD-9-CM?				

(continued)

Functional User Requirements/ Features*	Available	Custom Developed	Future Development	Not Available
Is the system compliant with the Version 5010 transaction standard?				
Health Record Output and Disclosure				
Does the system allow a unified view of all component subsystems of the EHR at the individual patient level and at the date of service encounter level for purposes of disclosure management (including the ability to print and generate electronic output)?				
Does the system provide the ability to define the records or reports that are considered the formal health record for a specified disclosure or disclosure purposes?				
Does the system allow VIP patients to be flagged and listed confidentially on corresponding reports (i.e., census)?				
Does the system produce an accounting of disclosure, reporting at a minimum the date and time a disclosure took place, what was disclosed, to whom, by whom, and the reason for disclosure?				

Functional User Requirements/ Features*	Available	Custom Developed	Future Development	Not Available
Does the system provide the ability to create hard copy and electronic output of report summary information and to generate reports in both chronological and specified record elements order?				
Does the system provide the ability to include patient identifying information on each page of electronically generated reports and provide the ability to customize reports to match mandated formats?				
Does the system allow for redaction and recording the reason, in addition to the ability to redact patient information from larger reports?				
Release of Information (Note: Administrative release of information functionality may or may not be an integral component of an EHR system.)				
Does the system support HIPAA management of non-TPO disclosures?				
Does the system track and report the date/time release of information requests received and fulfilled?				

(*continued*)

Functional User Requirements/ Features*	Available	Custom Developed	Future Development	Not Available
Does the system allow the ability to track whether the release of information consent/ authorization was adequate, in addition to a corresponding disposition?				
Does the system generate invoices with user-defined pay scales?				
Does the system allow tracking of payments received?				
Does the system generate template letters for standard correspondence (e.g., patient not found, date of service not valid)?				
Does the system allow information to be released electronically?				
Authentication				
Does the system authenticate principals (i.e., users, entities, applications, devices) before accessing the system and prevent access to all nonauthenticated principals?				

Functional User Requirements/ Features*	Available	Custom Developed	Future Development	Not Available
Does the system require authentication mechanisms and can the system securely store authentication data/information?				
If user names and passwords are used, does the system require password strength rules that allow for a minimum number of characters and inclusion of alphanumeric complexity, while preventing the reuse of previous passwords, without being transported or viewable in plain text?				
Does the system have the ability to terminate or lock a session after a period of inactivity or after a series of invalid log-in attempts?				
Access Controls				
Does the system provide the ability to create and update sets of access-control permissions granted to principals (i.e., users, entities, applications, devices) based on the user's role and scope of practice?				

(*continued*)

Functional User Requirements/ Features*	Available	Custom Developed	Future Development	Not Available
Does the system inactivate a user and remove the user's privileges without deleting the user's history?				
Does the system have the ability to record and report all authorization actions?				
Does the system allow only authorized users access to confidential information?				
Does the system prevent users with read and/or write privileges from printing or copying/writing to other media?				
Does the system define and enforce system and data access rules for all EHR system resources (at component, application, or user level, either local or remote)?				
Does the system restrict access to patient information based on location (e.g., nursing unit, clinic)?				
Does the system track restrictions?				

Functional User Requirements/ Features*	Available	Custom Developed	Future Development	Not Available
Does the system have the ability to track/audit viewed records without significant effect on system speed?				
Does the system allow for electronic access to specified patients/ encounters for external reviewers?				
Emergency Access Controls				
Does the system allow emergency access regardless of controls or established user levels, within a set time parameter?				
Does the system define the acceptable circumstances in which the user can override the controls for emergency access, as well as require the user to specify the circumstance?				
Does the system require a second level of validation before granting a user emergency access?				
Can a report be generated of all emergency access use?				

(*continued*)

Functional User Requirements/ Features*	Available	Custom Developed	Future Development	Not Available
Does the system provide the ability to periodically review/ renew a user's emergency access privileges?				
Does the system provide the ability to generate an after-action report to trigger follow-up of emergency access use?				
Information Attestation				
Does the system provide the ability for attestation (verification) of EHR content by properly authenticated and authorized users different from the author (e.g., countersignature) as allowed by users' scope of practice, organizational policy, or jurisdictional law?				
If more than one author contributed to the EHR content, does the system provide the ability to associate and maintain all authors/ contributors with their content?				

Functional User Requirements/ Features*	Available	Custom Developed	Future Development	Not Available
If the EHR content was attested to by someone other than the author, does the system maintain all authors and contributors?				
Does the system provide the ability to present (e.g., view, report, display, access) the credentials and the name of the author(s) and the attester, as well as the date and time of attestation?				
Data Retention, Availability, and Destruction				
Does the system provide the ability to store and retrieve health record data and clinical documents for the legally prescribed time or according to organizational policy and to include unaltered inbound data?				
Does the system provide the ability to identify specific EHR data for destruction and allow for the review and confirmation of selected items before destruction occurs?				

(continued)

Functional User Requirements/ Features*	Available	Custom Developed	Future Development	Not Available
Does the system provide the ability to destroy EHR data/ records so that data are not retrievable in a reasonably accessible and usable format according to policy and legal retentions periods, and is a certificate of destruction generated?				
Record Preservation				
Does the system provide the ability to identify records that must be preserved beyond normal retention practices and identify a reason for preserving the record?				
Does the system provide the ability to generate a legal hold notice identifying whom to contact for questions when a user attempts to alter a record on legal hold or an unauthorized user attempts to access a record on legal hold?				
Does the system provide the ability to secure data/records from unauditable alteration or unauthorized use for preservation purposes, such as a legal hold?				

Functional User Requirements/ Features*	Available	Custom Developed	Future Development	Not Available
Does the system provide the ability to merge and unmerge records?				
Does the system allow a record to be locked after a specified time so no more changes may be made?				
Minimum Metadata Set and Audit Capability for Record Actions				
Does the system capture and retain the date, time stamp, and user for every object/data creation, modification, view, deletion, or printing/ export of any part of the medical record?				
Does the system retain a record of the viewer?				
Does the system retain a record of the author of a change?				
Does the system retain a record of the change history?				
Does the system retain a record of the source of nonoriginated data?				
Does the system retain the medical record metadata for the legally prescribed time frame in accordance with the organizational policy?				

(*continued*)

Functional User Requirements/ Features*	Available	Custom Developed	Future Development	Not Available
Does the system include the minimum metadata set for a record exchanged or released?				
Pending State				
Does the system apply a date and time-stamp each time a note is updated (opened/ signature event)?				
Does the system display and notify the author of pending notes?				
Does the system allow the ability to establish a time frame for pending documents before administrative closing?				
Does the system display pending notes in a way that clearly identifies them as pending?				
Does the system allow the author to complete, edit, or delete (if never viewed for patient care) the pending note?				
Amendments and Corrections				
Does the system allow the author to correct, amend, or augment a note or entry?				
Does the system allow the author to indicate whether the change was a correction, amendment, or augmentation?				

Functional User Requirements/ Features*	Available	Custom Developed	Future Development	Not Available
Does the system record and display the date and time stamp of the change?				
Does the system provide a clear indicator of a changed record?				
Does the system provide a link or clear direction to the original entry/note?				
Does the system retain all versions?				
Does the system disseminate updated information to providers that were initially autofaxed?				
Documentation Succession Management and Version Control				
Does the system manage the succession of documents?				
Does the system retain all versions when a change is made?				
Does the system provide an indicator that there are prior versions (when appropriate)?				
Does the system indicate the most recent version?				
Retracted State				
Does the system allow for removing a record or note from view?				

(*continued*)

Functional User Requirements/ Features*	Available	Custom Developed	Future Development	Not Available
Does the system allow for access of a retracted note or record?				
Does the system allow the user to record the reason for retraction?				
Does the system allow for notification of the viewers of the data to present correct information (if applicable)?				
Data Collection and Reporting				
Does the system allow for real-time data collection and progress measurement against preset targets?				
Does the system produce reports on turnaround days, dollars pending, costs per chart by process, days to billing, and so on, as related to AR?				
Does the system have the ability to track clinical decision-making alerts (e.g., when they were added to the system or discontinued, used, ignored)?				
Does the system comply with meaningful use reporting requirements?				

Functional User Requirements/ Features*	Available	Custom Developed	Future Development	Not Available
Patient Financial Support				
Is your proposed solution fully integrated (or able to interface with the patient financial system), offering users an electronic form of the business office?				
Can patient information be placed in folders to easily identify those details that refer to the patient (guarantor) account(s)?				
Can you electronically capture, store, and retrieve computer-generated documents and reports, such as the UB-04 or the CMS 1500, which are HIPAA transaction standard compliant?				
Patient Portals				
Does the system allow for electronic patient access (e.g., Web portal)?				
Health Information Exchange				
Does the system enable participation in local health information exchange initiatives?				

* Also refer to certification requirements and Health Level Seven (HL7) EHR System Functional Model (EHR-S FM) for other key requirements/features.

b. System Requirements
Organizations should provide a list to vendors of what current technology needs to be supported. Vendors should then provide information on their system's available requirements.

Sample questions related to system requirements and features are provided below. This table is a *sample only*. Organizations must customize this RFP template to meet their needs.

System Requirements/ Features*	Available	Custom Developed	Future Development	Not Available
General System Requirements				
Is the system integrated or interfaced?				
Does the system provide the ability to archive via tape, CD, or DVD? Describe any other options.				
Are the COLD (computer output to laser disc) data streams available in ASCII (American Standard Code for Information Interchange)?				
Does the system support audit trails at the folder level for managing access, editing, and printing of documents?				
Does the system make audit trail logs available to the organization, including the date, time, user, and location?				
Does the system support an online help function/ feature?				
Is the proposed solution scalable (e.g., can it support 50 to 800 workstations, concurrent users)?				

System Requirements/ Features*	Available	Custom Developed	Future Development	Not Available
Does the system have the capability of recording change management logs related to platform upgrades and patches?				
Can the system identify or distinguish the facility location in a multi-entity environment?				
Can the system support a centralized database across multiple facilities?				
How compliant is your product with the HL7's EHR-S FM and EHR profiles? (Please provide us with your HL7 EHR-S FM and profile conformance statements.)				
System Security				
Does the system monitor security attempts for those without user rights and those logged in the audit trail/log?				
Does the system track all activity/functions, including where they change the database, and can they be managed through the audit trail/log?				
Does the system use encryption methods that render protected health information unreadable in compliance with the latest industry approaches and guidelines?				

(continued)

System Requirements/ Features*	Available	Custom Developed	Future Development	Not Available
Technical Requirements				
Do communication components include TCP/IP (transmission control protocol/internet protocol)?				
Does the system use CCITT Group III, IV for compression schemes?				
Does the system support standard HL7 record formatting for all input and output?				
Does the system support SQL for communication?				
Does the system support thin client PCs?				
Is the system sized for capacity to allow for planning? Describe your recommendations.				
Does the system support disk shadowing and system redundancy provisions? Please describe.				
Can your solution be supported as an Application Service Provider (ASP) hosted model?				
Does the system support browser-based options?				
Integration of Narrative Notes				
Does the system support HL7's Clinical Document Architecture Release 2				

System Requirements/ Features*	Available	Custom Developed	Future Development	Not Available
(CDA-R2) standard for the encoding of narrative, text-based clinical information?				
Does the system receive, display, transform, and parse CDA-encoded clinical documents as described in the HL7 CDA-R2 Implementation Guides for document types, such as History and Physical Note, Consultation Note, Operative Note, and Diagnostic Imaging Report?				
Does the system receive, display, transform, and parse CDA-R2-compliant documents with encoded headers (Level 1 encoding)?				
Does the system process CDA-R2-compliant documents that include Level 2 encoding?				
Does the system process CDA-R2-compliant documents that include Level 3 encoding?				

* Also refer to certification requirements and Health Level Seven (HL7) EHR System Functional Model (EHR-S FM) for other key requirements/features.

   c. Interfaces

   d. Organizations should provide a list of existing interfaces that will need to be supported, as well as new interfaces that will have to be created and supported, including any pertinent interoperability information that exists and will be needed in the future. Vendors should provide information regarding their system's ability to meet the organization's interface requirements.

4. Vendor Questionnaire
The organization should request information about the vendor and the product to assist with decision making.

a. Vendor Background and Financial Information

i. Company Name and Geography
The organization should request an address of a branch close to the facility, as well as the headquarters. Staff may want to visit both.

ii. Company Goals

iii. Year the Company Was Established, Significant Company Merges, Acquisitions, and Sell-offs

iv. Whether the Vendor Is Public or Privately Owned

v. Bankruptcy/Legal Issues (including under which name the bankruptcy was filed and when, or any pertinent lawsuits, closed or pending, filed against the company.)

vi. Research and Development Investment (expressed in a total amount or percentage of total sales)

vii. Status of Certification

b. Statement of Key Differentiators
The vendor should provide a statement describing what differentiates its products and services from those of its competitors.

c. Customer Base and References

i. Customer List (or total number of customers per feature or function, if a list of customers cannot be provided owing to confidentiality/privacy concerns)

ii. References that Can Be Contacted
The vendor should provide references the facility can contact/visit based on product features and functions most suitable to the facility, as well as those using the latest versions of the software.

d. Qualifications

i. The vendor should provide a list of qualifications and resume, including a sample list of similar projects and clients.

e. User Participation

i. User Groups
Organizations should provide a list of the user groups and ask whether it can attend a meeting or a call for review purposes.

ii. Requirements Gathering
The vendor should request information regarding customer participation in requirements-gathering stages of system

development. How is customer feedback, such as requests for new requirements, handled?

f. Technology
The vendor should provide technology specifications that support the product (for example, database, architecture, operating system, ASP versus in-house).

g. Services
The vendor should describe the services offered and corresponding fees (if applicable).

  i. Project Management

  ii. Consulting

  iii. MPI Cleanup

  iv. Integration

  v. Legal Health Record Definition

  vi. Process Reengineering

  vii. Other

h. Training
The vendor should outline the training provided during and after implementation.

i. Product Documentation
The vendor should specify the product documentation that is available and its formats.

j. Implementation/Migration
The vendor should provide detailed information about the implementation such as the timelines and resources required.

k. Data Conversion

  i. If the system is not currently ICD-10-CM/PCS or Version 5010 compliant, describe plans for becoming compliant by regulatory required dates.

  ii. How will the system handle both ICD-9-CM and ICD-10-CM/PCS data?

  iii. How long will the system support both ICD-9-CM and ICD-10-CM/PCS codes?

  iv. If the system uses General Equivalence Mappings (GEMs), such as between ICD-10-CM/PCS and ICD-9-CM, describe how the integrity of the maps is maintained.

  v. Describe other data conversions (for example, document imaging, platform conversions).

l. Maintenance

    i. Updates/Upgrades
The vendor should provide information on how the system is maintained, including how often the updates/upgrades are applied, methods used (for example, remotely, on site), and by whom.

    ii. Compliance with Meaningful Use Incentive Requirements
The vendor should provide its plan for addressing meaningful use on an ongoing basis, including plans for achieving corresponding certification requirements.

    iii. Expected Product Lifetime
The vendor should outline the expected time frame for the next version requiring a different platform or operating system upgrade

    iv. Customer Support
The vendor should outline the types of customer support packages offered (for example, 24/7, weekday only), methods of support (for example, help desk or tickets), and the tools used (for example, 800 number, e-mail, web-based).

    v. Expected Facility Support
The vendor should outline the number of full-time employees expected to support the product at the facility.

m. Pricing Structure

    i. Product Software Pricing

      1. Price

      2. The vendor should provide the price of the proposed solution, broken down by application/module, including licensing fees.

      3. Cost of Ownership (breakdown over a certain number of proposed contract years)

      4. Other Costs (maintenance, upgrades, consultation and support fees, post-implementation training and services, travel, and so on)

      5. Discounts (available discounts such as those based on participating as a beta site)

    ii. Invoicing (fee schedule and terms)

    iii. Return on Investment

    iv. Acceptance Period

    The vendor should outline the terms for validating the product after implementation and the refund policy

n. Warranty
The organization should request a copy of the warranty, as well as how it is affected by maintenance and support agreements after the implementation period

Sections 5 and 6 are to be completed by the facility.

5. Vendor Requirements and Instructions

a. RFP Questions

The facility should provide the name and contact information of one person to whom all questions concerning the RFP should be directed. Generally, questions about the RFP must be submitted in writing within a given time frame, and the questions and answers are distributed to all vendors responding to the RFP. Provide the preferred method of contact, such as fax number or e-mail.

b. Response Format, Deadline, and Delivery

c. Contract Duration

The facility should request the vendor to disclose how long the returned information will be considered valid.

6. Terms and Conditions

a. Confidentiality

State confidentiality rules in regard to the information the facility disclosed in the RFP as well as the rules pertaining to the information provided by the vendor.

b. Information Access

The facility should describe who will have access to the returned RFP and for what purpose.

c. Bid Evaluation and Negotiation

The facility should briefly describe the evaluation process and the deadlines and provide the appropriate information if vendors are allowed to negotiate after the evaluation is complete.

d. Formal Presentation

The facility should describe process and format requirements if the vendor is invited to present the software product suite.

e. Acceptance or Rejection

The facility should describe how the vendor will be notified regardless of whether the product is selected or not.

f. Contract Provisions

The facility should note the sections of the RFP response that can be included in the final contract.

g. Type of Contract

The facility should let the vendor know if this will be firm fixed price, cost plus fixed fee, a time and materials, or other type of contract.

Chapter 1
Check Your Understanding 1.1

1. The subjective nature of the information and the amount of information.

2. Patient information is used to measure quality and standardization is vital for the information to be reliable for use in making changes to how we deliver healthcare.

3. b

4. a

5. c

Check Your Understanding 1.2

1. Biomedical informatics incorporates methodologies applicable for managing data, information, and knowledge across the translational medicine continuum. Clinical informatics is part of the biomedical continuum but more specifically is the effective use of information for scientific study of patient care, clinical research, and medical education. Nursing informatics at the basic level is using technology to improve patient care with the more advanced level related to conducting research to validate practice and identify means to improve patient care.

2. Biomedical informatics incorporates methodologies applicable to managing data and translational medicine is then taking the scientific knowledge gained to support developing new procedures and modes of treatment to improve care.

3. The systematic application of information and utilization of computer technology to support public health initiatives as related to research, education, and delivery of public health services.

4. The issue of potential discrimination due to knowledge of genetic information.

5. Patient engagement and the increasing adoption of Internet and electronic media to connect providers and patients in new and innovative ways.

Check Your Understanding 1.3

1. Multiple terms that mean the same thing, the subjective nature of much of the clinical documentation, and the large amount of information all make it difficult to establish a standardized vocabulary.

2. b

3. d

4. a

5. c

Check Your Understanding 1.4

1. d

2. b

3. a

4. b

5. Understanding of and the ability to use computers and systems; understanding of the creation, maintenance, use, and storage of health information; recognition of roles and responsibilities of various employees who will be using a system.

Chapter 2
Check Your Understanding 2.1

1. e

2. d

3. b

4. a

5. c

Check Your Understanding 2.2

1. c

2. b

3. d

4. a

5. e

Check Your Understanding 2.3

1. c

2. b

3. c

4. b

5. c

Chapter 3
Check Your Understanding 3.1

1. a

2. c

3. d

4. e

5. c

Check Your Understanding 3.2

1. a

2. c

3. b

4. d

5. a

Check Your Understanding 3.3

1. b

2. a

3. c

4. b

5. d

Chapter 4

Check Your Understanding 4.1

1. b

2. c

3. b

4. a

5. a

Check Your Understanding 4.2

1. b

2. a

3. c

4. d

5. b

Check Your Understanding 4.3

1. c

2. b

3. a

4. d

5. d

Chapter 5
Check Your Understanding 5.1
1. d
2. b
3. c
4. a
5. b
6. c

Check Your Understanding 5.2
1. a
2. d
3. c
4. b
5. h
6. f
7. g
8. e

Check Your Understanding 5.3
1. u
2. s
3. s
4. u
5. s
6. u
7. s
8. u

Check Your Understanding 5.4
1. g
2. f
3. c
4. i
5. e
6. h
7. j
8. b

9. d
10. a
11. T
12. T
13. F

Check Your Understanding 5.5
1. a
2. c
3. v
4. a
5. v
6. a

Check Your Understanding 5.6
1. b
2. a
3. c
4. d

Chapter 6
Check Your Understanding 6.1
1. F
2. F
3. T
4. F
5. c

Check Your Understanding 6.2
1. T
2. F
3. F
4. F
5. e
6. c

Check Your Understanding 6.3
1. F
2. F

3. T
4. T
5. E

Chapter 7
Check Your Understanding 7.1

1. Everything in the model from supportive leadership, effective communication, and a trusting climate to expectations related to quality and productivity standards.

2. Information technology (IT) management and staff, and the manager or lead in release of information. Develop a project management team to lead the operation.

3. Some potential answers: Consider outsourcing some of the requests during the changeover. Work with release of information staff to determine how to avoid backlog.

4. Physician incomplete systems, reimbursement, data analytics.

Check Your Understanding 7.2

1. Answer to consider: Admitting your lack of experience and asking for help from the CEO or the Chief Information Office (CIO).

2. Answer will vary. Depending on your answer to #1, it may include the CIO, or a staff person in IT, or someone in the HIM department that is familiar with previous research done by the department.

3. Answer to consider: ED visits for last few years, patient satisfaction surveys about ED visits, revenue/loss information.

4. Answer to consider: Yes—they may provide insight into some of the ED issues that are not collected in data.

5. Answer to consider: Easily understood visual data such as graphs, figures, charts. Avoid lengthy written interpretations.

6. Answer to consider: IT, HIM, Marketing, healthcare provider, community clinic managers, home healthcare agency representative, public health workers.

7. Answer to consider: Patient survey to home addresses, survey when patients come to the community hospital or community clinics. Home healthcare workers, and public health workers that visit the home, may provide some insight as well. You may also want to contact local Internet services to determine where the black out spots are and work to improve systems.

8. Answer to consider: At a minimum provide patients with information about the portal, and access points in the community, such as a library or at the hospital. Provide patients with a copy of their health records upon discharge from the hospital.

9. Answer to consider: If a patient does not respond to reminders for preventive care, set up an alert to the physician that the patient may not have access. Alternatively, send out letters to patients about health reminders. For quality management, assess improvement of the system in six months.

10. Answer to consider: Ask the marketing department for ideas on this since that is their expertise. Work with the team to develop a patient survey. Within HIM, provide employees with information about informing individual patients about the patient portal. Work with the team to develop instructions for using the portal.

Check Your Understanding 7.3

1. Answer will vary on which criteria is chosen.

2. Answer to consider: You will need to discuss this with the committee as soon as possible. If the committee is not meeting soon, contact the committee chair for advice. Advice from legal counsel of faculty will be needed as well.

3. Answer to consider: You will need to discuss this with the committee as soon as possible. If the committee is not meeting soon, contact the committee chair for advice. The chief medical information officer should be contacted as well.

4. Answer to consider: Yes, since this is a legal and potentially a patient safety issue you need to report it.

5. Answer to consider: Yes, this is a legal issue and needs to be reported.

Chapter 8
Check Your Understanding 8.1

1. e
2. a
3. d
4. c
5. b
6. Providers are concerned about the reliability of the data, as well as the usability of the HIE and the incorporation of it into the workflow. The patients are most concerned about the privacy and security of their data and information.

Check Your Understanding 8.2

1. b
2. a
3. c
4. a

5. b

6. d

Chapter 9
Check Your Understanding 9.1

1. d

2. a

3. c

4. b

5. a

Check Your Understanding 9.2

1. a

2. b

3. T

4. F

5. T

Chapter 10
Check Your Understanding 10.1

1. T

2. F

3. T

4. F

5. F

Check Your Understanding 10.2

1. F

2. F

3. T

4. T

5. F

Check Your Understanding 10.3

1. F

2. T

3. F

4. F

5. T

Chapter 11
Check Your Understanding 11.1
1. c
2. d
3. b
4. a
5. F
6. T

Check Your Understanding 11.2
1. d
2. b
3. d
4. T
5. F
6. F
7. T
8. T

Check Your Understanding 11.3
1. F
2. T
3. F
4. F
5. F
6. F

Chapter 12
Check Your Understanding 12.1
1. F
2. F
3. T
4. F
5. a

Check Your Understanding 12.2
1. F
2. T

   3. F
   4. F
   5. T

Check Your Understanding 12.3

   1. T
   2. F
   3. T
   4. d
   5. a
   6. c
   7. b

Check Your Understanding 12.4

   1. d
   2. a
   3. d
   4. T
   5. F

Check Your Understanding 12.5

   1. e
   2. c
   3. a
   4. d
   5. b
   6. F
   7. F
   8. F
   9. T

Chapter 13

Check Your Understanding 13.1

   1. a
   2. a
   3. d
   4. There is a close correlation between higher incomes and increased use of consumer health informatics.

5. The spread is very important. Smart phones are the vanguard of the move of CHI from computers to other and newer technologies.

6. African Americans, Latinos, adults living with a disability, elderly (over 65 years old), high school or less education, low-income households

7. Food, product, or drug recalls

8. A digital divide is the disadvantage or isolation of those populations without access to the Internet.

9. The use of mobile phones with web-browser functionality.

Check Your Understanding 13.2

1. d

2. The toilet could monitor your weight, calculate your BMI, and monitor blood pressure and glucose.

3. Existing or being everywhere at the same time; constantly encountered and widespread.

4. Answers to consider: The US National Library of Medicine, the Texas Medical Center Library, American Cancer Society, American Diabetes Association, numerous other sites, such as WebMD, pharmacies, grocery stores, and health organizations.

Check Your Understanding 13.3

1. Validity is being logically or factually correct and reliability is being consistently good in quality.

2. It is an organization to help ensure ethical standards for healthcare sites.

3. Yes. HON will conduct a thorough investigation of the site and if the site meets the ethical standards of HON, a HONcode seal is placed on the site.

4. Yes. The reputable sites will have a hyperlink to a policy statement.

5. Yes. Cookies are small bits of data sent from a website. They can be used to track a user's activities and can be a privacy concern.

6. Yes. The Office of the National Coordinator for Health Information Technology (ONC), primarily through the Office of the Chief Privacy Office, is taking steps to meet the challenges of privacy and security issues related to mobile and online health information.

Chapter 14
Check Your Understanding 14.1

1. d

2. b

3. c

4. a

5. d

Check Your Understanding 14.2

1. b

2. c

3. a

4. Computer science core, and courses related to statistics and research methods, management, and legal, ethical, and social issues.

5. To validate the profession and define the body of knowledge, develop best practices, and find new applications in healthcare for the outcomes related to the intersection of information and technology.

Glossary

Access: The right to inspect and obtain a copy of protected health information about the individual in a designated record set, for as long as the protected health information is maintained in the designated record set

Accountable Care Organization (ACO): An organization of healthcare providers accountable for the quality, cost, and overall care of Medicare beneficiaries who are assigned and enrolled in the traditional fee-for-service program

Accounting of disclosures: A listing of all of the disclosures made outside of the entity holding the protected health information

Addressable implementation specifications: Standards under the HIPAA Security Rule that should be implemented unless an organization determines that the specification is not reasonable and appropriate. If this is the case, then the organization must document why it is not reasonable and appropriate and adopt an equivalent measure if it is reasonable and appropriate to do so

Ad hoc standards: Standards established by a group of stakeholders without a formal adoption process

Administrative safeguards: Administrative actions such as policies and procedures and documentation retention to manage the selection, development, implementation, and maintenance of security measures to protect electronic protected health information and manage the conduct of the covered entity's or business associate's workforce in relation to the protection of that information

Administrative Simplification: The category of provisions in Title II of HIPAA, in addition to the HIPAA Privacy, Security, and Enforcement Rules, Title II or the HIPAA Administrative Simplification Rule also includes rules and standards for transactions and code sets, and identifier standards for employers and providers

Aggregated health information exchange (HIE): Combines all of the data into a centralized repository with a MPI or record locator service. The different HIE participants query, or send a request to, the repository to obtain demographic, clinical, or other information

Alert fatigue: A commonly observed condition among physicians overwhelmed with large numbers of clinically insignificant alerts, thus causing them to "tune out" and potentially miss an important drug-drug or drug allergy alert

American National Standards Institute (ANSI): The US representative to the International Organization for Standardization (ISO)

American Recovery and Reinvestment Act (ARRA): An economic stimulus bill created to help the United States recover from the downturn of the economy with a total amount of $787 billion allocated to the recovery

Any and all records: A phrase frequently used by attorneys in the discovery phase of a legal proceeding. Subpoena-based requests containing this phrase may create a situation where the record custodian or provider's legal counsel can work to limit the records disclosed to those defined by a particular healthcare entity's legal health record. Typically, this is only during a subpoena phase, unless the information is legally privileged or similarly protected; the discovery phase of litigation probably can be used to request any and all relevant materials

Application service provider (ASP): A third-party service company that delivers, manages, and remotely hosts standardized applications software via a network through an outsourcing contract based on fixed, monthly usage, or transaction-based pricing

Architectural models: A framework or structure for the flow of data and information within information systems

Audit logging: Refers to metadata kept on each transaction or event that occurs within an EHR system

Authorization: Must be obtained under the HIPAA Privacy Rule for the disclosure of PHI unless the PHI meets an exception stated in the Privacy Rule where an authorization is not required. The authorization must be written in plain language and must contain certain core elements, one of which is a statement that specifies that treatment, payment, enrollment, or eligibility for benefits cannot be denied because an individual declines to sign an authorization

Biomedical informatics: Incorporates a core set of methodologies that are applicable for managing data, information, and knowledge across the translational medicine continuum, from bench biology to clinical care and research to public health

Availability: Under the HIPAA Security Rule, the concept of ensuring electronic protected health information can be accessed as needed by authorized users. Encompassed in the concept of availability are many safeguards such as the data backup and storage specification

Blue Button: A big, virtual button on existing patient portals in order to give patients access to their health information

Breach: The acquisition, access, use, or disclosure of protected health information in a manner not permitted, which compromises the security or privacy of the protected health information

Break the glass: A method that allows users to access data that they may not otherwise be allowed to access. The users are alerted in advance that their actions are being monitored giving them an opportunity to halt their actions, if inappropriate

Broad network access: Any capabilities available over the network can be accessed by a wide variety of interface devices (laptops, smart phones, and so on) using standard mechanisms

Business associate (BA): All entities that are not members of the workforce, but are providing a service or performing a task on behalf of a covered entity with the expectation or possibility that they will have access to protected health information

Business associate agreement (BAA): Clearly documents the requirements of the business associate "to implement administrative, physical, and technical safeguards that reasonably and appropriately protect the confidentiality, integrity, and availability of the PHI that it creates, receives, maintains, or transmits on behalf of the covered entity" (45 C.F.R. § 164.308(b)(1) and 164.314)

Business continuity planning (BCP): Includes the recovery and use of the technology as in disaster recovery planning as well as the ability of the organization to continue the processes required for ongoing business operations. Sometimes requires operational procedures in the absence of information technology

Business impact analysis: A method for evaluating and prioritizing the risks that face a business. The goal of the is to identify any gaps in current recovery capability and to develop a strategy for meeting the identified recovery time and recovery point objectives

Cardinality: Describes the relationship between two data tables by referring to the number of elements in each table of a database

Categorical data: Data elements that represent mutually exclusive categories or labels

Centralized: A system in which the systems processing functions occur on a single computer

Certification: An evaluation performed to establish the extent to which a particular computer system, network design, or application implementation meets a prespecified set of requirements

Certification Commission for Health Information Technology (CCHIT): An industry-wide initiative engaging a diverse group of stakeholders in a voluntary, consensus-based process that began certifying EHRs in 2006

Characteristics of data quality: Part of the Data Quality Management Model from AHIMA. The 10 characteristics are accessibility, accuracy, consistency, comprehensiveness, currency, definition, granularity, relevancy, precision, and timeliness

Chief information officer (CIO): A senior manager responsible for the overall management of information resources in an organization

Chief knowledge officer (CKO): The person who oversees the entire knowledge acquisition, storage, and dissemination process and identifies subject matter experts to help capture and organize the organization's knowledge assets

Chief medical information officer (CMIO): An emerging position, typically a physician with medical informatics training, that provides physician leadership and direction in the deployment of clinical applications in healthcare organizations

Chief nursing informatics officer (CNIO): A position emerging in larger healthcare facilities and organizations. The typical responsibilities in this position are related to the implementation and utilization of HIT systems for clinical care

Civil penalties: Generally fines or money damages used to sanction violators

Classification system: A system that arranges or organizes like or related entities for easy retrieval

Client-server: A network distribution method that involves multiple servers dedicated to different functions with workstations running the application and retrieving data from a server as needed

Clinical analytics: Mining discrete patient healthcare data such as laboratory results, medication, and genetics to make clinical decisions or to aid in translating data for research or further healthcare treatment

Clinical data repository (CDR): A centralized database focused on clinical information that usually contains a controlled medical vocabulary

Clinical data warehouse: Snapshots of a variety of clinical databases found throughout a healthcare organization that are combined for the purpose of reporting and analysis

Clinical decision making: The process of utilizing information to formulate a diagnosis

Clinical decision support (CDS): Software processes and algorithms that use codified information from a patient record and aid in diagnosis and treatment

Clinical decision support system (CDSS): A special subcategory of clinical information systems that is designed to help healthcare providers make knowledge-based clinical decisions

Clinical documentation: The functionality of electronic capture of clinical notes

Clinical informatics: Part of the biomedical continuum. It is focused on information systems to ensure that they support patient care that is safe, efficient, effective, timely, patient-centered, and equitable. Also, the scientific study of patient care, clinical research, and medical education and the effective use of information to support these activities, establish standards, and set policy

Clinical information systems (CIS): Systems designed to facilitate the management of the activities of various clinical departments and to provide electronic charge capture and results reporting

Clinical phenotyping: Determining which observable characteristics are applicable for a given subset of patients

Cloud computing: A model for enabling ubiquitous, convenient, on-demand network access to a shared pool of configurable computing resources (such as networks, servers, storage, applications, and services) that can be rapidly provisioned and released with minimal management effort or service provider interaction

Code set: Any set of codes used to encode data elements, such as tables of terms, medical concepts, medical diagnostic codes, or medical procedure codes. A code set includes the codes and the descriptors of the codes

Cold site: A type of data backup facility. Equipment must be brought in, but the site is powered and secure. This is much less expensive than other options, but could take up to a month to operationalize

Column-delimited data: A flat file database format where information is stored in text files as columns of data. The data must be accompanied by documentation that lists the order and position of the variables so that the data may be interpreted

Comma-separated values (CSV): A flat file database format where fields are delimited by a comma. May include the variable names in the first row. If not, then they require documentation to identify the variables in each position

Community cloud: This cloud is supported for use by a community of users who share a trait, such as security needs, in common. One or more of the community may own and operate the cloud, or it may be operated by a third party or a combination of the two. A healthcare example of a community cloud might be the data infrastructure needed for an accountable care organization or that required by a health information exchange

Comparable and consistent: Data that has been normalized or transformed so that they conform to the designated standards

Computer-aided diagnosis (CAD): The incorporation of computer images with aspects of artificial intelligence to detect and identify potential disease factors

Computer-assisted coding (CAC): Software that extracts and translates transcribed or computer-generated free-text data into diagnosis and procedural codes for billing and coding purposes

Computer-based patient record (CPR): A historical term for an electronic patient record that provides complete and accurate data, alerts, reminders, clinical decision support, links to medical knowledge, and other aids

Computer literate: Having sufficient knowledge and skill to be able to use computers, familiar with the operations of a computer

Computerized provider (physician) order entry (CPOE): Applications that allow providers to write orders for medications or other treatments and transmit them electronically

Computers-on-wheels (COWs): Self-contained rolling carts containing a computer for access to the EHR on each unit

Concept: An idea or unique unit of knowledge or thought created by a unique combination of characteristics

Concept identification: A text processing method that maps the text to standardized concepts using clinical terminologies

Concurrent processes: Processes which run simultaneously and access shared resources such as databases

Confidentiality: A legal and ethical concept that establishes the healthcare provider's responsibility for protecting health records and other personal and private information from unauthorized use or disclosure. In the context of the HIPAA Security Rule, it means that electronic accessible health information is accessible only by authorized people and processes

Consensus standards: Standards are those that are developed through a formal process of comment and feedback by interested stakeholders

Consolidated Health Informatics (CHI): The initiative to adopt existing health information interoperability standards throughout all federal agencies

Consumer: A person who purchases goods and services for personal use

Consumer informatics: The focus is on the interest of the consumer. A goal is to support and inform consumers to facilitate the management and participation in their own care

Continuous data: Numerical data where there is an equal interval between the data points

Cost of ownership: A benefit of cloud computing. Using cloud computing can be more cost effective than maintaining a server onsite. Additional savings may be realized by reducing the number of employees and contractors needed for server maintenance, legacy system conversions, and upgrades

Covered entity (CE): A healthcare provider, health plan, or healthcare clearinghouse that transmits health information in electronic form in connection with healthcare transactions

Criminal penalties: A fine or imprisonment, whether suspended or not

Crosstabs: Serve to highlight any errors where there is an expected or explicit relationship between two data elements

C-suite: Executive management, such as the chief operating officer (COO), chief information officer (CIO), and so on

Data: Disparate components of information including dates, numbers, images, symbols, letters, and words that represent basic facts and observations about people, processes, measurements, and conditions

Data analytics: Use of statistical analysis of data to make business decisions

Data cleaning: Sometimes termed data scrubbing, this involves examining the data thoroughly to detect wrong or inconsistent data

Data dictionary: A tool that provides metadata or information about data

Data flow diagram: A method to map out a data model; it maps out the database's boundary and scope

Data governance: Making decisions and exercising authority for data-related matters; establishing a culture where quality data is obtained and valued to drive the business

Data-interchange standards: Establish the means by which a sender transmits or communicates data or information to a receiver (also known as transaction standards)

Data liquidity: The ubiquitous sharing of healthcare data and information

Data mapping: The process of associating concepts or terms from one coding system to concepts or terms in another coding system and defining their equivalence in accordance with a documented rationale and a given purpose

Data mining: Involves searching, analyzing, and summarizing large data sets from different perspectives to identify trends and other useful information

Data model: A representation of the data to be stored in a database and the relationships between the tables and data fields

Data Quality Management Model: A model presented by AHIMA covering the different processes of data handling during which data quality should be addressed. The data handling processes are categorized as application, collection, warehousing, and analysis

Data set standards: Established to assist in the tracking and understanding of important events such as births, deaths, hospital discharges, and so on. Such standards establish the data elements or data variables to be collected and define each data element

Data standards: Standards may be related to the data set, such as the data elements specified for the Uniform Hospital Discharge Data Set, or the allowable data values, such as a selection list being provided for the address data element of State. Standards such as the allowable data elements within a data set, the definitions of the different data elements, or the allowable data values, which constrain the data that can be entered into a field, ensure that the data is as accurate as possible

Data table: Grouping of data organized with records or rows and fields or columns

Database: A collection of data tables

Database management system (DBMS): A system installed locally on each machine that is designed to keep track of data locations and coordinate data modifications; creates and maintains a database. Provides a method for adding or deleting data and also supports methods to extract data for reporting

Decentralized: A system in which the processing functions are split or distributed, among one or more machines in the network system

Decision analysis: A systematic approach to decision making under conditions of imperfect knowledge; a practical application of probability theory that is used to calculate the optimal strategy from among a series of alternative strategies

Decision support database: A common example of a clinical data warehouse. These databases are found in many healthcare entities and may include claims data, financial data, and quality data combined in one database to support both internal and external reporting

Decision support systems (DSS): A computer-based system that gathers data from a variety of sources and assists in providing structure to the data by using various analytical models and visual tools in order to facilitate and improve the ultimate outcome in decision-making tasks associated with nonroutine and nonrepetitive problems

De facto standards: Standards that have evolved over time to become universally used without a government or other mandate

Deidentified health information: Health information that neither identifies nor provides a reasonable basis to identify an individual

Dependability: A benefit of cloud computing. They are up and running 24 hours a day, 7 days a week, every day of the year, which ensures access to much needed items such as business applications, financial data, and help desk personnel

Descriptive statistics: Also known as summary statistics, this is a category of methods for describing and summarizing the features of a collection of data, including frequencies, mean, mode, range, and standard deviation

Designated Record Set: A group of records maintained by or for a covered entity that is (1) the medical records and billing records about individuals maintained by or for a covered health care provider; (2) the enrollment, payment, claims adjudication, and case or medical management record systems maintained by or for a health plan; or (3) used, in whole or in part, by or for the covered entity to make decisions about individuals

Diagram 0: A data flow diagram expanding on the context diagram and adds details regarding the data tables and their relationships

Digital Imaging Communication in Medicine (DICOM): A standard that promotes a digital image communications format and picture archive and communications systems for use with digital images

Digital immigrant: An individual who lived before the advent of the digital age but has adapted more or less to the digital age

Digital native: A person who has only known a world of digital toys and tools

Disaster recovery planning (DRP): Defines the resources, actions, tasks, and data required to manage the business recovery process in the event of a physical disaster

Disclosure: The output and release upon request of appropriate health record documents

Discrete data: Data elements that represent mutually exclusive categories or labels

Distributed system: A collection of independent computers connected through a network and managed by system software that enables the computers to coordinate their activities and to share system resources such that the users perceive the system as a single, integrated system

Document and data nonrepudiation: Characteristics that defend against charges questioning the integrity of data or documents. They delineate the methods by which the data are maintained in an accurate form after their creation, free of unauthorized changes, modifications, updates, or similar changes

E-discovery: The process of discovering what parts of the patient's records may be used for litigation or further legal proceedings. It is an opportunity for opposing counsel to obtain relevant information. It is named to reflect an emphasis on electronic records; however paper–electronic hybrids may also be included

E-health: An emerging field at the intersection of medical informatics, public health, and business, referring to health services and information delivered or enhanced through the Internet and related technologies

eHealth literacy: The ability to seek, find, understand, and appraise health information from electronic sources and apply the knowledge gained to addressing or solving a health problem

Electronic media: (1) Electronic storage material on which data is or may be recorded electronically, including, for example, devices in computers (hard drives) and any removable or transportable digital memory medium, such as magnetic tape or disk, optical disk, or digital memory card; (2) transmission media used to exchange information already in electronic storage media. Transmission media include, for example, the Internet, extranet or intranet, leased lines, dial-up lines, private networks, and the physical movement of removable or transportable electronic storage media

Electronic medical record (EMR): An electronic record of health-related information on an individual that can be created, gathered, managed, and consulted by authorized clinicians and staff within a single healthcare organization

Electronic medication administration records (eMAR): Use of technology and bar coding to track medications from when ordered to when given to the patient

Electronic patient portals: Provide access to personal health information from a patient's healthcare organization. These portals provide patients with opportunities to view results of exams and treatment, and also provide alerts for preventive care

Electronic protected health information (ePHI): Individually identifiable health information that is transmitted by electronic media or maintained in electronic media

Encryption: The process of transforming text into an unintelligible string of characters that can be transmitted via communications media with a high degree of security and then decrypted when it reaches a secure destination

Entity-relationship diagram (ERD): Displays the relationship between tables in a relational database

Episode of care: The specific instance of a condition or illness with a defined time frame with the beginning and ending times of care identified

E-prescribing: Allows practitioners to use electronic devices to write and submit prescription orders directly to a participating pharmacy rather than faxing or providing the patient with a written prescription that must then be taken to the pharmacy

Equivalence: In a data mapping, determined by the distribution of map relationships for a given map

Evidence-based medicine: The use of the current best evidence in making clinical decisions about the care of individual patients by integrating individual clinical expertise with the best available clinical evidence from systematic research

Expressivity: How well a note conveys the patient's and provider's impressions, reasoning, and thought process; level of concern; and uncertainty to those subsequently reviewing the note

Fault tolerant: Systems that are highly available and remain in operation even when hardware, software, or network failures occur

Federal Rules of Civil Procedure (FRCP): The guidelines that govern the procedures for civil trials

Federal Rules of Evidence (FRE): Governs what and how electronic records may be used and the roles of record custodianship for purposes of evidence in a trial

Federated health information exchange (HIE): Designed as provider-to-provider networks using the Internet for connectivity, with no central repository of data. A central entity maintains the master patient index or record locator service, which is used to determine where patients have been treated previously and where their health information might exist

Field: Data elements representing attributes of the information being collected

File Server: A distribution method where the system runs entirely on the end user's workstation and transfers entire files

Firewall: Monitors and controls all communication in to and out of an intranet. It is implemented by a set of processes that act as a gateway to a network applying the organizational security policy

Flat file: A text file, usually delimited by a comma or tab, with one record found on each row. It has only one table of data

Foreign key: A variable in one table that is a primary key in another table

Forward maps: Those that map from an older source code or data set to a newer target code or data set

Frequency: The number of times that a particular observation or value occurs in a dataset

Functionality: An aspect of an EHR that should be evaluated. It addresses the features of the EHR product, including patient encounter documentation, automating and facilitating office workflow, decision support during patient encounters, and reporting that supports care management and template customization

Future-proofing: A benefit of cloud computing. Computer hardware, software, and networking solutions begin their move toward obsolescence almost as soon as they are implemented, which can be costly. Cloud computing moves the cost of updating certain parts of the technology from the customer to the cloud provider, a substantial benefit given the rapid pace of the growth of Internet and other technologies

Genetic Information Nondiscrimination Act of 2008 (GINA): This law provides the legal standard to be followed for the collection, use, and disclosure of genetic information

Genome: All the genetic information present in a given organism

Genomics: A branch of biotechnology concerned with the genetic mapping and DNA sequencing of sets of genes or the complete genomes of selected organisms

Government mandate: Standards that are specified or established by the government for certain purposes

Health: The state of being free from illness or injury

Health informatics: The field of information science concerned with the management of all aspects of health data and information through the application of computers and computer technologies

Health Information and Management Systems Society (HIMSS): A cause-based not-for-profit organization exclusively focused on providing global leadership for the optimal use of IT and management systems for the betterment of healthcare. The HIMSS mission is to lead healthcare transformation through the effective use of health information technology

Health information exchange (HIE): As a noun HIE refers to an organization that supports, oversees, or governs the exchange of health-related information among organizations according to nationally recognized standards. As a verb health information exchange refers to the actual exchange of health information electronically between providers and others with the same level of interoperability, such as labs and pharmacies

Health information system (HIS): A set of components and procedures organized with the objective of generating information that improve healthcare management decisions at all levels of the health system

Health information technology (HIT): The technical aspects of processing health data and records including classification and coding, abstracting, registry development, and storage

Health Information Technology for Economic and Clinical Health (HITECH) Act: One part of ARRA. Designated funding to modernize the healthcare system by promoting and expanding the adoption of health information technology. HITECH provided $20 billion in Medicare and Medicaid incentive payments to physicians and hospitals for meaningful use of EHRs and $2.6 billion to support ONC initiatives

Health Insurance Portability and Accountability Act (HIPAA): Legislation that addresses standards for transactions and code sets for electronic exchange of health-related information to perform billing or administrative functions; standards for terminologies related to medications including the Food and Drug Administration's names and codes for ingredients, manufactured dosage forms, drug products, and medication packages; and additional standards for privacy and security of patient information

Health IT Standards Committee: An official federal advisory committee established by the Health Information Technology for Economic and Clinical Health (HITECH) Act enacted as part of the American Recovery and Reinvestment Act (ARRA) of 2009. The committee makes recommendations to the National Coordinator for Health IT on standards, implementation specifications, and certification criteria for the electronic exchange and use of health information

Health Level 7 (HL7): An international organization of healthcare professionals dedicated to creating standards for the exchange, management, and integration of electronic information

Health literacy: The degree to which individuals have the capacity to obtain, process, and understand basic health information and services needed to make appropriate health decisions

Health plan: An individual or group plan that provides, or pays the cost of, medical care

Healthcare clearinghouse: A public or private entity, including a billing service, repricing company, community health management information system, or community health information system, and value-added networks and switches, that do either of the following functions: (1) processes or facilitates the processing of health information received from another entity in a nonstandard format or containing nonstandard data content into standard data elements or a standard transaction; (2) receives a standard transaction from another entity and processes or facilitates the processing of health information into nonstandard format or nonstandard data content for the receiving entity

Healthcare Common Procedure Coding System (HCPCS): Consists of two levels or systems. Level I is CPT, a large, well-curated catalog of clinical and surgical procedures maintained by the American Medical Association as a proprietary and copyrighted resource. Level II of the HCPCS is maintained by CMS. CMS creates and administers the Level II HCPCS codes as alphanumeric identifiers for products, supplies, and services not included in CPT

Healthcare provider: Any person or organization who furnishes, bills, or is paid for healthcare in the normal course of business

HIPAA Enforcement Rule: 45 CFR 160, subparts C, D, and E. This Rule spells out the authority of the Office for Civil Rights (OCR) related to the enforcement of the HIPAA Privacy and Security Rules

HIT Policy Committee: A federal advisory committee established under the HITECH Act

Hot site: A type of data backup facility for critical applications and operations, which can be online within hours. This option is the most expensive

Human Gene Nomenclature (HUGN): A system for exchanging information regarding the role of genes in biomedical research in the federal health sector

Hybrid cloud: This consists of two totally separate cloud infrastructures (private, community, or public) that are unique, but share standardized or proprietary technology facilitating data and application portability

Hybrid (health) record: A type of patient record that is maintained in both paper and electronic formats. It may be part of a mixture of paper and electronic or multiple electronic systems that do not communicate or are not logically architected for record management

Imaging informatics: Synonymous with radiology informatics or medical imaging informatics, it utilizes the radiology information gathered from individual patients to enhance patient care by finding ways to efficiently and reliably use the collected data

Imputation: A process that uses special statistical methods to provide missing values in data records. Imputation methods must be described fully and imputed values clearly labeled

Informatics: Using technology to acquire, manage, maintain, and use information as a basis for the plethora of decisions that must be made in a cost-effective manner. Also, the study of collecting, organizing, storing, and using electronic information

Information infrastructure: Processing, tools, and technologies to support the creation, use, transport, and storage of information

Infrastructure as a service (IaaS): This is the most minimal level of cloud computing where the infrastructure is provided, but the consumer controls the operating systems, storage, and applications. The consumer may also have control over networking components such as the firewall

Institute of Medicine (IOM): An independent, nonprofit organization that works outside of government to provide unbiased and authoritative advice to decision makers and the public

Integrated: Designed to bring together multiple information systems, and allow them to communicate in a timely and effective manner and work together as one system

Integrity: Under the HIPAA Security Rule, this means that electronic protected health information is not altered or destroyed in an unauthorized manner

Interfaces: Hardware or software that enable disparate CIS and HIS software systems to communicate with each other

International Classification of Functioning and Disability (ICF): Classification of health and health-related domains that describe the body functions and structures, activities, and participation

International Organization for Standardization (ISO): A worldwide, nongovernmental, internationally recognized standards development body

Interoperability: Standards that allow different health information systems to work together within and across organizational boundaries in order to advance the effective delivery of healthcare for individuals and communities

Interval data: A category of continuous data that do not have a true zero and can have negative numbers. An example of interval data is temperature, which can be negative or positive

Join: Combine data from two or more tables in a database

Knowledge management (KM): The process of capturing and disseminating information so it can be used for decisions at multiple levels of an organization

Laboratory information system (LIS): A system that provides a hub to integrate laboratory information, including orders with results; there may be user access to the information. Other functionality includes scheduling, billing, and other information needed by the lab; rarely is all of this information integrated with an EHR

Legal health records: A concept created to describe the data, documents, reports, and information that comprise the formal business record(s) of any healthcare organization that are to be utilized during legal proceedings

Legal hold: A legal concept that requires special, tracked handling of patient records to ensure no changes can be made to a record involved in litigation. Common in the paper record environment to substantiate the integrity of the record, this is less common in the electronic environment where audit logs are the standard

Linearization: A subset of the ICD-11 foundation component, that is fit for a particular purpose (reporting mortality, morbidity, or other uses); jointly exhaustive of the ICD universe (foundation component); composed of entities that are mutually exclusive of each other; and each entity is given a single parent

Litigation response: Typically the term used to describe the processes and procedures invoked if the potential for lawsuits or litigation is detected. It is a set of procedures that, when instituted, protects the relevant records. Litigation response is not only triggered by atypical record disclosure requests but by any sign or action that shows a potential for a lawsuit

Logical Observation Identifiers Names and Codes (LOINC): A dictionary of laboratory codes and clinical test descriptors, originated by Regenstreif Institute and funded by federal support grants as a public resource for the common good. It is publicly usable without any fees or license

Legacy data: Existing data, some of which are on paper, and some of which may already be digital. Whatever the current format, they must be converted to a format that is compatible with the new product or system

Limited data set: Protected health information from which certain specified direct identifiers of individuals and their relatives, household members, and employers have been removed

Local area network (LAN): A network that connects various devices together via communications within a small geographic area such as a single organization

Meaningful use: The use of a certified EHR in a meaningful manner such as for e-prescribing; clinical decision support; maintenance of a problem list of current and active diagnoses; the exchange of health information; and the submission of quality or other measures. This is evaluated as part of the EHR Incentive Program of CMS

Meaningful use of information: Using systems with certified software to enhance the use of data obtained from health records

Measured service: Use of resources in the cloud can be monitored, controlled, and reported, allowing for better management

Medical identity theft: The assumption of a person's name and sometimes other parts of his or her identity—such as insurance information or Social Security Number—without the victim's knowledge or consent to obtain medical services or goods, or when someone uses the person's identity to obtain money by falsifying claims for medical services and falsifying medical records to support those claims

Medical informatics: Both the information and data parts as well as the controlling and automatic nature of data processing itself

Medical scribe: A medical student, nurse practitioner, or physician's assistant who assists the physician with the required documentation in the patient's medical record

Metadata: Data that provides information about another piece of data. Essentially, data about data

Method: A piece of information stored about an object in an object-oriented database. It describes how to use the stored data

Middleware: A bridge between two applications or the software equivalent of an interface

Minimum necessary: Requires covered entities to evaluate their practices and enhance safeguards as needed to limit unnecessary or inappropriate access to and disclosure of protected health information

Mobility: A benefit of cloud computing. Data streaming from the clouds allows for greater mobility because the Internet is accessible from multiple mobile devices, such as smart phones and tablets, PDAs, virtual desktops, or traditional laptops or PCs

Morbidity: Diseases or conditions for which patients seek treatment

Mortality: The cause of death on death certificates. Mortality data are used to present the characteristics of those dying, determine life expectancy, and compare mortality trends with other countries

Narrative-text string: A type of search are similar to the find functionality used every day in programs such as Microsoft Word or Adobe Reader

National Drug File–Reference Terminology (NDF-RT): A data set created by the Veterans Administration for specific drug classifications

National Institute of Standards and Techonology (NIST): An agency of the US Department of Commerce, founded in 1901 as the nation's first federal physical science research laboratory

Natural language processing (NLP): A technology that converts human language (structured or unstructured) into data that can be translated then manipulated by computer systems

Negation: An issue with the widespread use of NLP in the real-time clinical domain. Negation involves the ability of the processor to detect the differences between "no chest pain," meaning it is absent, and "chest pain," meaning it is present

No-consent: A model for HIE that does not require any agreement on the part of the patient to participate in an HIE. HIEs that have adopted this model operate in states that explicitly allow this model via legislation

Nominal data: Those data where the categories are simply names. For example, a data element often collected for healthcare consumers is gender

Notice of Privacy Practices (NPP): An essential document regarding an individual's right to receive adequate notice of how a covered entity may use and disclose his or her PHI. The notice also must describe the individual's rights and the covered entity's legal duties with respect to that information

Numeric (computational) literacy: The ability to calculate or reason numerically. An example of the need for this can be found in an understanding of body-mass index calculations or if drug dosing may call for calculations

Nursing informatics: Where the practice of nursing intersects with computers and information science. At the basic level it is using technology to improve patient care. The more advanced level is with the nurse scholar conducting research to validate practice and identify means of improving nursing practice to achieve enhanced outcomes and greater patient satisfaction

Object-oriented databases: Designed to handle data types beyond text and numbers. An object-oriented database stores two types of information about the object, the data itself and the method

Office for Civil Rights (OCR): The enforcement agency for the HIPAA Privacy and Security Rule. Since April 14, 2003, the Privacy Rule has been enforced by the OCR. The OCR has enforced the Security Rule since July 26, 2009

Office of the National Coordinator for Health Information Technology (ONC): Principal advisor to the Secretary of the Department of Health and Human Services on the development, application, and use of health information technology

ONC-Authorized Testing and Certification Bodies (ATCBs): Empowered to perform complete EHR or EHR module testing and certification. They utilize conformance testing requirements, test cases, and test tools developed by the NIST to determine whether the software complies with the EHR Incentive Program requirements for establishing meaningful use of an EHR

On-demand self-service: Anyone with the appropriate permissions can make use of the resources without additional intervention

Online diagnosers: Individuals who use the Internet to determine a diagnosis or identify a medical condition

Ontology: A system of categories used as a method for combining data; a common vocabulary organized by meaning that allows for an understanding of the structure of descriptive information that facilitates a specific topic or domain

Openness: Flexibility to extend and improve the existing system with minimal impact

Operations: In the context of HIPAA, any of the following activities: (a) quality assessment and improvement activities, including outcomes evaluation, patient safety activities, population-based activities, protocol development, and case management and care coordination; (b) competency assurance activities, including provider or health plan performance evaluation, credentialing, and accreditation; (c) conducting or arranging for medical reviews, audits, or legal services, including fraud and abuse detection and compliance programs; (d) specified insurance functions, such as underwriting, enrollment, premium rating, related to the creation, renewal, or replacement of health insurance or benefits, along with risk rating and reinsuring risk relating to healthcare claims; (e) business planning, development, management, and administration; and (f) business management and general administrative activities of the entity, including but not limited to deidentifying protected health information, creating a limited data set, and certain fundraising for the benefit of the covered entity

Opt-in: A model for HIE that requires patients to specifically affirm their desire to have their data made available for exchange within an HIE. This option provides up-front control for patients since their data cannot be included unless they have agreed

Opt-in with restrictions: A model for HIE that allows patients to make all or some defined amount of their data available for electronic exchange. Patients may restrict how their data is used by allowing access only to specific providers, by allowing only specific data elements to be included, or by allowing data to be accessed only for specific purposes

Opt-out: A model for HIE that allows for a predetermined set of data to be automatically included in an HIE, but a patient may still deny access to information in the exchange. This model allows the consumer to prevent their data and information from inclusion in the HIE

Opt-out with exceptions: A model for HIE that makes the patient's information available in the exchange, but enables the patient to selectively exclude data from an HIE, limit information to specific providers, or limit exchange of information to exchange for specific purposes

Ordinal data: Data where the names or labels have an order to them with meaning attached. For example, a patient may be diagnosed with cancer, which is often represented as Stage I, Stage II, Stage III, or Stage IV

Patient portal: A secure method of communication between the healthcare provider and the patient

Payment: Encompasses activities of a health plan to obtain premiums or to determine or fulfill its responsibility for coverage and provision of benefits under the health plan, and furnish or obtain reimbursement for healthcare delivered to an individual and activities of a healthcare provider to obtain payment or be reimbursed for the provision of healthcare to an individual

Personal health record (PHR): An example of consumer informatics. It is an electronic or paper health record maintained and updated by an individual for himself or herself, a tool that individuals can use to collect, track, and share past and current information about their health or the health of someone in their care

Physical models: Capture the hardware composition of a system in terms of the computer and other devices. The model is a pictorial representation of the arrangement of the different pieces and connection points

Physical safeguards: Physical measures, policies, and procedures to protect a covered entity's electronic information systems and related buildings and equipment, from natural and environmental hazards, and unauthorized intrusion

Physician champion: A physician tasked with the responsibility of representing the views of the physician users

Picture archiving and communication systems (PACS): Provides storage of electronic images and reports

Platform as a service (PaaS): At this intermediate level of capability consumers create or acquire applications using programming languages and tools supported by the cloud computing service provider. While the consumer does not control the underlying infrastructure they do exercise more control over the applications

Point-of-care testing (POCT): Where the diagnostic tests are performed at or near where the patient care is taking place

Population health: The level and distribution of disease, functional status, and well-being of a defined group of people with specified characteristics

Post-hoc text processing: Using algorithms after the data is entered to structure the data for processing

Practicality: An aspect of an EHR that should be evaluated. It addresses costs including goals about price, internal resources to maintain the EHR, whether the EHR is integrated or interfaced with the practice management systems, and interfaces with labs

Practice management system (PMS): Supports scheduling, financial, and billing activities. PMSs generally include patient registration, scheduling, eligibility verification, charge capture, electronic claims processing, billing, and collections

Predictive modeling: Where multiple data points are analyzed utilizing sophisticated software programs to identify the one characteristic that results in a problem or provides the solution

Primary data use: Use of healthcare data for direct patient care

Primary key: Uniquely identifies the row in a database

Private cloud: Accessible to only one customer and can be operated by the organization, a third party, or a combination of the two, at the customer's location or offsite. Healthcare organizations, especially larger ones, may choose this option due to the need for patient information security or if sensitive research is being conducted

Probability: Using patient-related data to determine the likelihood of various occurrences in the disease process and modes of treatment

Protected health information (PHI): Individually identifiable health information that is transmitted by electronic media, maintained in electronic media, or transmitted or maintained in any other form or medium

Public cloud: This cloud is open to the general public and owned by an academic institution, the government, or some other organization for the benefit of the public. The owner or a third party or some combination thereof can operate it, at any location

Public health: The level and distribution of disease, functional status, and well-being of all of the inhabitants of a given neighborhood, city, region, state, country, or the world

Public health informatics: The systematic application of information and utilization of computer technology to support public health initiatives as related to research, education and delivery of public health services

Quality improvement (QI): A set of activities that measures the quality of a service or product through systems or process evaluation and then implements revised processes that result in better healthcare outcomes for patients, based on standards or care

Rapid elasticity: Service is provided on demand, meaning that more can quickly be provided when needed and reduced just as fast, so the consumer only pays for what they need and use

Ratio data: In addition to the equal intervals between data points seen in continuous data, ratio data have a true zero (0) point. An example of ratio data in healthcare would be "patient weight"

Record: In database terminology, a collection of fields that are related in a database

Record custodians: Also known as record stewards, they are commonly charged with leading multidisciplinary definition projects for both the HIPAA-required Designated Record Set and the legal health record. They are also expected to develop proper organization, management, guidelines, and processes related to the use of business records as a protective legal defense tool

Recovery point objective (RPO): The length of time that you can operate without a particular application

Recovery time objective (RTO): The maximum amount of time tolerable for data loss and capture

Red flags: Suspicious documents, information, or behaviors that indicate the possibility of identity theft. Examples of red flags include inconsistencies in documents (driver's license and insurance card), documents that appear to be altered, and not having more than one form of ID (insurance card but no other form of ID)

Regional Extension Centers (RECs): Established by the ONC to assist primary care providers in quickly becoming adept and meaningful users of EHRs. RECs provide training and support services to assist doctors and other providers in adopting EHRs, share information and guidance to help with EHR implementation, and give technical assistance as needed

Relational database: In such a database, data with a common purpose, concept, or source are arranged into tables. The relationship between the tables is displayed in an entity-relationship diagram (ERD)

Reliability: A measure of consistency of data items based on their reproducibility and an estimation of their error of measurement

Rendition: The act of rendering data into documents, usually in report form. Report writers are the most common form of rendering, but there are others such as the creation of documents for continuity of care based on preprogrammed routines as required by meaningful use

Reputation: The reputation of the vendor should also be evaluated when purchasing an EHR, including how established the vendor is, references from other clients, and confirmation that their software is certified

Request for information (RFI): The RFI is used to ask vendors for information about their products and services. It is often used to obtain information from a large number of vendors to narrow the field of vendors to whom a request for proposals will be issued

Request for proposal (RFP): The RFP is a formal request to vendors to provide specific information about how they can meet the organization's specific requirements. In the RFP, the organization should describe the goals and priorities for the IT acquisition including technical and functional requirements

Required implementation specifications: Standards under the HIPAA Security Rule that are not optional, but must be implemented in conformance with the regulation

Resource pooling: The cloud computing provider resources serve multiple consumers, usually independent of location, though these can be specified by the consumer

Resource sharing: Being able to use the hardware, software, or data anywhere in the system

Reverse map: Goes from a newer source code or data set to an older target code or data set

Risk: The probability of incurring injury or loss, the probable amount of loss foreseen by an insurer in issuing a contract, or a formal insurance term denoting liability to compensate individuals for injuries sustained in a healthcare facility

RxNORM: A system created by the National Library of Medicine, for describing clinical drugs. RxNorm is the meaningful use specification for pharmaceutical names and codes in the United States

Sanctions policy: Under the HIPAA Security Rules, this must outline how cases of noncompliance will be addressed within the organization knowing that even with a strong risk management plan, the potential for noncompliance (either intentional or nonintentional) still exists

Scalability: The ability to support growth while maintaining the same level of service

Seamless care: Consistent, coherent, logical, without discontinuities or disparities, and of uniform quality care

Secondary data use: The nondirect care use of personal health information and other healthcare data

Security: A benefit of cloud computing. The security of the cloud application is paramount for healthcare providers to be able to ensure the privacy of individually identifiable healthcare data. Cloud computing service companies working with providers and others would be subject to all aspects of the HIPAA Privacy and Security Rules

Security incident: The attempted or successful unauthorized access, use, disclosure, modification, or destruction of information or interference with system operations in an information system

Security Risk Analysis: Provides covered entities and business associates with the structural framework upon which to build their HIPAA Security Plan. Covered entities and business associates are required to conduct a Security Risk Analysis to evaluate risks and vulnerabilities in their environment and to implement reasonable and appropriate measures to protect against reasonably anticipated threats or hazards to the security or integrity of electronic protected health information

Select query: The purpose of a select query in SQL is to pull records that meet a certain criteria from a particular table or combination of tables

Semantic interoperability: The ability to exchange data and information with its original meaning intact and understood by all receivers

Software as a service (SaaS): The highest level of cloud computing service models, SaaS enables access to the cloud computing provider's applications via a variety of devices, usually through an interface such as a web browser

Source: the code or data set from which the data map originates

Spoliation: The malicious alteration, concealment, or destruction of evidence

Standards development organizations (SDOs): An organization involved, in the healthcare context, in creating and maintaining healthcare standards. In order to promulgate a recognized standard, SDOs must be accredited by ANSI and, if applicable, the ISO

Structured data: Binary, machine-readable data in discrete fields, with limitations on what can be entered into the field. The structured entry of healthcare data involves the use of templates and on-screen forms with the possible entry fields and the potential entries in those fields controlled, defined, and limited. Structured data can have many benefits including completeness, quality, and accessibility of the data for a variety of purposes

Structured Query Language (SQL): The programming language that is used to manipulate data in a relational database. SQL is sometimes pronounced "sequel"

Systematized Nomenclature of Medicine–Clinical Terms (SNOMED-CT): A processable collection of medical terminology covering most areas of clinical information such as lab results, nonlab interventions and procedures, anatomy, diagnosis and problems, and nursing. It is a logically organized and massive terminology, mostly ordered by a formal description logic, which permits SNOMED-CT to benefit from the classifying reasons developed by computer science and the fields of formal ontology and logic

Target: The code or data set in which one is attempting to find a code or data representation with an equivalent meaning

Technical safeguards: The technology and the policy and procedures for its use that protect electronic protected health information and control access to it

Technology literacy: Entails having some basic knowledge about technology, some basic technical capabilities, and the ability to think critically about technological issues and act accordingly

Telehealth: Used interchangeably with telemedicine, although this term tends to include both medical and nonclinical elements of care to include education, monitoring, and administration to facilitate the prevention or exacerbation of medical conditions

Telemedicine: The remote delivery of healthcare services over a telecommunications network

Temporal: An issue with the widespread use of NLP in the real-time clinical domain. Temporal means the computer can detect any time frames included when the concept is identified. For example, "past history of cancer" is very different from simply "cancer"

Terminal emulation software: Used on a personal computer to allow a user to connect to a host as if the user is on a dumb terminal

Terminology: A set of terms representing the system of concepts of a particular subject field

Terminal-to-host: The application and any data stay on a host computer with the user connecting either via a dumb terminal or using terminal emulation software on a personal computer to connect as if the user is on a dumb terminal. Sometimes this arrangement is also termed a thin client, with most of the actual processing taking place on a central computer

Threat: The potential for exploitation of a vulnerability or potential danger to a computer, network, or data

Three-tiered architecture: Expands on the two-tier system with the addition of an application server that contains the software applications and the business rules. Clients in this architecture are called "thin clients" because most of the processing is done on the server, and the client has very little software installed on it

Topology: The network's physical layout. Types of cabled network topologies include point-to-point, star, bus, tree, or ring

Transaction: The transmission of information between two parties to carry out financial or administrative activities related to healthcare

Transaction set: The data required to complete a specified communication

Transaction standards: Establish the means by which a sender transmits or communicates data or information to a receiver (also known as data-interchange standards)

Translational medicine: Taking the scientific knowledge gained from basic advances in research to the bedside by developing new procedures and modes of treatment to improve healthcare

Transparency: The end user sees the distributed system as a single machine

Treatment: The provision, coordination, or management of healthcare and related services for an individual by one or more healthcare providers, including consultation between providers regarding a patient and referral of a patient by one provider to another

Two-tiered model: A model composed of several client computers that are used to capture and process the data. The servers in this configuration are powerful machines that have application software installed on them and in turn store the data captured by client machines

Uniform Rules for e-Discovery: Amendments to the FRCP specifically designed for electronically stored information

Unintended consequences: Unanticipated and undesirable issues or problems

Unstructured data: Unstructured data entry is the use of free text or string data in the health record. This does not mean that there is no organization to the data, just that it is not structured with specific data elements, allowable values, and so on. In the paper record a large amount of the data, especially the day-to-day progress notes, were unstructured

Usability: An aspect of an EHR that should be evaluated. It addresses the speed and ease of use, including goals about tasks that must be done fast, computer literacy of the practice staff, and the methods by which data will be entered

Validity: (1) The extent to which data correspond to the actual state of affairs or that an instrument measures what it purports to measure. (2) A term referring to a test's ability to accurately and consistently measure what it purports to measure

Virtual private networks (VPNs): Extend the firewall protection boundary beyond the local intranet by the use of cryptographically protected secure channels at the IP level. A VPN is a private network that uses a public network (usually the Internet) to connect remote sites or users together privately

Vital statistics: Statistics on events such as birth and death important enough that a government collects information on them through certain registration procedures

Visual literacy: The ability to understand graphs or other visual information. For example, the consumer may need to understand a graph trend line of laboratory results

Vocabulary: A dictionary of terms; that is, words and phrases with their meanings

Vulnerability: An inherent weakness or absence of a safeguard that could be exploited by a threat

Warm site: A type of data backup facility. IT provides basic infrastructure, but takes time, possibly a week, to activate. This is less expensive than a hot site

Wide area network (WAN): A computer network that connects devices across a large geographical area

Workforce: Employees, volunteers, trainees, and other persons whose conduct, in the performance of work for a covered entity or business associate, is under the direct control of such covered entity or business associate, whether or not they are paid by the covered entity or business associate

World Wide Web (WWW): A global network of networks offering services to users with web browsers

Index

A

Access, 231

Access control standard, 263–64

Accessibility, data, 113, 116

Accountability implementation specification, 263

Accountable Care Organization (ACO), 132, 192, 216, 350–51

Accounting of disclosures (AOD), 241–42, 312

Accredited Standards Committee (ASC) X12 5010, 106

Accuracy, data, 113, 116

Accurate documentation in health record, 314

ACO. *See* Accountable Care Organization (ACO)

ACS. *See* American Cancer Society (ACS)

Ad hoc standards, 101

ADA. *See* American Diabetes Association (ADA)

Address Discrepancy Rule, 273

Addressable implementation specifications, 251

Administrative functions and EHR, 32

Administrative processes and reporting, healthcare delivery functions, 35

Administrative safeguards
  business associate contracts, 258–59
  contingency plan standard, 257–58
  evaluation standard, 258
  information access management standard, 255–56
  security awareness and training standard, 256
  security incident procedures standard, 257
  security management process standard, 254–55
  security officer, 255
  workforce security standard, 255

Administrative simplification, 222, 223

Agency for Healthcare Research and Quality (AHRQ), 139, 146, 173
  CHI definition, 323

Health Information Technology Evaluation Toolkit, 147

Aggregated HIE, 184

Aggregating health information
  population health, 191–92
  public health, 192–97

AHIMA. *See* American Health Information Management Association (AHIMA)

AHRQ. *See* Agency for Healthcare Research and Quality (AHRQ)

Alert fatigue, 176

Ambulatory EHR, 36–38

Amendments, health record documentation, 314

American Cancer Society (ACS), 331

American Diabetes Association (ADA), 331

American Health Information Management Association (AHIMA), 7, 171, 174
  Bill of Rights, 243–44
  Body of Knowledge, 365
  myphr.com website, 335

American Hospital Association (AHA) 2009 survey, 30, 35–36

American Medical Association, 212

American Medical Informatics Association (AMIA), 7, 323

American Medical Informatics Association Board Position Paper, 144

American National Standards Institute (ANSI), 102

American Recovery and Reinvestment Act (ARRA), 7, 17, 31, 102, 133, 182, 222, 224, 259, 290

AMIA. *See* American Medical Informatics Association (AMIA)

Amoxicillin, 213

Analysis phase in SDLC processes, 136–37

ANSI. *See* American National Standards Institute (ANSI)

Any and all records, concept of, 318

AOD. *See* Accounting of disclosures (AOD)

Application Programming Interface (API), 60

Application server, 51

Application service provider (ASP), 140